The Complete
Guide to
Breast
Reconstruction

The Complete Guide to Breast Reconstruction

Choosing the Best Options after Your Mastectomy

FIFTH EDITION

Kathy Steligo

JOHNS HOPKINS UNIVERSITY PRESS
BALTIMORE

Note to the Reader: This book is not meant to substitute for medical care of people with breast cancer, and treatment should not be based solely on its contents. Instead, treatment must be developed in a dialogue between the individual and their physician. Our book has been written to help with that dialogue.

Drug dosage: The author and publisher have made reasonable efforts to determine that the selection of drugs discussed in this text conform to the practices of the general medical community. The medications described do not necessarily have specific approval by the US Food and Drug Administration for use in the diseases for which they are recommended. In view of ongoing research, changes in governmental regulation, and the constant flow of information relating to drug therapy and drug reactions, the reader is urged to check the package insert of each drug for any change in indications and dosage and for warnings and precautions. This is particularly important when the recommended agent is a new and/or infrequently used drug.

© 2023 Johns Hopkins University Press
All rights reserved. Published 2023
Printed in the United States of America on acid-free paper
9 8 7 6 5 4 3 2 1

Johns Hopkins University Press
2715 North Charles Street
Baltimore, Maryland 21218
www.press.jhu.edu

Library of Congress Cataloging-in-Publication Data

Names: Steligo, Kathy, author.
Title: The complete guide to breast reconstruction : choosing the best options after
  your mastectomy / Kathy Steligo.
Other titles: Breast reconstruction guidebook
Description: Fifth edition. | Baltimore : Johns Hopkins University Press, 2023. | Series:
  A Johns Hopkins Press health book | Includes bibliographical references and index.
Identifiers: LCCN 2022059440 | ISBN 9781421447599 (paperback ; acid-free paper) |
  ISBN 9781421447605 (ebook)
Subjects: LCSH: Mammaplasty—Popular works. | Musculocutaneous flaps—Popular works. |
  Mammaplasty—Complications—Popular works. | Women—Health and hygiene—Popular works. |
  Breast—Cancer—Surgery—Popular works. | Breast—Cancer—Patients—Rehabilitation—
  Popular works.
Classification: LCC RD539.8 .S73 2023 | DDC 618.1/90592—dc23/eng/20230119
LC record available at https://lccn.loc.gov/2022059440

A catalog record for this book is available from the British Library.

Special discounts are available for bulk purchases of this book. For more information, please contact Special Sales at specialsales@jh.edu.

Contents

Foreword, by Sue Friedman, DVM ix

Introduction 1

Part I
Mastectomy and Breast Reconstruction Basics 4

1. Why Mastectomy?   7
Inside the Breast   9
Surgeries to Diagnose, Treat, and Reduce the Risk of Breast Cancer   11
Lumpectomy or Mastectomy?   19

2. Considering a Risk-Reducing Mastectomy   23
Should You Have Genetic Testing?   25
How Real Is Your Risk?   26
Risk-Reducing Mastectomy   28
Paying for Genetic Counseling, Testing, and Risk-Reducing Surgeries   30

3. Going Flat: Mastectomy without Reconstruction   33
What to Expect   34
The Goldilocks Option   38
The Prosthesis Alternative   38
Paying for a Mastectomy and Prostheses   42

4. How a Mastectomy Affects Reconstruction   44
Mastectomy Cause and Effect   44
Losing and Regaining Sensation   46
Skin-Sparing Mastectomy   49
Nipple-Sparing Mastectomy   50

5. Breast Reconstruction Basics   **59**
Sorting Through the Options   60
Timing Your Reconstruction   64
Health Matters   68
Coordinating Reconstruction with Treatment   70

Part II
Rebuilding the Breasts   76

6. Reconstruction with Breast Implants   **79**
Implants Inside and Out   80
Prepectoral and Subpectoral Placement   83
Tissue Expander-to-Implant Reconstruction   85
Direct-to-Implant Reconstruction   87
Are They Safe?   91
Recovery   95
Potential Problems and Fixes   97

7. The Expander Experience   **106**
Getting Your Fill   107
Minimizing Discomfort   109
Living in Limbo   111
Exchange Surgery   112
Potential Problems and Fixes   114

8. Autologous Tissue Flaps   **116**
Tissue Flap Basics   117
Muscle-Sparing and Muscle-Sacrificing Flaps   120
Borrowing from the Abdomen   124
Other Donor Sites and Procedures   132
Potential Problems and Fixes   144

Part III
Procedures to Improve Symmetry, Shape, and Appearance   148

9. Revision Procedures   **151**
Making a Good Reconstruction Better   152
Revisions for Reconstruction with Implants   152
Revisions for Autologous Reconstruction   159
Fixes with Fat   160

10. Modifying Your Opposite Breast — 166

Breast Augmentation — 167
Breast Lift — 170
Breast Reduction — 173

11. Final Touches: Recreating Your Nipple and Areola — 178

The Icing on the Cake — 178
Building the Nipple — 180
A Colorful Finish — 182
Problems and Fixes — 187

Part IV
What to Expect from Prep, Post-op, Recovery, and Beyond   192

12. Preparing for Surgery — 195

Countdown: Four Weeks to Surgery — 195
Two Weeks before Surgery — 200
One Week to Go — 204
The Day before Surgery — 207
Reconstruction Day — 210

13. What to Expect in the Hospital — 212

Admitting and Pre-op — 212
In the Operating Room — 213
A Peek into Post-op — 214
The Rest of Your Hospital Stay — 218

14. Back Home — 219

A Timetable for Healing — 219
Managing Medication — 225
Dealing with Drains — 226
Tips for an Easier Recovery — 230
Optimism Helps You Heal — 235
Seeing Your New Breasts for the First Time — 236

15. Dealing with Unexpected Problems — 237

Inherent Risks of Surgery — 238
Lingering Pain — 242
Improving Scars — 244
Lymphedema — 247
Reconstruction Do-Overs — 248

Strategies for Minimizing Complications 252
Managing Depression, Anxiety, and Unsettled Emotions 254

16. Life after Reconstruction 258
Getting Back to Ordinary 258
Returning to Work 262
Dating, Intimacy, and Sex 262
Surveillance and Follow-Up after a Mastectomy 266

Part V
Finding Answers, Making Decisions   268

17. Shopping for Surgeons 271
Five Characteristics of an Ideal Plastic Surgeon 273
Where to Start 276
Pre-appointment Footwork 278
Making the Most of Your Consultation 279
The Value of a Second (or Third) Opinion 281
Tips for Travelers 282

18. Payment and Insurance Issues 286
Are You Covered? 288
Appealing When the Answer Is No 289
Help for the Underinsured and the Uninsured 294

19. A Road Map for Making Difficult Decisions 298
Moving in the Right Direction 299
Sources of Information and Inspiration 304
A Checklist for Making Decisions 307

20. Information for Family and Friends 308
Hints for Family Members 308
Food for Thought for Partners and Spouses 309
Issues for Caregivers 312
Do's and Don'ts for Friends 313

Acknowledgments 317
Glossary 319
Resources 327
Notes 329
Index 337

Foreword

Sue Friedman, DVM

At age 28, as a new veterinarian—with a thoroughness I typically reserved for canine patients—I performed my first breast self-exam, only to find a lump. The biopsy revealed a benign fibroadenoma. However, the resulting scar tissue made my breasts hard to examine, and mammograms became part of my wellness routine. My mammogram at age 33—the one that may have saved my life—led to a diagnosis of breast cancer. I was shocked. I took excellent care of myself, and I had no family history of breast cancer.

Although my cancer was caught early, it was scattered throughout my breast; my surgeon recommended a mastectomy and reconstruction. She told me that I was the perfect candidate for a type of reconstruction they had just begun doing at her hospital, using my abdominal fat to reconstruct my breast. While I didn't look forward to losing my breast, I was grateful that it could be recreated. But there were no other patients for me to speak with, and my surgeon dismissed any other reconstructive option. Despite my medical background, I was lost trying to negotiate the decisions and emotional impact of what was before me. I never got a second opinion, blindly trusting my surgeon's recommendations. After my quick recovery, my doctors told me I was "cured" and that, as a young survivor, I should live my life without further worry. Two successive setbacks taught me otherwise.

First, I experienced a recurrence of cancer in my lymph nodes just nine months later. Then I learned from a magazine article, not my doctors, that I had several red flags for an inherited mutation in a *BRCA1* or *BRCA2* gene. Genetic testing revealed that I had a *BRCA2* mutation and a very high risk for cancer in my remaining breast. I wanted to do whatever I could to avoid another cancer diagnosis, so I chose a risk-reducing mastectomy of my healthy breast. At that time, a mastectomy was typically done to treat breast cancer rather than to prevent it. But the advent of genetic testing was changing that.

I wanted the new reconstruction to match my other breast, but I couldn't have a second TRAM flap, since my abdominal fat had been used for my original reconstruction. Were there other options? This time, I did my research, learned about alternatives, and got second and third opinions. I settled on reconstruction using fat from my buttock. The procedure was new, and only a handful of surgeons were performing it, so I traveled out of state for my surgery. I made the choice that felt right for me. I had no regrets, although I wished for a guide to help me understand the implications of each option and to prepare for surgery and recovery.

After completing treatment and risk-reducing surgeries, I started the organization Facing Our Risk of Cancer Empowered (FORCE) to support and educate other people with inherited high-risk mutations. With a lifetime risk for breast cancer as high as 80 percent, women with these mutations were beginning to explore their options for a risk-reducing mastectomy and reconstruction. During FORCE's early days, genetic testing was new and risk-reducing surgery was considered extreme. FORCE became a lifeline for women who had nowhere else to turn for support and resources. Questions about risk-reducing surgery, requests to see photos of reconstructed breasts, and peer support from other women who had navigated these decisions were our most requested resources. That was why, in 2002, when Kathy Steligo, an established writer who had just had her first breast reconstruction, emailed me about a book she was writing about mastectomy and breast reconstruction, I was enthusiastic about helping in any way I could. This was a topic of huge interest, and there was a tremendous need for a comprehensive, objective resource that would help women make informed decisions and prepare for surgery and recovery.

More than 20 years later, this book is more relevant than ever. Women have the right and the opportunity to consider their priorities and preferences when making decisions about a mastectomy with or without breast reconstruction. They can consider a nipple-sparing mastectomy, advanced methods of reconstruction, and procedures that potentially encourage the return of sensation in the new breast. These options were not available 25 years ago when I struggled to make my decisions. Along the way, the first four editions of *The Breast Reconstruction Guidebook* (now titled *The Complete Guide to Breast Reconstruction*) have been FORCE's trusted companions; each edition staying current on the latest developments and presenting options in plain language.

At FORCE, the first piece of advice we give to everyone considering a mastectomy is to read this book. And we will continue to do so with this new edition.

It is an honor to write the foreword to an exceptional book that has had a profound impact on so many women. As an advocate, I have shared hundreds of copies with patients, colleagues, and friends who are navigating the breast cancer experience. As I tell everyone I meet who is facing cancer, I am sorry that you need to be here but I'm glad that you have found your way to FORCE. The same sentiment applies to this book. *The Complete Guide to Breast Reconstruction* is the most important resource for anyone who is considering a mastectomy to treat or reduce their breast cancer risk. The information, insight, and stories within will explain, support, inform, and show you that you are not alone.

Be empowered and be well!

Sue Friedman, DVM
Founder and Executive Director,
Facing Our Risk of Cancer Empowered (FORCE)

Introduction

We often hear about the speed of technology—how fast it moves and how the pace of change keeps accelerating. We seem to be constantly updating our computers and smartphones to take advantage of faster, more powerful chips and new features. The same is true of breast reconstruction. In the early days of modern breast reconstruction, major innovations could be identified by decades. Breast implants were introduced in the 1960s. In the '70s and '80s, "natural" reconstruction with fat and muscle from the back or abdomen offered alternatives to implants. During the 1990s, the game-changing DIEP procedure, which rebuilds breasts with fat while preserving the muscle, was introduced. Several innovations occurred in the 2000s: oncologically safe nipple-sparing mastectomy; new generation silicone "gummy bear" breast implants that hold their shape; and acellular dermal matrix, a tissue replacement material that made one-stage breast reconstruction possible. Fat grafting—liposuctioning excess fat and carefully injecting small amounts into a reconstructed breast—is now routinely used to refine the shape, increase the volume, and improve the contour of reconstructed breasts.

Men and women who have a mastectomy benefit from reconstructive procedures that continue to improve and offer new possibilities. Illustrating the ever-increasing pace of change, advancements since the last edition of this book have been impressive:

- More plastic surgeons routinely provide advanced breast reconstruction procedures.
- Improved procedures shorten recovery time and develop fewer complications compared to traditional methods.
- Placing implants above the chest muscle where breast tissue was removed (instead of the traditional placement under the muscle)

shortens the reconstructive timeline and reduces time needed for recovery.

- More ways have been developed to rebuild breasts with your own excess fat while preserving muscle.
- Three-dimensional nipple and areola tattoos create the illusion of having nipples where there aren't any.
- Improved protocols before, during, and after surgery reduce pain, time in the hospital, and recovery.
- Health insurance companies more often acknowledge breast reconstruction as more than a cosmetic procedure and cover the costs accordingly.

One thing that hasn't changed in the 20 years since this book was first published is that individuals who face a mastectomy have common dilemmas: "Should I have reconstruction?" and "What is the best option for me?" Perhaps the most significant change, however, is that people now have choices regarding mastectomies and reconstruction. Because no single method is right for everyone, it's important to learn about and carefully consider each of these alternatives before deciding which one, if any, meets your personal preferences and priorities. You may not be able to change your need for a mastectomy, but you can make decisions about whether to restore your breasts; how, when, and where it should be done; and who should do it for you. Ultimately, you may decide to have breast reconstruction or you may decide not to have it.

If you determine that reconstruction is right for you, you'll have several decisions to make. Do you want the shortest procedure with the quickest recovery or a method that will give you the most natural breasts possible? Does keeping your own nipples and areolas appeal to you? Do you have excess fat that you'd like to be rid of in the process? You may not be a candidate for all procedures, and some choices may not be available in your area or within your health insurance network. Others may not interest you because of the investment in time or recovery.

Whether a mastectomy will treat your breast cancer or reduce your high risk of having a cancer diagnosis, choosing to stay flat after your mastectomy or replacing your breasts is your right and your choice. The breast cancer surgery decisions you face are profoundly personal. There is no single "right" or "best" reconstructive method. You may know exactly what you want or feel confused about what you should do. What's most important to know, particularly if you're feeling that you'll never be the same after losing your breasts, is that after your mastectomy, you can have soft, symmetrical breasts. Although plastic surgeons can't restore every aspect of your natural breasts, the days of creating replacement "lumps" on the chest are far behind us. The goal now is to rebuild breasts with natural-looking contour and shape, whether you're clothed or not. Reconstruction isn't perfect, and it isn't always easy. But it can restore your premastectomy profile and profoundly affect your self-image and peace of mind so that you can get on with your life.

When you face a mastectomy, you need hugs, support, understanding, and knowledge. Like preceding versions, this new edition was written to provide you with three of those four essentials. The information here will objectively explain your options, answer your questions, and demystify confusing terms and concepts. If you're looking for answers, this information will help you ask the right questions, approach reconstruction with hope and confidence rather than worry and fear, and ultimately make informed decisions that are best for you.

As a survivor who has twice confronted breast cancer and twice had reconstruction and several revision procedures, I understand how you feel. I know firsthand that sorting through the various reconstructive opportunities can be a confusing, time-intensive, and frustrating experience. By the time you've read through this book, I hope that you'll feel more confident in your understanding of mastectomies and reconstruction. You may decide to go ahead with reconstruction. You may not. Either way, you'll know what to expect. And even if you decide that reconstruction is not for you, you'll know what to expect from a mastectomy and the recovery.

Someday, science may lead us to a time when mastectomies are archaic, and this book is obsolete. But discovery isn't easy, and the development process isn't quick. Sooner or later, researchers will discover how to repair defective genes that cause breast cancer. Men and women may undergo gene therapy to eliminate breast cancer or the threat of it. We'll move breast cancer to the list of diseases we no longer need to fear, and mastectomies will no longer be needed. Until then, reconstruction is our best option for replacing lost breasts.

Part I
Mastectomy and
Breast Reconstruction
Basics

If you're facing a mastectomy, you might think that every aspect of losing your breasts is out of your control. In fact, there are different types of mastectomy surgeries, and each one has room for choices. Making choices, however, requires understanding your options. You may consider keeping your nipples, for example, or prefer a particular incision placement. If you have a choice between a lumpectomy with radiation or a mastectomy, you'll need to decide which one is best for you.

All mastectomy procedures have one thing in common: they remove the breast tissue that makes up the bulk of the breast. Breast reconstruction replaces that lost tissue. Whether you have a mastectomy to treat or prevent breast cancer and whether you ultimately decide to have reconstruction, this section will help you understand the basics of both. You'll find answers to five important issues:

- why a mastectomy is recommended and what it involves
- how preventive mastectomy reduces your risk if you have an inherited predisposition to breast cancer
- what to expect from a mastectomy if you decide not to have breast reconstruction
- how a mastectomy affects breast reconstruction
- why, when, and how breast reconstruction is done

Chapter 1

Why Mastectomy?

No words can describe the stress and anxiety that unexpectedly creep up about having mastectomy. I wish I could tell someone, "This is how I feel," but I can't. Anything I say about it, any way I describe it, is inadequate. I love and appreciate each and every person who supports me and cares about me more than anyone will ever know. But this is something that no one would truly understand unless they've been there.

—MARIA

As women, our breasts nourish our babies, provide pleasure, and define much of our physical profile. It's heartbreaking to lose a part of us that is so uniquely feminine, and it's natural to have concerns about losing one or both breasts: Will a *mastectomy*, removing one or both breasts, eliminate our cancer? How will we look afterward when we are clothed and when we are not? Will we ever feel normal again? In most situations, removing breast tissue (often combined with other treatment) does eliminate breast cancer. Afterward, talented plastic surgeons can restore breast volume and shape with manufactured implants or your own tissue.

Although early Egyptians are generally credited with the initial written description of breast cancer, Greek physicians in AD 180 may have been the first to recommend surgery to remove a breast tumor.[1] By the 1700s, surgery was considered to be the most appropriate breast cancer treatment. A letter in 1811 written by English novelist Fanny Burney to her sister describing how her breast was removed by one of Napoleon's surgeons is believed to be the first documented evidence of a mastectomy during the "modern" era. Fortified with just a single wine cordial, Burney had a successful operation and lived for another 29 years.

In 1894, renowned surgeon William Halsted introduced the *radical mastectomy* as an aggressive way to contain breast cancer. He performed this surgery with two benefits that his predecessors didn't have: anesthesia and sterilized surgical instruments. At the time, the biology of breast cancer wasn't understood sufficiently to address individual condition and tumor size or to provide treatment choices. Breast cancer was recognized as a local disease that could best be contained with aggressive treatment: removing the entire breast, the muscles of the chest wall, and the underarm lymph nodes. The procedure left women with a flat or concave chest, arm weakness, and, in some cases, lingering pain. In the absence of other effective, more conservative methods, Halsted's procedure became the standard treatment for most women diagnosed with breast cancer; and, although it was disfiguring, the procedure saved many of their lives. In the late 1970s, surgeons discovered that, for most cases of breast cancer, removing only the tumor and breast tissue was just as effective and far less debilitating.

Surgeons are still key players in almost all breast cancer treatment plans, and they now participate in multidisciplinary medical teams that assess and coordinate each patient's overall treatment. Despite encouraging advances that find more breast cancers at an early stage when they're easier to treat, we still haven't cracked the cancer code. While we're beginning to understand the nature of certain breast cancers, we don't yet know how to prevent or cure all of them. We've learned that breast cancer is not one but many different diseases that must be approached in different ways. That realization has helped experts replace the one-size-fits-all treatment approach with more effective treatment choices that are less invasive and more personalized.

In the United States, breast cancer is the second most common diagnosed cancer in women (after skin cancer) and the second most common cause of cancer death (after lung cancer). Annually, 1 in 8 women are diagnosed with breast cancer; and, although most women survive treatment, more than 43,000 lose their lives to this disease each year.[2] Many more—even those diagnosed in the early stages of breast cancer—lose their breasts because of this dreaded disease or in an effort to prevent it. More than 100,000 mastectomies are performed each year by *general surgeons* or *breast surgeons*.

FIGURE 1.1 Breast skin covers fatty tissue, ducts, and lobes (*left*). Lymph nodes filter impurities from the breast (*right*).

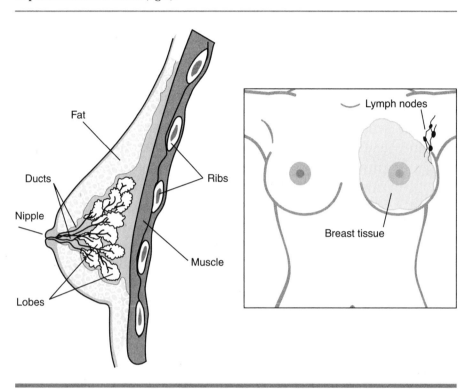

Inside the Breast

Positioned over the pectoralis major chest muscles, breasts consist of *lobes*, *ducts*, connective tissue, and fat. Women have 15 to 20 lobes, each containing multiple small *lobules* that produce milk, which is delivered through ducts to the nipple. Fatty tissue covering the lobes gives the breast its size and shape. Clear, watery *lymph fluid* circulates through the breasts (and the rest of the body). Along the way, lymph fluid collects and then transports cellular debris, as well as bacteria and viruses that cause disease, to a network of small, bean-shaped *lymph nodes*, where these materials are destroyed or filtered (figure 1.1). Cleansed lymph fluid then returns to the blood system.

Breasts contain no muscle, which is why no amount of exercise makes them bigger. In our twenties and thirties, our breasts have more dense glandular tissue than fat. This tissue makes the youthful breast firm. It's also the reason *mammograms* aren't routinely recommended for women before the age of 40. Mammograms cannot always find abnormalities in dense tissue and tend to produce more false positive results, meaning that additional testing or a biopsy shows that the suspicious area is not cancer. *Magnetic resonance imaging (MRI)* is more sensitive and can better distinguish suspicious areas in dense tissue; it finds more abnormalities, both harmless and harmful. MRIs may also locate small breast irregularities that are missed by mammography.

Some research shows that a combination of digital mammography, MRI, and ultrasound is the most effective screening method for dense breasts. As we age—particularly after menopause—our breasts consist of more fat, and our once-firm breasts begin to sag. Though not usually welcomed or desired, aging breast tissue bodes well for early detection; on a mammogram, fat stands out in contrast to abnormalities.

What Is Breast Cancer?

We all dread the "C" word. But what, exactly, is it? Cancer occurs when environmental, lifestyle, or hereditary factors cause healthy cells—in this case, breast cells—to mutate and grow uncontrollably until they form *malignant* (cancerous) tumors. Breast tumors continue to develop, usually without symptoms, until they form a spot that shows up on a mammogram or a lump that can be felt.

Breast cancer is a term that encompasses different types of malignancies in the breast. *Noninvasive breast cancers* remain in situ, or "in place," within the confines of the ducts or lobules where they begin. (Most breast cancers begin in the ducts.) *Ductal carcinoma in situ (DCIS)* is contained within the ducts. Too small to be felt, DCIS is the earliest form of breast cancer (stage 0) and the most common noninvasive type of the disease. DCIS isn't life threatening, and treatment is successful in almost all cases. However, DCIS increases the chance of developing *invasive breast cancer*, which is more worrisome because it can spread beyond the breast to other parts of the body and is more difficult to treat. While fast-growing DCIS tumors may be more likely to mutate into invasive cancer, research suggests that some slow-growing DCIS tumors do not affect a person's survival; close surveillance rather than treatment may be appropriate, in the same way early-stage prostate cancer is now viewed. Until experts can reliably predict which DCIS cases are likely to become invasive, surgery with or without radiation and/or hormonal therapy is still recommended.

Invasive or *infiltrating ductal carcinoma (IDC)* is the most common type of breast cancer. It begins in the lining of the milk ducts and spreads to the surrounding breast tissue. *Invasive lobular carcinoma (ILC)* begins in the lobules. Unlike other types of breast cancers that form a lump, ILC spreads through the breast tissue, making it more difficult to detect. Like invasive ductal carcinoma, ILC increases the risks of a recurrence and a new cancer in the breast. *Inflammatory breast cancer* and other less common types of breast cancer can develop in the breast skin, nipple, or *areola* (the darker skin around the nipple). The American Cancer Society (www.cancer.org) provides detailed information about screening, diagnosis, and treatment for different types of breast cancers.

Surgeries to Diagnose, Treat, and Reduce the Risk of Breast Cancer

A breast *biopsy*—a small sample of tissue or cells that is removed surgically or with a special needle—helps to determine whether cancer is present. Most biopsies prove to be *benign* (noncancerous). When a biopsy reveals cancerous cells, your medical team will design the best course of treatment based on the type of cancer, how far it has progressed, whether it's likely to recur, and other factors. Treatment may include *chemotherapy* or *radiation therapy* to destroy cancer cells, medication to block the hormones that some tumors need to grow, *targeted therapy* that restricts or blocks proteins or other substances that certain cancers need to thrive, or *immunotherapy* that stimulates your own immune system to destroy cancer cells.

Some type of surgery is usually involved when breast cancer is diagnosed. Thankfully, the days of routine radical mastectomy are behind us. We live in an age of patient participation; and, when prudent, procedures that preserve most of the breast are often effective.

Lumpectomy

Individuals with a single, small tumor that hasn't spread beyond the breast are often candidates for a *lumpectomy* (also called partial mastectomy). A lumpectomy is an outpatient surgery that removes just the tumor and a margin of surrounding tissue (which must be clear of cancer cells). In most cases, a lumpectomy is followed by radiation treatment to eliminate any remaining cancer cells in the breast. This *breast-conserving therapy (BCT)*—lumpectomy

Breast Cancer Surgeries

- Breast-conserving surgery (lumpectomy) removes the cancerous area of the breast along with a margin of healthy tissue.

- Breast-conserving therapy includes lumpectomy and radiation.

- Unilateral mastectomy removes one breast.

- Bilateral mastectomy removes both breasts.

- Total mastectomy removes the breast tissue and may include the nipple, areola, and sentinel lymph node.

- Modified radical mastectomy removes breast tissue, the lining of the chest muscles, and some underarm lymph nodes.

- Radical mastectomy removes the entire breast, the underarm lymph nodes, and the pectoral muscles. This is rarely performed, unless cancer is found in the pectoral muscles.

- Sentinel lymph node biopsy removes one to four underarm lymph nodes.

- Axillary lymph node dissection removes multiple underarm lymph nodes.

and radiation—is standard treatment for most early-stage breast cancers to re-duce the risk of recurrence and improve survival. Cancer is less likely to return in the breast after radiation. If it does return, then the entire breast needs to be removed.

A lumpectomy may be a reasonable choice if you have any of the following circumstances:

- your tumor is smaller than 5 centimeters (2 inches) and is small relative to your breast size
- you have a single area of cancer or close multiple areas that can be removed without greatly distorting your breast
- you don't have inflammatory breast cancer
- you haven't had a previous lumpectomy or radiation on the affected breast
- you're in the second or third trimester of pregnancy
- you're not at high risk for a second breast cancer
- you're able and willing to complete all necessary radiation therapy sessions
- you don't have scleroderma, lupus, or any other connective tissue disease that might increase your sensitivity to radiation side effects

Mastectomy

When a lumpectomy can't eliminate all of the cancer, treatment usually includes a mastectomy. *Unilateral* mastectomy removes one breast and takes about two hours; *bilateral*, or double, mastectomy removes both breasts and can take up to four hours (figure 1.2). Both operations are performed under general anesthesia.

Depending on your diagnosis, you may have a choice between a lumpectomy or a mastectomy. Small, early-stage tumors can be treated with a lumpectomy and radiation or with a mastectomy with similar survival rates. Mastectomy may be recommended if

- your tumor is larger than 5 centimeters (2 inches) or large relative to your breast size. (Chemotherapy or hormone therapy given before surgery may shrink the tumor enough so that it can be removed with a lumpectomy.)

- you have multiple areas in different quadrants of the same breast that cannot be removed without greatly distorting your breast
- you have inflammatory breast cancer
- clear surgical margins can't be obtained after a lumpectomy
- your affected breast has previously been treated with radiation therapy
- you can't have or prefer not to have radiation therapy
- you have a high risk for a second breast cancer
- you're unable to have radiation therapy

The type of mastectomy you have depends on the nature of your breast cancer. A *total mastectomy* removes the entire breast tissue and may include the nipple and areola (figure 1.3). This surgery is commonly used to treat DCIS in multiple areas of the breast or when the cancerous area extends beyond the edges of the biopsy. It's also performed to greatly reduce high risk in individuals who have an inherited predisposition to breast cancer. A *modified radical mastectomy* is similar but also removes some or all underarm lymph nodes and the lining over the chest muscle (figure 1.3). Radical mastectomy is performed only when advanced tumors are found in the chest muscle.

FIGURE 1.2 A unilateral mastectomy removes one breast (*left*). Bilateral mastectomy removes both breasts (*right*).

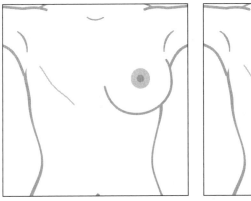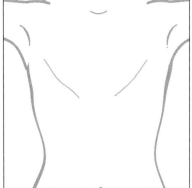

FIGURE 1.3 Total mastectomy (*left*) and modified radical mastectomy (*right*).

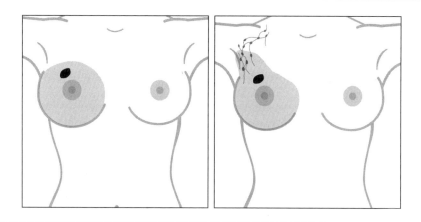

Lymph Node Surgeries

While most small, early-stage breast tumors are detected while they're still confined to the breast, invasive cancer cells that break away can then travel to other parts of the body through the *lymph system*. Without intervention, these cells can hitch a ride straight to the bloodstream and *metastasize* (spread) to healthy tissue and organs elsewhere in the body, requiring chemotherapy or other drugs that treat the entire body. Because cancer cells in any of the lymph nodes indicate that the malignancy has spread beyond the breast, some of the lymph nodes are removed and examined whenever invasive breast cancer is diagnosed.

Sentinel Lymph Node Biopsy

Checking the nearby lymph nodes for any sign of cancer can help indicate whether metastasis has occurred. If you've been diagnosed with early-stage invasive breast cancer and your nodes appear to be normal during surgery, then your breast surgeon will perform a minimally invasive *sentinel lymph node biopsy (SLNB)*. In this procedure, a small amount of harmless blue dye, with or without a radioactive tracer, is injected near the breast tumor. Lymph nodes then take up the dye as it travels through the lymph system. The *sentinel lymph node*, the one closest to the tumor, is removed and examined under a microscope; sometimes, one or two adjacent nodes are removed, as well. A sentinel node

Same-Day Mastectomy

Thanks to improved hospital protocols, pain management, and patient education, more mastectomies are being performed as outpatient procedures. After a *same-day mastectomy*, you might be on your way home a few hours after your surgery. You may be a candidate for this early discharge from the hospital if your mastectomy doesn't include lymph node removal (or removes only a sentinel lymph node), you don't have immediate breast reconstruction (or you have reconstruction with breast implants immediately after your mastectomy), and you don't develop a postoperative complication. Same-day programs that successfully prepare patients for what to expect when they get home result in high patient satisfaction and no statistical differences in emergency visits, reoperation, and readmission. Before you're discharged from the hospital, you'll receive instructions about postoperative home care, how to manage pain, who to call if problems develop, and when you should have a follow-up appointment with your surgeon.

Source: Specht MC, Kelly BN, Tomczyk E, et al. One-year experience of same-day mastectomy and breast reconstruction protocol. *Annals of Surgical Oncology.* 2022;1–9. https://doi.org/10.1245/s10434-022-11859 -9; Shelby M, Byrum S, Billar J, et al. Shared decision-making to foster same-day discharge for patients with breast cancer undergoing mastectomy with or without immediate implant-based reconstruction. *Journal of Clinical Oncology.* 2021;39(28):supplement 65; Jogerst K, Thomas O, Kosiorek HE, et al. Same-day discharge after mastectomy: breast cancer surgery in the era of ERAS®. *Annals of Surgical Oncology.* 2020;27:3436–45. https://doi.org/10.1245/s10434-020-08386-w.

that is clear of cancer cells is great news: the rest of your lymph nodes are also presumed to be clear. (Any lymph nodes that look or feel enlarged or unusual will be removed during your lumpectomy or mastectomy.) The American Society of Clinical Oncology (ASCO) guidelines for early-stage breast cancer recommend offering SLNB to patients who

- have DCIS that is treated with mastectomy
- previously had breast cancer surgery or axillary lymph node surgery
- were previously treated with chemotherapy or other systemic treatment
- have multicentric tumors (multiple tumors that develop separately)

ASCO guidelines state that SLNB should *not* be offered to patients who[3]

- have a tumor that is 5 centimeters (2 inches) or larger or has spread in the breast or to lymph nodes
- have inflammatory breast cancer
- have DCIS and plan to have lumpectomy with radiation
- are pregnant

Axillary Lymph Node Dissection

When cancer cells are found in the sentinel node, an *axillary lymph node dissection (ALND)* is subsequently performed. During an ALND, the surgeon removes a pad of fat that contains some or all of the lymph nodes in the axilla (armpit) to determine whether chemotherapy or other systemic treatment is needed. This is usually, but not always, performed during a lumpectomy or a mastectomy. Because studies show that overall survival and the risk of recurrence in the breast or axilla (armpit) are similar regardless of whether additional lymph nodes are removed, ALND is performed less often than it was in the past. ALND isn't necessary when sentinel nodes are found to be clear of cancer cells or if you have one or two positive sentinel nodes and you plan to have a lumpectomy and radiation. If you have one or more positive sentinel nodes and plan to have a mastectomy without radiation, then talk to your doctor about the benefits and limitations of ALND. It's still used when

- three or more sentinel nodes contain cancer cells
- cancer has spread beyond the lymph nodes

The Risk of Lymphedema

While ALND is a critical diagnostic step, removing multiple lymph nodes can impair the lymph system's ability to adequately filter body fluids. The fluids may then collect in the arm, causing mild to severe *lymphedema*, a lifelong condition characterized by chronic swelling and numbness that can occur months or years after nodes are removed. Up to 30 percent of people who have axillary node dissection are believed to develop lymphedema, as opposed to the 5 to 17 percent for those who have the less invasive sentinel node procedure.[4] Radiating lymph nodes also increases the risk for lymphedema.

- enlarged lymph nodes can be felt before surgery or seen on imaging and a needle biopsy shows cancer
- cancer cells are found in the sentinel lymph node even after chemotherapy was given before surgery to reduce the size of the tumor

Male Mastectomy

Everyone, regardless of the sex assigned at their birth, has breast tissue and is at risk for developing breast cancer. The risk, however, is much greater in people who were assigned female at birth, but the danger extends to men, as well. The estimated lifetime risk of breast cancer for men is quite low: about 1 in 833 compared to 1 in 8 women.[5] Breast cancer is more common in men over the age of 60, although men of any age can be diagnosed. The risk is greater for men who have a family history of the disease or an inherited pre-disposition to breast cancer. It is also believed to be higher for trans women who take estrogen as part of hormone therapy (chapter 2). Most male breast cancers are one of the following types: DCIS, invasive ductal carcinoma, invasive lobular carcinoma, or Paget's disease of the nipple.

Because men have far less breast tissue than women, proportionately, male tumors tend to involve more of the breast than the same size tumor in a woman. Depending on the nature of the cancer, a total mastectomy or a modified radical mastectomy is usually recommended, followed by radiation if the cancer is advanced when diagnosed. Some men may be candidates for a mastectomy, while a lumpectomy and radiation may be reasonable for others. Radiation, chemotherapy, hormone therapy, and/or targeted therapy may also be recommended.

Men often don't need reconstruction after mastectomy because the amount of tissue removed isn't disfiguring. Men may opt for one or more of the reconstructive options described in part II, "Rebuilding the Breasts." Men are also entitled to health insurance coverage for breast reconstruction that is mandated by the Women's Health and Cancer Rights Act, even if the name of the law implies that it's just for women.

Lumpectomy or Mastectomy?

Depending on the nature of your cancer, you may have a choice between BCT or a mastectomy. You may opt for BCT if your priority is to preserve your breast. (A mastectomy would likely be recommended if your cancer returns after BCT because generally, radiating the same area of a breast more than once is believed to be unsafe.) Choosing a mastectomy also adds more complexity to decision-making and lengthens recovery. Should you have breast reconstruction? And, if so, are you prepared to have it at the same time as your mastectomy or sometime in the future? This is another layer of decision-making that requires additional research and careful consideration of the advantages and disadvantages of each choice.

If you have stage I or stage II breast cancer that can be treated with breast-conserving therapy or a mastectomy, then your doctor will likely leave the choice up to you. Where you're being treated in the United States may make a difference: decisions about breast conservation vary in different regions of the country. Lumpectomies are more common in the Northeast and in the West,

TABLE 1.1 Comparing Lumpectomy and Mastectomy

LUMPECTOMY	MASTECTOMY
preserves most of the breast	removes the breast
may need additional surgery	less likely to need additional surgery
outpatient procedure	outpatient or overnight hospital stay
radiation therapy usually required	radiation not required if lymph nodes are clear
shorter recovery	longer recovery
slightly higher risk of local recurrence*	slightly lower risk of local recurrence**
continued mammograms advised	mammograms no longer needed***
reconstruction not usually needed	reconstruction is always an option

*Depending on the hormone receptor status of the tumor. The risk of a distant recurrence (elsewhere in the body) is the same for BCT and mastectomy.

**When lymph nodes are clear.

***After unilateral mastectomy, routine mammograms of the remaining breast are recommended.

while mastectomies occur more often in the South and in the Midwest.[6] Physicians in metropolitan areas and locations where radiation facilities are plentiful are more likely to recommend BCT. The age and medical training of surgeons may also influence their treatment recommendations.

Your feelings, preferences, and priorities will also affect your decision. You may be unable to accommodate the schedule of radiation appointments, or you might simply prefer to avoid the potential side effects of radiation. Understandably, you may be anxious to get rid of the source of your cancer—your breast—and feel safer when you do. While the likelihood of a recurrence is slightly higher after a lumpectomy and radiation than after a mastectomy, a lumpectomy with radiation is as effective as a mastectomy in terms of survival. If you're uncomfortable with your risk for recurrence, you may feel that removing your breast will give you greater peace of mind. If you have a high risk of recurrence or another new tumor, removing your breast may give you greater peace of mind. It's a difficult decision that is best made by taking time to understand all of the facts, considering all of your options, and weighing the pros and cons of both surgeries before making the informed decision that is best for you (table 1.1).

Unless you have a very aggressive cancer, taking two or three weeks to get a second opinion will be well worth your time. (See "The Value of a Second (or Third) Opinion," chapter 17.) Another perspective can help you make an informed decision, and it just might save your breast. If you decide that a mastectomy is your best course of action, you have choices about how you'll look after your breast is removed.

Contralateral Mastectomy

If you're diagnosed with cancer in one breast, it's natural to fear a future diagnosis in the opposite breast. That's why many people who face unilateral mastectomy choose to remove their opposite, healthy breast, as well. *Contralateral prophylactic mastectomy (CPM)* isn't recommended for most breast cancer patients because the risk for a new cancer in the opposite breast is low, and CPM doesn't improve survival. CPM is generally recommended only for a small subset of individuals who have a very high risk of developing a second breast cancer (more on this in chapter 2). Yet despite the lack of benefit for most breast cancer patients, the rate of CPM has increased substantially in the past 20 years in all age groups, particularly among women who are younger than age 39, even though the majority of women who choose the procedure don't meet clinical guidelines for removing both breasts.[7] So why remove a perfectly healthy breast and have additional surgery that you don't need? There may be several reasons:

- People who are planning to have a unilateral mastectomy might decide to have CPM instead to gain peace of mind based on their overestimated risk for a future cancer in the opposite breast.
- Premastectomy MRIs, which are increasingly used, sometimes show early-stage abnormalities in the opposite breast. Individuals who have premastectomy MRIs are more likely to choose a contralateral mastectomy.[8]
- Widespread media coverage of celebrity mastectomies might influence a person's decision.
- Some people want to avoid future breast screenings.
- Some individuals prefer to have reconstruction of both breasts at the same time for better symmetry.

Questions for Your General Surgeon or Breast Surgeon

- What are my surgical options?
- Which procedure do you recommend for me and why?
- What are the benefits and risks of a lumpectomy compared to a mastectomy?
- Will I need radiation therapy?
- What is my risk of recurrence with either surgery?
- What is my expected survival with either surgery?
- What is my risk of contralateral breast cancer with either surgery?
- Can neoadjuvant (before surgery) chemotherapy, hormone therapy, or targeted therapy shrink my tumor enough so that lumpectomy is an option?
- How long can I take to make a decision?

Chapter 2

Considering a Risk-Reducing Mastectomy

My mother has breast cancer again; one of her sisters is in stage IV, and another is in remission. My grandmother and my mother's other sisters died of cancer. Even with this history, having my breasts removed was the hardest decision I've ever had to make. Though I had many breakdowns, I knew after all the crying that the decision I made was the right one. My breasts were precious to me but not as precious as my children. I wanted to make sure I'll be here to see them go off to life. Believe me when I say it's a relief.

—NORA

People who develop breast cancer are often surprised that no one else in their family has been diagnosed, but most cancers aren't hereditary. Most are *sporadic*; they develop from genetic damage we acquire as we age, rather than inherit. A small percentage of breast cancers are familial—they tend to run in families—with diagnoses of breast or ovarian cancers that occur across many generations and lead to the suspicion that hereditary factors may be the cause. Only 5 to 10 percent of breast cancers are caused by known inherited *gene mutations*—changes in genes that are passed from parent to child. About half of these are caused by mutations in the *BReast CAncer1* (*BRCA1*) and *BReast CAncer2* (*BRCA2*) genes. These genetic changes have been identified in almost every country and culture, but they're more common in certain ethnic populations. For example, about 1 in 40 people of Ashkenazi (Eastern European)

Other High-Risk Genes

The link between *BRCA* mutations and breast cancer is well-established, but harmful mutations in other genes, including *ATM*, *CDH1*, *CHEK2*, *PALB2*, *PTEN*, *STK11*, *TP53*, and others, elevate breast cancer risk, as well. The estimated increase varies, depending on which gene has the mutation. Other, as yet unidentified, genes may also affect breast cancer risk. Every parent with an inherited gene mutation has a 50 percent chance of passing it to their children. Having a family history of cancer, even when family members don't appear to have an inherited mutation, can also elevate cancer risk. Researchers don't know why some *previvors*—people who inherit a high risk for cancer but haven't been diagnosed—develop cancer and others don't.

Jewish ancestry carry a mutation in one of these genes, compared to about 1 in 500–1,000 individuals in the general population.

Although researchers haven't found all of the reasons that breast cancer runs in some families, discovering the relationship between *BRCA* genes and breast cancer gave them an unprecedented insight into the biology of hereditary breast cancer. While we often hear about people who decide to have genetic testing to see whether they have the "breast cancer gene," this is a misnomer. We all have two copies of *BRCA1* and *BRCA2* genes that, when healthy, produce proteins that repair cell damage and suppress tumor growth. When mutations damage these genes, their protective function is lost, and the risk of developing breast, ovarian, and certain other cancers increases. In some cases, the increase is significant. Inherited mutations in other genes also increase the risk of developing breast cancer as well as other cancers.

Should You Have Genetic Testing?

A small blood sample can be used to trace an individual's ancestry, identify DNA in crime scene evidence, and determine genetic predisposition to disease. *Genetic testing* is the only way to tell whether you've inherited a mutation that makes you prone to breast cancer. But testing isn't right for everyone, and not all families with breast cancer test positive for a mutation in a cancer-causing gene. Most have negative test results. You might wonder whether you, too, should be tested for an inherited gene mutation. Hereditary red flags aren't always obvious, and recognizing and interpreting them requires particular training and skill. If you're concerned that the cancer in your family is inherited and you're considering genetic testing to find out whether you carry a mutation, consulting with a specially trained *genetic counselor* is an important first step.

A genetic counselor will interpret your personal and family medical history to determine whether your family has a pattern of hereditary cancer, explain the benefits and limitations of genetic testing, and advise whether testing is appropriate for you or other family members. If you test positive for a mutation, the counselor will explain how different risk-management actions can reduce your chance of diagnosis. If your test is negative, the counselor will help you understand the implications of that result. Your primary physician or oncologist can refer you to a genetic counselor or genetics expert. You can also use the online directory of the National Society of Genetic Counselors (www.nsgc .org). If genetics experts are not accessible in your area, InformedDNA (www .informeddna.com) provides genetic counseling by telephone and video.

You may benefit from genetic testing if your family's medical history shows the following:

- a blood relative has tested positive for an inherited gene mutation linked to cancer

or

- you or a family member has had
  - pancreatic, ovarian, fallopian tube, primary peritoneal, or male breast cancer at any age
  - breast, colorectal, or endometrial cancer at age 50 or younger

- breast or prostate cancer at any age and Eastern European Jewish ancestry
- triple-negative breast cancer at any age
- prostate cancer at age 55 or younger or metastatic prostate cancer
- two separate cancer diagnoses
- rare or young-onset cancers (typically diagnosed before age 50)
- more than 10 colon polyps
- colorectal or endometrial cancer at any age with tumor testing that suggests Lynch syndrome (an inherited predisposition to colorectal and other cancers)
- tumor testing that shows a mutation in a gene associated with hereditary cancer

or

• more than one family member on the same side of the family has had a combination of breast, colorectal, ovarian, fallopian tube, primary peritoneal, endometrial, pancreatic, prostate, or stomach cancer; melanoma; a rare cancer; or young-onset cancer

How Real Is Your Risk?

Even as researchers continue to make great strides in understanding breast cancer, much about it remains an enigma. The science of risk assessment is far from perfect, and too many unknowns prevent genetics experts from predicting who will or won't get breast cancer or accurately pinpointing an individual's exact level of risk.

For the average woman in the United States, breast cancer risk is based on the rate of diagnosis among the entire population—hence, the familiar 1-in-8 statistic. Calculating risk for someone who has an inherited mutation in a *BRCA* gene or other high-risk gene is not as simple (table 2.1). For this, experts use estimates based on studies of breast cancer rates among high-risk families. Because these studies have found varying levels of risk, a high-risk individual's probability of developing breast cancer is often expressed as a range of estimated risk. Because every person's situation is unique, your risk assessment is influenced by the mutation you've inherited, the risk factors you can control

TABLE 2.1 Estimated Lifetime Risk of Breast Cancer (%)

	GENERAL POPULATION	BRCA1 MUTATION	BRCA2 MUTATION	OTHER HIGH-RISK MUTATIONS
Women*	13.0	65.0	61.0	15–60
Men**	0.1	0.1–1.5	1.9–7.7	unclear

Source: Li S, Silvestri V, Leslie G, et al. "Cancer risks associated with *BRCA1* and *BRCA2* pathogenic variants." *Journal of Clinical Oncology* 40, no. 14 (2022): 1529–41; Chen J, Bae E, Zhang L, et al. "Penetrance of breast and ovarian cancer in women who carry a *BRCA1/2* mutation and do not use risk-reducing salpingo-oophorectomy: An updated meta-analysis." *JNCI Cancer Spectrum* 4, no. 4 (2020): pkaa029.

Note: Estimates may change as more research is completed.

*To age 70.

**To age 80.

(smoking, weight, birth control, breast-feeding, and others), and those you cannot control (race, gender, age, family history, and others).

Regardless of the imprecise nature of risk assessment, experts agree that having a high-risk gene mutation or a strong family history of breast cancer doesn't guarantee that you'll also be diagnosed one day; but it significantly raises your risk. Whether you're a man or a woman, having a mutation in a *BRCA* gene or other high-risk gene raises the likelihood of breast cancer and increases the chance of receiving a diagnosis at a younger age, of having an aggressive type of breast cancer, and of developing breast cancer in both breasts. The risk for certain other cancers is also higher, depending on which gene has the mutation. If you're a breast cancer survivor with an inherited gene mutation, your risk of recurrence and another primary tumor is greater than other breast cancer survivors who don't have an inherited mutation.

While understanding and confronting unusually high cancer risk can be perplexing and frightening, there are opportunities to do something about it. Someday scientists may discover ways to repair defective genes. Until that time, if you're predisposed to developing breast cancer, you have options to manage your high risk or increase surveillance:

- risk-reducing medication with increased surveillance
- preventive mastectomy

- increased breast screening with a physical exam, mammogram, MRI, and/or ultrasound, which won't lower your risk of developing breast cancer but may find a future malignancy at an early, more treatable stage

Risk-Reducing Mastectomy

If genetic testing shows that you've inherited a mutation in a *BRCA1*, *BRCA2*, *PALB2*, *PTEN*, *TP53*, or another gene that increases your risk for breast cancer, your genetic counselor or doctor may recommend a *risk-reducing mastectomy (RRM)* (also called *prophylactic bilateral mastectomy*)—preemptively removing both breasts—as the most effective way to lower your risk. It isn't advised for women with average or slightly increased risk or for high-risk men. RRM decreases the odds of a diagnosis by at least 95 percent.[1] (A small risk remains because it's not possible to remove every bit of breast tissue.) If your estimated risk for breast cancer is 65 percent, RRM will reduce it to about 3 percent—about one-quarter of the risk for women who don't have a *BRCA* mutation. (Other lifestyle and behavioral factors also increase or further decrease your level of risk.) Your doctor may also recommend considering RRM if you

- have a strong family history of breast cancer
- have been diagnosed with breast cancer in one breast, which raises the risk for a diagnosis in your opposite breast
- have been diagnosed with lobular carcinoma in situ, especially with a family history of breast cancer
- had radiation to your chest before age 30

Some experts argue that many women who preventively remove their breasts do so needlessly because not all of them will develop breast cancer. Clinically, that may be an understandable hypothesis. You might not have the same point of view, though, if you're extraordinarily prone to developing breast cancer or you've seen loved ones struggle with a cancer diagnosis and treatment, and you're willing to lose your breasts to avoid the same fate and potentially save your life. Even with its impressive risk-reducing benefit, RRM is a deeply personal choice. It isn't right for everyone, and it shouldn't be considered lightly because once it's done, it can't be undone. However, if you're prepared to do whatever you can to reduce your elevated chance of being diagnosed with breast cancer and dealing with a mastectomy and/or chemotherapy, radiation, or other treatments, it's the most effective alternative.

Making a Decision

A risk-reducing mastectomy may be an easy decision for some women. Others would never consider removing their healthy breasts. Whatever your circumstances, the decision can be torturous. Should you? Shouldn't you? No one can answer that question for you. If you have a high risk of breast cancer, talk with your healthcare team about all of your options before deciding what is right for you. If you decide RRM is the best way to have peace of mind as you live your life, you'll have a skin-sparing or nipple-sparing total mastectomy followed by immediate breast reconstruction. Breast reconstruction after RRM produces exceptional cosmetic results, particularly if your healthy breasts are unscarred from biopsies or previous surgeries. If you're unsatisfied with the shape, size, or position of your natural breasts, reconstruction can improve those issues, although your new breasts may not look or feel the same. If you prefer to forego reconstruction, your chest will remain flat after your surgery.

Additional Surgeries to Further Reduce Breast Cancer Risk

Removing both ovaries and both fallopian tubes also reduces the high risk of breast cancer. Experts also recommend *risk-reducing salpingo-oophorectomy (RRSO)* between ages 35 and 40 or when you complete childbearing if you have a *BRCA1* mutation, and between ages 40 and 45 if you have a *BRCA2* mutation (*BRCA2*-related breast cancer is less likely to develop before age 50). RRSO before natural menopause reduces ovarian cancer risk by up to 90 percent; it also lowers breast cancer risk by about half.[2] Having both RRM and RRSO lowers overall breast cancer risk by 95 percent. Less is known about the beneficial effects of RRSO in women with other high-risk mutations. The decision to have RRSO deserves careful consideration because it can cause serious side effects. If you're still having menstrual periods, it will push your body into menopause, and you may prematurely experience hot flashes, insomnia, vaginal dryness, and other change-of-life symptoms. Your gynecologist or oncologist can discuss these issues with you and let you know what to expect.

Ultimately, whether you proceed with a prophylactic mastectomy or not is your decision. Friends and family might consider breast removal to be extreme. Unless they've had to make the decision themselves, people may not understand why you would deliberately remove your perfectly healthy breasts. Take the time you need to consider what each risk-reducing option involves, how it affects your current and future level of risk, and the potential side effects. Speak with your healthcare team, including a genetics specialist, to gain a clear sense of your own risk. Carefully consider your tolerance for risk, your lifestyle, and other factors before deciding which alternative is the best for you. Facing Our Risk of Cancer Empowered (FORCE), the foremost nonprofit education and support group for the hereditary cancer community, provides information online (www.facingourrisk.org), by phone, and through outreach coordinators in most states. The organization's message boards offer a supportive, safe, and empowering place to learn, share, and just vent about genetic high risk, prophylactic surgery, mastectomy, and reconstruction. *Living with Hereditary Cancer Risk*, the organization's decision-making resource for previvors and survivors of hereditary cancer, is a comprehensive road map for living in a high-risk body.

> I do think prophylactic bilateral mastectomy is pretty extreme but so is cancer. It's all a matter of how much risk you're willing to live with day to day, compared to your willingness to undergo major surgery to reduce that risk to as close to zero as possible. You do as much research as you can by reading and talking to people who have the appropriate knowledge and experience, then you do what's right for you. I didn't want RRM. However, in examining my own personal and family history, my temperament, and life goals, I couldn't not have it.
>
> —*Jill*

Paying for Genetic Counseling, Testing, and Risk-Reducing Surgeries

Most public and private health insurance plans cover the cost of genetic counseling and testing if you meet certain criteria and your doctor recommends the test. Some insurers may require that you have genetic counseling before being tested and that you provide a letter from your genetic counselor or referring physician stating the medical necessity of the test.

Coverage and out-of-pocket costs vary depending on your situation, the test involved, and the terms of your plan. Medicare only pays for genetic testing for inherited mutations if you have been diagnosed with cancer. Medicaid coverage of genetic counseling and testing varies by state. Some Medicaid programs may cover testing fees if you meet state requirements. Under the Affordable Care Act, most health plans must pay for the entire cost of genetic counseling and testing for a *BRCA* mutation with no *out-of-pocket* costs to patients, but this coverage has limitations.

Testing can be costly, so it's important to know in advance what your health insurer will cover and under what terms. Your genetic counselor will review your coverage, help you obtain preauthorization, and, if necessary, help you appeal if your insurance denies payment for counseling or testing. If your request for coverage is denied, ask your primary care physician, oncologist, or medical geneticist to write a supportive letter explaining how your high-risk status meets nationally recognized guidelines for these services. The FORCE website has several sample appeal letters. If you're uninsured or underinsured, your genetic counselor can determine whether you're eligible for discounted or no-cost testing offered by some labs.

If you test positive for an inherited mutation that raises your risk of breast cancer, most health insurers will cover the costs for recommended increased surveillance, risk-reducing medication, and a preventive mastectomy with or without reconstruction. Out-of-pocket expenses depend on the specific service performed and the details of your policy. Several states require this coverage when it's "medically necessary," although insurance companies may define it in different ways. (Federal law doesn't require health insurers to cover a mastectomy solely to reduce the risk of breast cancer.) Some health insurance providers will pay some or all of the costs with either a letter from your doctor recommending a mastectomy to lower your high risk or a second confirming opinion. Contact your local affiliate of the American Cancer Society or Susan G. Komen about donated surgical services.

Questions for Your Genetic Counselor

- Does my family history show a pattern of inherited disease?
- Should I have genetic testing to see if I have an inherited predisposition to cancer?
- For which mutations should I be tested?
- How reliable are genetic test results?
- What are my options if I test positive?
- What are the implications of a negative test?
- Will my test results influence my cancer treatment?
- What does genetic testing mean for me and my family members?
- Will my insurance pay for testing? If not, what are my options for low-cost testing?

Chapter 3

Going Flat: Mastectomy without Reconstruction

I had an epiphany when I woke up after my mastectomy: I thought I would lose my sex appeal and femininity without my breasts, but that didn't happen. I spent many years with a knock-out curvaceous body, but now I'm okay with the new me and I've never regretted my decision. I found my spirit, my beauty, my confidence . . . myself. I've never worn breast forms. I go flat and I'm not embarrassed. I look great, and I'm still turning heads; most people don't even know I have no breasts. A surprising benefit to having no breasts is that when I hug my husband, we are chest to chest, skin to skin—closer than we ever were before when my breasts were "in the way." It's a nice feeling.

—SANGRIA

Discussions about whether women should have breast reconstruction after a mastectomy are like politics: everyone has an opinion. Wander around the internet and you'll find vehement blogs against reconstruction, arguing why women should stay flat after a mastectomy. You'll also find the polar opposite view: strongly worded tributes to the physical, emotional, and psychological benefits of breast reconstruction. As women, we are all different. We have distinct goals, varying likes and dislikes, and decidedly contrasting opinions of what is right for each of us. Some of us feel the breast reconstruction journey is worth the effort, and that is fine. Others consider it a waste of time and effort, and that's also okay because what is right for one isn't necessarily right for all.

You might decide against reconstruction if you

- are comfortable not having breasts
- want to avoid additional surgery and recovery
- don't want breasts that aren't "real" and have little or no feeling
- want to try going flat before committing to reconstructive surgery
- are unsure about reconstruction at the time of your mastectomy
- have a health condition or pending treatment that precludes having reconstructive surgery

What to Expect

The goal of a mastectomy is always to remove as much breast tissue as possible, regardless of whether you have reconstruction. If you don't have reconstruction at the time of your mastectomy, a broad elliptical incision is made across your breast, through which the tumor (if you have breast cancer), your breast tissue, and most of the skin, including the nipple and areola, and any previous biopsy scars are removed (figure 3.1). The edges of skin on either side of the incision are pulled together and closed around a *surgical drain*, which remains in place for two to three weeks to drain fluids away from your chest as you heal (read more about drains in chapter 14).

Before your surgery, it's important to speak with your general surgeon or breast surgeon about how your incision will be made and how your chest will look after your mastectomy. To avoid *dog ears* (puckered skin at the ends of the incision), uneven scars, bulges of excess skin, and a concave chest that often remain after a mastectomy without reconstruction, talk to your surgeon about an *aesthetic flat closure*. It's a procedure that removes all excess breast skin and fat so that the postmastectomy chest is smooth and flat against the chest wall. If your surgeon is unable or unwilling to accommodate this, consider seeing a different surgeon. If you're unhappy with the way your chest looks after a mastectomy, you can then consult with a plastic surgeon who can revise your scar, improve your chest contour by transferring fat from elsewhere on your body, and make other cosmetic improvements (figure 3.2). If you change your mind about breast reconstruction, it's an option at any time in the future.

FIGURE 3.1 Mastectomy without reconstruction is performed through an elliptical incision that spans the breast.

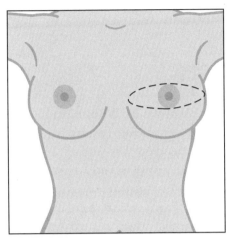 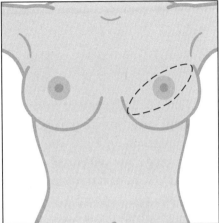

FIGURE 3.2 Scar revision and fat grafting can improve unsatisfactory mastectomy scars (*left*), creating aesthetic flat closures instead (*right*).

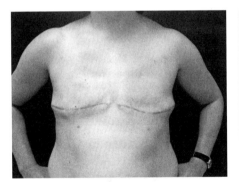 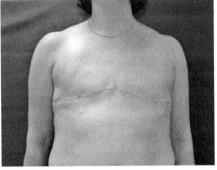

Flat Denial

Going flat isn't right or wrong. It's a personal choice. While most plastic surgeons support patients who prefer to forego breast reconstruction, some women report experiencing "flat denial," meaning that their surgeons assume that they want or should have breast reconstruction after a mastectomy. Most respondents to a survey of 931 women who decided against reconstruction after a unilateral or bilateral mastectomy said that they were satisfied with their surgical outcome and their surgeons' support and empathy for their decision to go flat. Yet 22 percent said they had experienced flat denial—their surgeon didn't offer information about going flat, didn't support their decision to do so, or left excess skin after a mastectomy, in case the woman "changed their mind" later. Women with this experience were more likely to be dissatisfied with the results of their surgery. If your surgeon doesn't offer you the option to go flat, isn't receptive to your decision, or insists that you'll later change your mind, consider finding another breast surgeon who supports your decision.

Source: Baker JL, Dizon DS, Wenziger CM, et al. "Going flat" after mastectomy: patient-reported outcomes by online survey. *Annals of Surgical Oncology.* 2021;28(5):2493–2505.

A mastectomy is performed in a hospital or other medical facility under general anesthesia. A unilateral mastectomy lasts 1–2 hours; a bilateral procedure lasts longer, depending on the nature of your mastectomy and your hospital's protocol. You'll be up and walking around soon after your surgery. In many hospitals and surgery centers, patients go home the same day. Once you return home, you'll need extra rest for several days. A nurse will demonstrate gentle (but important) movements to prevent stiffness in your shoulder and arm. Performing these exercises daily will gradually restore full range of motion and strength in your chest, shoulders, and arms. While you'll become a bit stronger each day, you may need four to six weeks before you're fully healed and able to resume your normal routine.

Unless complications occur, you may be surprised to feel minimal pain after your mastectomy, because nerves in the breast are severed when the tissue is removed. Your chest will be numb and may feel heavy, and you may feel a pulling sensation under your arm; this improves as your chest heals. Prescribed medication will control any discomfort in the first few days after your surgery, and then you can use over-the-counter medication as needed. Initially, your mastectomy incision will be red and prominent. It will fade noticeably after several months but remain on your chest, even if you have reconstruction later on. As more than one patient has said, mastectomy scars are a reminder that you've lost a breast; they're also a reminder that you've survived.

Having a *BRCA1* mutation, my risk-reduction plan included preventive mastectomies without reconstruction. As a physician and a caregiver for a cancer patient, I wanted to quickly get back to my life. I felt lucky that my lifestyle, personality, and relationships weren't focused on my breasts, and I didn't want to bother with mastectomy bras and prostheses. With no reconstruction to worry about, I had only minor issues with healing. But I worried about what people would think about my choice and how I would cope with prominent scars that run unevenly across my chest with an inch gap in-between, which isn't the ideal cosmetic appearance. After a year, the scars faded to my natural skin color. Three years later, I'm proud and pleased to have acted so quickly and adapted so well to this big challenge and major surgery. I've moved forward with my life, and I never worry about how my activities will affect my chest. I'm confident in my ability to do a self-exam of my chest to find any future cancer. My scars sometimes attract my attention when I look in the mirror—often I just see me. No one has ever commented about noticing that I go flat. I wouldn't have done anything differently.

—Margaret

The Goldilocks Option

If you don't want or can't have breast reconstruction but you prefer not to be completely flat, you might want to consider a *Goldilocks mastectomy*. In this procedure, the breast tissue is removed, the nipple is preserved, and the fat that remains under the breast skin is shaped into a breast.[1] The premise of this type of mastectomy is that it's just right for some individuals: it doesn't leave them too flat like a traditional mastectomy, and it's not as complex nor as involved as breast reconstruction. Instead, it's somewhere in between.

Unlike a traditional mastectomy that is performed through an incision across the breast or around the areola, Goldilocks mastectomy involves incisions that are similar to those made for a breast reduction (described in chapter 10). The newly shaped breast is smaller than the person's natural breast; the size depends on the amount of fat that remains after the mastectomy. Women who are obese or who have very large breasts tend to have more subcutaneous fat, which can provide the best results. No additional surgeries are needed, although subsequent fat grafting can add volume and improve contour, if needed.

Not all breast surgeons offer this procedure. If you're interested in a Goldilocks mastectomy, look for a breast surgeon, general surgeon, or surgical oncologist who has experience with this procedure and ask to see their before-and-after patient photos. No large studies have yet identified appropriate candidates for this procedure or determined its predictability and safety.

The Prosthesis Alternative

With a flat chest, you may need to discover new ways to dress. Many of your premastectomy clothes may continue to fit well; others may not. These challenges may differ depending on whether you had one or both breasts removed. Fortunately, you have lots of options. Postmastectomy bras, lingerie, camisoles, athletic wear, and swimsuits are designed to be feminine and fashionable. After bilateral mastectomy, you may prefer to remain flat under your clothes or wear *breast prostheses*, breast-shaped forms that temporarily attach to your chest or fit into the pockets of special bras, lingerie, swimsuits, and camisoles to temporarily restore shape and profile. If both of your breasts are removed, your new "breast" size is limited only by the prostheses you choose. Unilateral mastectomy presents a more practical problem. Because one breast is missing, you may feel unbalanced or lopsided and find it difficult to fit into clothes. When you're dressed, one side of your chest will be flat; if you wear a bra, one cup will be empty. You can balance your remaining breast and regain symmetry with a weighted prosthesis that will provide equilibrium and help you to maintain proper posture. (Weighted prostheses aren't necessary after bilateral mastectomy because your chest, although flat, is balanced.) If you're undecided about reconstruction or you need to delay it until you've completed your postmastectomy treatment, a prosthesis can serve as a temporary breast during the in-between interval.

Some prostheses adhere to your chest and can be worn without a bra. Consider trying one before you buy several, just in case the adhesive irritates your skin. Prostheses can be worn in or under your clothes to help keep your shoulders in proper alignment, balance your posture, and provide symmetry when you're dressed. You can also buy sew-in pockets to modify bras to hold prostheses. If you're handy with a needle and thread, you can alter just about any bra yourself (search the internet for "sew-in mastectomy pockets"). Partial prostheses are also available to fill out postlumpectomy indentations in the top, bottom, or side of your breast.

If you contact Reach to Recovery (www.cancer.org; search for "Reach to Recovery") several weeks before your mastectomy, a volunteer will bring a lightweight starter prosthesis and a mastectomy camisole or bra to the hospital and show you how to use them. When your mastectomy scar heals sufficiently—generally in about four to six weeks—your surgeon will give you a prescription for mastectomy bras and more balanced, better designed prostheses. Be sure to get a written prescription; otherwise, your insurance may not cover the cost. It's a good idea to be measured by a qualified fitter—one who is certified by the American Board for Certification in Orthotics, Prosthetics, and Pedorthics—for your first postmastectomy bra and prosthesis to ensure they fit properly on your chest and aren't too light or too heavy. Try on different styles to see which ones look and feel the best.

FIGURE 3.3 Triangular prostheses fill in missing tissue at the sides and top of the breast (*left*). Teardrop prostheses add extra fullness at the bottom (*center*). Some prostheses are adjustable (*right*).

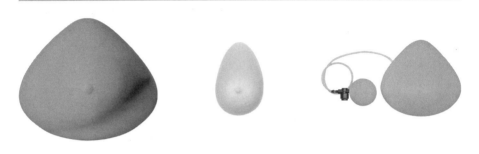

Images courtesy of Amoena USA Corporation

A Plethora of Prostheses

Prostheses are available in different shapes (figure 3.3), skin tones, and materials; and they vary in cost. Although inexpensive cotton, foam, and fiberfill prostheses are comfortable and fill a bra, they provide minimal shape. Soft gel prostheses are lighter. Silicone breast forms feel and look the most natural—they're also more expensive—and most closely mimic the weight of a natural breast (the silicone used is different from the filling of breast implants). You can buy them with or without nipples; you can also purchase stick-on nipples. Silicone prostheses are heavier than cotton, foam, or gel and can be uncomfortably hot in the summer or when a menopausal hot flash occurs. Lightweight silicone prostheses are also available. Very light breast forms made of thousands of plastic microbeads and covered with soft fabric are another alternative; they're like beanbags with tiny beads that mold to your body. Visit the BreastFree website (www.breastfree.org) or Knitted Knockers (www.knittedknockers.org) for details about making your soft breast forms.

Where to Shop

Nordstrom and JCPenney sell mastectomy garments and prostheses online, from catalogs, and in their store lingerie departments, where specially trained fitters will help you find exactly what you need. Postmastectomy boutiques are often listed online or in the phone directory under "mastectomy forms and supplies" or "prosthetics." You'll also find a wide selection online (try www.amoena.com, www.landsend.com, www.tlcdirect.org, and www .mastectomyshop.com). Your hospital or breast care clinic may also have a qualified fitter or may refer you to a local boutique. If you'd like to explore the possibility of a prosthesis made to your exact specifications, visit www .newattitudebreasts.com or search online for "custom breast prosthesis." It's a more expensive option and may not be fully covered by insurance.

Tips for Buying Prostheses

- Let a qualified fitter in a mastectomy boutique or department store help you find the right size and fit you correctly.
- Take someone with you for a second opinion about how you look wearing different prostheses.
- After unilateral mastectomy, it's important to match the weight and size of your remaining breast.
- Consider prostheses of different weights and fabrics for different activities or occasions.
- If you like to swim, choose a prosthesis that won't be damaged by salt water or chlorine.

More Information and Support

Looking for more insight into what it's like to go flat after a mastectomy? Three helpful and informative sources are BreastFree (www .breastfree.org), Flat & Fabulous (www.flatandfabulous.org), and Not Putting on a Shirt (www.notputtingonashirt.org).

Paying for a Mastectomy and Prostheses

The Women's Health and Cancer Rights Act (WHCRA) requires insurance companies that pay for a mastectomy to also cover the cost of breast prostheses. Coverage varies, so check with your health insurer to see what your policy covers and what information is required for a claim. Some insurers base their coverage on Medicare guidelines: With a doctor's prescription, coverage typically includes one non-silicone prosthesis (two after bilateral mastectomy) every six months and one silicone prosthesis every two years (two after bilateral mastectomy). Medicare coverage also includes four to six mastectomy bras annually or more if your doctor says they are medically necessary—if you have additional surgery or lose or gain weight, for example. (Bras aren't usually covered until after a mastectomy surgery.) These guidelines sometimes change, so it's a good idea to check with your insurance company to see what your coverage allows.

You'll need to pay out-of-pocket costs, such as any health insurance co-pays and additional costs if you haven't yet met your required deductible for the year. Many retailers will bill your insurance company directly after you pay a small co-payment. Other vendors may require full payment at the time of purchase; you can then request reimbursement from your insurance company. (Medicare requires a reimbursement claim directly from the supplying vendor; the reimbursement payment is then forwarded directly to you.) If you don't have insurance and can't afford a prosthesis, contact your local and state cancer organizations or the following sources to explore financial assistance or the possibility of getting prostheses at no charge:

- American Cancer Society (www.cancer.org)
- CancerCare (www.cancercare.org)
- Patient Advocate Foundation (www.copays.org)

Questions for Your General Surgeon or Breast Surgeon

- Where will my incisions be on my chest?
- Can you give me an aesthetic flat closure?
- How many of these have you done?
- May I see your patient photos of this procedure?
- How long will my mastectomy take?
- Will this be an outpatient procedure?
- What should I expect from recovery?
- What if I'm not happy with the way my chest looks after the mastectomy?

Chapter 4

How a Mastectomy Affects Reconstruction

My reconstructed breasts look fabulous, but I can't feel a thing except along the outside. Most of my breasts feel as though they've been shot through with Novocain. When I'm sitting down, I can lean forward and not even feel the edge of the table pressing into my new boobs. They could be on fire, and I wouldn't know it! You get used to it.

—ANGEL

If you're considering reconstruction, two questions are probably foremost in your mind: How will my new breasts look? And how will they feel? Even though reconstruction isn't perfect, and not all women have optimal outcomes, it can be a remarkable process. But even the best plastic surgeons can't replace what a mastectomy takes away: your natural breasts. A mastectomy and immediate reconstruction are two distinct procedures by different surgeons that are performed during one visit to the operating room. It's important to understand how certain aspects of a mastectomy influence your reconstruction.

Mastectomy Cause and Effect

Before your operation, your surgeon will draw the incision lines on your breast. If you've chosen to have immediate reconstruction with your mastectomy, the surgeon will also mark around any previous biopsy scars where the cancer was found; they'll be *re-excised* during surgery. This means cutting around the scar and removing it, in case any cancerous cells remain.

Each step of the mastectomy procedure affects your breast reconstruction:

Mastectomy: Once you're anesthetized on the operating table, the surgeon makes incisions along the markings made on your breast.

Effect: The placement of your incision(s) depends on how much tissue must be removed and your plastic surgeon's preference to facilitate your reconstruction. Incisions leave permanent scars. Although your mastectomy scar may be hidden in the *inframammary fold* (the crease under your breast) or camouflaged by tattoos, incisions made on the breast remain. Scars fade considerably within several months after surgery and become less visible after a year or two.

Mastectomy: The breast skin within the incisions, including the nipple and areola, may be removed. There are exceptions to this, as you'll see later in this chapter.

Effect: New nipples can be created, but they will lack sensory nerves, which means they won't respond to touch or temperature as natural nipples do.

Effect: Amputating the nipple and areola and then closing the incision flattens the natural projection of the breast. The location or size of a tumor often requires the removal of additional skin, which also reduces projection, particularly when skin is taken from the front of the breast. A reconstructed breast tends to have better projection when the mastectomy incision runs vertically from the bottom of the areola to the inframammary fold, rather than horizontally across the nipple.

Mastectomy: All visible breast tissue from the collarbone to the underarm and across to the middle of the rib cage is separated from the underlying muscle and overlying skin and is removed.

Effect: Because breast tissue blends with the thin layer of tissue beneath the skin and is intimately attached to the chest wall, it's not possible to remove every bit of it. Some residual breast tissue is left behind, regardless of the type of mastectomy. That's why a small chance of recurrence remains after a mastectomy.

Effect: Removing breast tissue eliminates the milk ducts and lobules. Breast-feeding isn't possible after a mastectomy, even if your breast and nipple are reconstructed, because the mechanisms to produce and deliver milk have been eliminated.

Effect: Removing breast tissue severs nerves that travel throughout the breast and provide sensation. Although women often retain or recover some feeling in the upper, outer, or lower perimeters of their breasts and in between their breasts, much of the breast typically remains numb after a mastectomy. Reconstruction can recreate breast shape and volume, but it doesn't restore the degree and dimension of sensation you had before a mastectomy.

Losing and Regaining Sensation

Sensory nerves send electrical impulses (messages) to the spinal cord and brain. (These nerves differ from motor nerves, which carry information from the brain and spinal cord to muscles.) Sensory nerves run throughout breast tissue: nipples and areolas are a bonanza of nerve endings. Sensory nerves become casualties of mastectomy when they're severed as breast tissue is removed, and they can no longer send messages to the spinal cord and brain. With the sensory system down, sensation is lost.

Understanding the Nature of Sensation

After a mastectomy, nerves may regenerate and provide varying degrees of sensation in areas of the breast. Patches of pressure sensation in the skin may return in time and continue to improve for a year or more after surgery, but it won't be the same discrete sensitivity to light touch, temperature (cold and heat), or pain that you're used to. Because nerves typically grow unpredictably and at a snail's pace—about one inch per month and more slowly after radiation or chemotherapy—it can take several months or several years before they grow enough to reach the breast skin. Compared to reconstruction with implants, *autologous flap reconstruction* (with your own tissue) offers a better chance of regaining some sensation if nerve endings in the chest spontaneously connect with nerves in the flap. As nerve endings grow into the tissue of the new breast, areas may become hypersensitive; you might feel that you have too much sensation or experience tingling, burning, or other strange sensations. These unusual feelings gradually subside. Some women have *phantom sensations* similar to those experienced by people who have lost an arm or a leg. This occurs when the brain temporarily continues to receive sensory impulses from nerves in the breast, even though the nerves have been severed or removed.

Can Sensation in the Skin be Restored?

Neurotization, restoring sensation, is one of the last remaining frontiers in breast reconstruction, and perhaps one of the most important. For the most part, it's been an elusive goal because the focus of a mastectomy has tradition-ally been to remove breast tissue rather than preserve sensory nerves, and neurosurgical technology has not yet advanced enough to reliably repair and restore function in tiny nerves like those found in breast tissue. Neurotizing a reconstructed breast can be addressed in four ways:

- preserving sensory nerves during a mastectomy (without compro-mising oncologic safety)
- nerve regrowth that occurs naturally after reconstruction, without surgical intervention
- repairing sensory nerves that are cut during a mastectomy
- reconnecting a nerve in an autologous flap to a sensory nerve in the chest

Most surgeons who offer breast reconstruction don't pursue nerve restora-tion; it's an exacting procedure that requires meticulous skill, extra time, and hasn't been proven to work. Increasingly, however, it's gaining interest among patients and surgeons. Some surgeons attempt to improve sensation in the skin with *microneurorrhaphy*, which involves reconnecting a sensory nerve in an autologous flap (your own tissue) to a nerve in the chest that was cut during a mastectomy. This is an unpredictable and unreliable process that isn't possible if the recipient nerve in the chest is damaged during a mastectomy. (Sensation is minimal at best after reconstruction with breast implants because implants don't have nerves and they can block growing nerves from reaching the skin.)

Attempting to improve sensation with *nerve grafts* or *nerve conduits* are newer approaches in breast reconstruction that have been successful with other types of reconstructive surgeries. A nerve graft is a segment of donated or processed nerve that connects two cut nerves, similar to the way a dam-aged electrical cord is repaired. A nerve conduit is a bit different (figure 4.1). Rather than directly providing sensation, it supports growth between two

FIGURE 4.1 Nerves run throughout breast tissue (*left*). Nerve conduits support growth between two severed nerves (*right*).

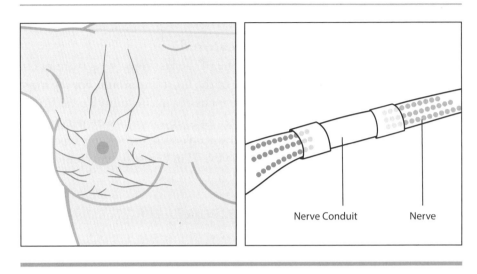

Nerve Conduit   Nerve

severed nerves. Ideally, new nerve fibers grow through the conduit from one end of a nerve and into the other, reestablishing some level of sensation. Although studies of nerve reconnection with autologous reconstruction are encouraging, objective results are difficult to measure, and these procedures don't guarantee sensation or the type of feeling that might be restored.[1] Autologous tissue reconstruction that is buried beneath intact breast skin (skin-sparing and nipple-sparing mastectomies) is not likely to produce a meaningful benefit to sensation in the overlying skin. Some degree of sensation in the skin might be improved with autologous reconstruction that involves large areas of exposed flap skin (delayed reconstruction). Larger, well-controlled studies with standardized design and methods of measuring sensation are needed to objectively evaluate whether nerve grafts and connectors can reliably and predictably speed up and/or improve sensation that would spontaneously develop without intervention.

Neurotization is typically viewed as experimental by many health insurance companies and may not be covered. For now, the best hope for maximized sensation is a meticulous mastectomy technique, with attention to protecting sensory nerves when possible, combined with autologous tissue reconstruction.

Skin-Sparing Mastectomy

If you have immediate reconstruction, a *skin-sparing mastectomy* will remove as much breast tissue as possible while preserving most of your breast skin to hold an implant or a flap of your own tissue to form your new breast. Your breast surgeon and plastic surgeon will work together to plan where your mastectomy incision(s) should be made to accomplish both of these goals and to camouflage the incisions on your reconstructed breast as much as possible. Your nipple and areola will be removed through a circular or elliptical incision, leaving a hole through which the entire mastectomy and reconstruction will be performed (figure 4.2). An additional incision to the side or below the nipple may be needed to remove biopsy scars and breast tissue. If your mastectomy is being performed to treat breast cancer, any skin involving or near the tumor will also be removed. If you have reconstruction with your own tissue, a portion of the flap skin will fill this opening. If you have implant reconstruction, the opening will be closed, usually with dissolvable stitches. Later tattooing of the nipple and areola will mask the scar.

Compared to delayed breast reconstruction, skin-sparing mastectomy with immediate reconstruction produces a new breast with minimal scarring. If you begin a mastectomy and immediate reconstruction without breast scars from previous biopsies or other operations, you have a good chance of emerging from the operating room in much the same way. Skin-sparing mastectomies aren't

FIGURE 4.2 Skin-sparing mastectomy may be performed through a periareolar incision (*left*) or a cat's eye incision (*center*). An additional vertical or horizontal incision may also be required (*right*).

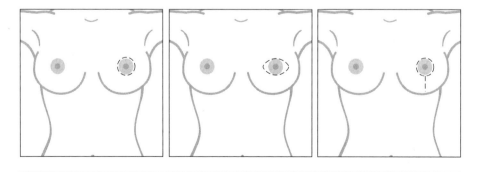

recommended if you have inflammatory breast cancer or cancer in or near your breast skin.

Nipple-Sparing Mastectomy

Nipple-sparing mastectomy (NSM) represents the evolution of breast removal—from Halsted's radical mastectomy that took the entire breast, chest muscle, and lymph nodes, to a procedure that removes breast tissue but preserves most of the visible breast, including the skin, nipple, and areola. With an NSM, your incision will be minimized and positioned to be less obvious and may be completely hidden on your reconstructed breast. NSM produces superior cosmetic results, concealing your mastectomy scar, without compromising cancer treatment. What lies beneath the skin is different (an implant, a tissue flap, or both), yet your breast appears natural, intact, and virtually unchanged. Studies of NSM show that the rate of local–regional recurrence is low among carefully selected candidates: between 1.8 and 2.3 percent of women who have NSM experience a local or regional recurrence of their breast cancer.[2]

Compared to skin-sparing mastectomy, which removes the nipple and areola, an NSM requires meticulous surgical skill to carefully remove the tissue at the base of the areola and nipple without damaging the delicate supportive blood vessels. If this vital blood supply is compromised, some or all of the nipple may die. Placing the incision under the breast or along the outer contour, rather than around the nipple, reduces the odds of that happening and avoids severing small nerves that serve the nipple and areola (figure 4.3).

FIGURE 4.3 Nipple-sparing mastectomy incisions are often made under the breast (*left*), beneath the areola (*center*), or horizontally from the areola to the outer breast (*right*).

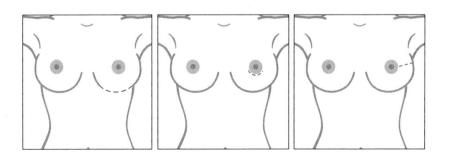

I decided on nipple-sparing mastectomy with immediate reconstruction because my breasts were important to my sexuality, and I was concerned about losing erogenous sensation. My surgeon performed a nerve reconnection, even though it is controversial. It took a year and a half, but my right breast now has nearly normal sensation, and the nipple has some erogenous feeling. It's not as pleasurable as before, but it is thrilling to have some feeling back. My left nipple senses touch and temperature, although it has no erogenous response. I know many women regain feeling without the extra two-hour procedure to reconnect nerves, so it's hard to know if my sensation would have returned anyway. I feel lucky and just like the same old me, which was all I really wanted.

—Lisa

After my nipple-sparing surgery my breasts were bruised and dented, with the nipples pointing in opposite directions. Week by week the bruising disappeared and the nipples evened out. After a few months, I was very pleased with my results, and within six months I was thrilled. It took about a year for my breasts to settle permanently. Now the scars under my breasts have faded to practically nothing. I went from an A-cup to a small C-cup, my projection looks natural, and I can go braless without a problem. It was important to me to come out of surgery looking essentially the same, and that is what keeping my nipples did for me. My new breasts look like my own, and they are fantastic! I do not have sensation on or around my nipples; however, I went into surgery well aware of this probability, and I accept it as part of the trade-off to vastly reduce my breast cancer risk. I would make the same decision, with the same surgeons, in a heartbeat.

—Andrea

— EXPERT INSIGHT —

Blood Flow is Critical for Nipple-Sparing Mastectomy

DAVID J. WINCHESTER, MD, FACS

One of the concerns with nipple-sparing mastectomy is that much of the blood supply to the nipple is derived from the underlying breast tissue and not the surrounding skin. It is necessary to divide these blood vessels to separate the tissue from the overlying nipple. Everyone has different anatomic variations; until this step is taken, it's difficult to determine whether the nipple will survive. If it can immediately get enough blood flow from the surrounding skin, it will remain healthy. When the incision is placed right next to the nipple, a significant portion of the necessary blood flow is temporarily divided; blood flow is usually better when the incision is placed either along the outer breast or the lower portion of the breast.

During NSM, the nipple and areola remain attached to the breast (figure 4.4). The underlying tissue is removed and examined; if cancer is found, the nipple and areola are then also removed. (NSM isn't the same as *subcutaneous* mastectomies performed in the 1970s that intentionally left behind breast tissue—and sometimes cancer cells—to preserve adequate blood supply to the

FIGURE 4.4 Before (*left*) and after (*right*) bilateral nipple-sparing mastectomy and immediate reconstruction.

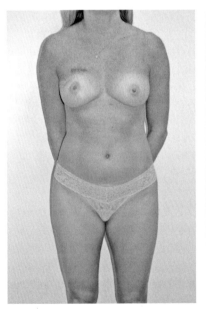 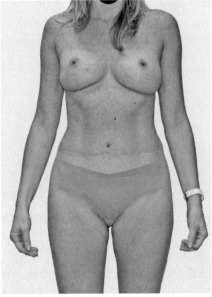

Images provided by Joshua Levine, MD, Center for Breast Reconstruction

Are You a Candidate for NSM?

Most people can have a nipple-sparing mastectomy, but it isn't right for everyone. NSM is not recommended if you have inflammatory breast cancer, Paget's disease, or cancer cells directly below the nipple ducts. Generally, you're a candidate if

- you plan to have immediate breast reconstruction
- your breast skin, nipple, and areola are free of cancer cells
- your tumor is small and not close to your nipple and areola
- you're having a preventive mastectomy to reduce your high risk of breast cancer
- you understand that your nipple may not retain the same sensation it had before your mastectomy

nipple.) Some surgeons core the interior of the nipple, replacing the tissue with a bit of rib cartilage or synthetic surgical material; this leaves the nipple permanently erect. Radiation therapy before or after NSM, smoking, circulatory problems, and other factors may increase the chance of losing some or all of the nipple. If the nipple dies, it must be removed, and a new one, if desired, can be reconstructed.

NSM and Ptotic Breasts

If your breasts are *ptotic* (meaning they're oblong rather than round and they head south so that the nipples point downward or hang below the

FIGURE 4.5 Ptotic breasts before (*upper and lower left*) and after (*upper and lower right*) nipple-sparing mastectomy with immediate reconstruction.

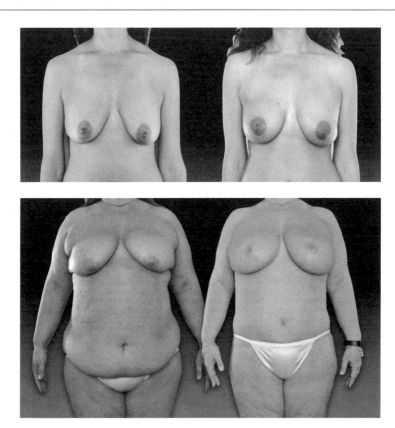

Images provided by Dr. Frank J. DellaCroce, Center for Restorative Breast Surgery, LLC

inframammary fold), your surgeon might recommend a skin-sparing mastectomy rather than nipple-sparing mastectomy because your nipples won't be well-positioned after reconstruction. One way to get around the problem is to perform a breast lift (chapter 11) a few months after the NSM with immediate tissue flap reconstruction to ensure proper nipple placement.[3] Alternatively, a breast reduction can be performed several weeks before a mastectomy to better position the nipples before your reconstruction. If you have sagging breasts, ask how your surgeon will approach these issues so that you can preserve your nipples if you want to and so that they end up where they should be after reconstruction: centered on your new breasts (figure 4.5).

What Can You Expect?

If, like many women, you consider your nipples to be the focal point of your breasts, keeping them intact preserves a much-appreciated part of your natural breasts. But will they be the same? Cosmetic superiority aside, NSM is not without challenges and doesn't guarantee that your nipples will look, feel, or react as they did before. Some women find that their preserved nipples are permanently flattened after NSM; others have permanently erect nipples. After a unilateral mastectomy, the nipple on your reconstructed breast may not line up exactly with its counterpart on your opposite breast.

Although a nipple-preserving mastectomy preserves the physical integrity of the nipple and areola, sensation after NSM is unpredictable and varies; women retain or regain sensation to differing degrees, and not everyone perceives or defines it in the same way. Some women report improved sensation and erectile function within six months to a year after their surgery. For others, nipple sensation and reaction are minimal or lost altogether. Even though sensation and response are typically diminished after NSM and may not be the same as they were before a mastectomy, women often say it's a comfort and a boost to their self-image to retain their nipples. Others admit they wouldn't have chosen NSM if they knew in advance that their nipples wouldn't be the same. Some women find that their concept of sexual stimulation on the reconstructed breast is redefined. They may have no nipple sensation, but they can be somewhat stimulated by feeling their partner's touch on another part of the breast where they do have some feeling.

Nipple Delay

For some patients, performing a minor *nipple delay* procedure a few weeks before the mastectomy boosts the chance that the nipple will survive the subsequent NSM. Often performed as an in-office procedure under local anesthesia, a nipple delay involves an incision that is made under the areola or in the inframammary crease under the breast. (Your mastectomy will be performed through the same incision.) The nipple and areola are separated from the breast tissue, and the small blood vessels to the nipple are disconnected. As a result, blood vessels in the surrounding skin grow stronger so that the nipple has a more robust blood supply when the mastectomy is performed. A small sample of breast tissue beneath the areola is removed at the same time. If that tissue is clear of cancer cells, the NSM can proceed. If cancer cells are found, a skin-sparing mastectomy will be done instead, and the nipple and areola will be removed.

Nipple Banking

Nipple banking is another nipple-sparing option, although it's seldom used in the United States. In this procedure, the nipples are removed during a mastectomy and checked for cancerous cells. If they're clear, they're stored in the groin for several months until they can be transferred to the newly reconstructed and healed breast mounds. Banked nipples are flat and have little or no sensation.

> I decided not to keep my nipples because I inherited a nasty family mutation, and my father developed breast cancer near his nipple. I told my surgeon to "take everything." At 51 years old, I still had a pretty good intimate life with my husband, and I was not going to sacrifice my life for those nipples.
>
> —*Debra*

— EXPERT INSIGHT —

Early Mastectomy Planning Permanently Affects Your Reconstructive Outcome

FRANK J. DELLACROCE, MD, FACS

Back in 1894, Dr. Halsted revolutionized the treatment of breast cancer with the first mastectomy. His approach was called radical, but he did push for progress in the field. Since then, breast cancer treatment has evolved in nearly every way, from genetic testing to dramatic leaps forward in plastic and reconstructive surgery. Nothing is the same as it was 100 years ago, except for one thing: the football-shaped, side-to-side, across-the-breast incision design that removes the breast in a wedge. This takes away the tip of the breast and flattens it into a permanent and irreversible dome, leaving an empty space in your bra and complicating clothing options for obvious reasons. But it's completely avoidable, and it's simpler than you might think.

An elliptical, flattening incision design may be reasonable in three situations:

1. when you decide not to have reconstruction
2. if you have advanced disease and immediate reconstruction isn't advised
3. if, after doing all your homework, you're still unsure about having reconstruction and you want to put that decision off until later, understanding that you will lose the advantage of appearance and touch sensation that are enhanced when we carefully preserve your outer breast skin

The goal today is to hide incisions, reduce or eliminate scarring, and preserve and even enhance shape. The art of modern mastectomy incision planning overcomes the 100-year-old problem. Newer designs can be used for all breast sizes and shapes and can be applied to all situations, whether we're treating active disease or performing preventive mastectomies for high-risk patients. These carefully planned incisions (figures 4.2 and 4.3) work for reconstruction with implant placement and when we rebuild breasts with natural living tissue on the same day as your mastectomy, otherwise known as immediate reconstruction:

- The side incision is used for compact breasts that aren't saggy. This is nice because it's hidden from the midline and can't be seen in even the lowest cut garments. It's used for NSM as well as non-NSM procedures.
- The vertical incision can be used for women with large or sagging breasts. It allows for lifting the nipple position and reshaping the overall breast. This incision can do some incredible things for women with even the largest breasts. It also works for NSM and non-NSM plans.
- The underneath incision is used for breasts of moderate size. It is particularly appealing because we can hide it completely. Generally used only for women who have NSM, it can leave the reconstructed breast with an untouched look.

Your reconstructive outcome begins at the beginning. Early decisions are important. Be encouraged, be your own advocate, and seek a second opinion if you need to. There's no need to live 100 years in the past. When the best modern techniques are combined with an experienced team, your opportunity for a quality outcome increases greatly. Remember, not every situation is the same and the skillset and experience of every team are different. Consult with your physician for individual advice and care planning.

Questions for Your Breast Surgeon

- Am I a candidate for an NSM?
- How many NSM procedures have you done?
- Where will my incisions be and how will they affect my nipple reaction and sensation?
- How much sensation and reaction can I expect to retain in my nipple?
- Will my nipple remain attached during NSM?
- If I keep my nipple, will it be flat?
- Will my nipple be centered on my reconstructed breast?
- What complications might occur and how will you address them?
- May I see photos of your reconstructions after a nipple-sparing mastectomy?
- May I speak to other patients who have had an NSM?

Chapter 5

Breast Reconstruction Basics

At 31, I just couldn't deal with having no breasts. If I had to have a mastectomy, I wanted to restore my breasts as closely as possible, and that meant reconstruction.
—RILEY

Until we know how to prevent breast cancer or develop treatments that could make needing a mastectomy obsolete, reconstruction is our best antidote to breast loss. Plastic surgeons can improve birth defects, repair severe burns, and rebuild facial features. They can also recreate breasts after a mastectomy, complete with nipples and areolas. (Breast reconstruction can also help people who are born with Poland syndrome, a condition characterized by little or no breast tissue; sometimes the chest muscle is also missing or highly underdeveloped.) Breast reconstruction is more complex and requires more surgical skill than *breast augmentation*, which uses implants or fat to increase the size of healthy breasts.

The goal of breast reconstruction is no longer only to restore your shape when you're dressed; the bar is now much higher. Surgeons now strive to create soft, gently sloped breasts that look natural when you're clothed and also when you're not. Creating natural-looking breasts is what good reconstruction does. Although some results are better than others, your outcome depends on your surgeon's expertise, the procedure you choose, and your physical makeup. While breast reconstruction is imperfect—it can't erase mastectomy scars, fully restore premastectomy sensation, or reestablish your ability to breastfeed—it can soften the harshness of a mastectomy and restore your feeling of physical wholeness. In the right surgeon's hands, reconstructed breasts are much more than the sum of their parts. Breast reconstruction can be a work of art that is customized to your anatomy and preference. Because bilateral reconstruction starts with a "clean slate," some women find that their reconstructed breasts have better shape, size, position, and symmetry than their natural breasts. With your breast volume restored, you can wear many of the same clothes you wore before your mastectomy, including lingerie, T-shirts, and swimwear, without special bras or prostheses.

Women say they choose reconstruction because it

- makes them feel whole again
- is not a constant reminder of their mastectomy, unlike a flat chest or prostheses
- is a more permanent way to restore breast shape than prostheses
- restores their self-image and confidence in their physical appearance
- gives them a sense of control they didn't have with their treatment
- brings a sense of closure to the physical and emotional struggle of breast cancer diagnosis and treatment
- softens the difficult decision to have a preventive mastectomy (for high-risk individuals)

Reconstruction can produce good and often excellent results. While problems can occur, research shows that women are generally satisfied with their breast reconstruction regardless of the technique used.[1] This doesn't mean that every woman thinks her recreated breasts are perfect, but overall, women who have breast reconstruction say that it has positively impacted their post-mastectomy lives.

Sorting Through the Options

No breast reconstruction is one-size-fits-all. Missing breast tissue can be replaced by using different procedures of varying lengths and intensity of recovery; each has advantages and disadvantages. About 80 percent of all breast reconstruction is accomplished with FDA-approved *breast implants* (chapter 6).[2] Reconstruction with implants usually begins with a *tissue expander*, which is a temporary implant that stretches the remaining breast skin and/or chest muscle to make room for the size implant you want (chapter 7).

TABLE 5.1 Comparing Breast Implant and Autologous Flap Procedures

IMPLANTS	FLAPS
don't require blood supply	require blood supply
shorter surgery, longer timeline*	longer surgery, shorter timeline
less intense, shorter recovery	more intense, longer recovery
incision/scar at mastectomy site	incision/scar at mastectomy and donor sites
retain size	size may fluctuate with weight changes
fixed shape	can be sculpted and shaped
replacement eventually required	lifelong
future operations likely	future operations unlikely
rare link to ALCL**	not linked to disease

*Procedures that include tissue expansion.

**Some textured tissue expanders and implants.

Autologous flaps of your own fat, skin, and sometimes muscle can also be used to create breasts after a mastectomy (chapter 8). These natural tissue flaps form full-sized breasts during the initial operation. Compared to implant reconstruction, autologous procedures are more complex and require greater surgical skill (table 5.1). Although recovery is longer, the overall reconstruction timeline is shorter than reconstruction with tissue expansion. A combination of implants and autologous flaps can also be used for breast reconstruction.

Although some procedures shorten the overall reconstruction timeline, most still involve traditional methods that include two or more operations over several months (figure 5.1). The initial surgery forms the *breast mound*—a breast without a nipple or an areola—with implants, your own tissue, or a combination of both (figure 5.2). This first stage of reconstruction is the most complex, and it involves the most recovery. The second stage, performed three months or more after the initial operation, is *revision surgery* to correct problems, refine cosmetic imperfections, improve symmetry, and rebuild the nipple. Optional tattooing of the new nipple and areola completes the reconstructive process.

Reconstruction: Your Right. Your Choice.

Everyone who faces a mastectomy has the right to know about reconstructive procedures, understand what they involve, and make their own decision about whether to have a new breast after a mastectomy. Most people are candidates for breast reconstruction, even though many are still unaware that it's an option or don't have access to a plastic surgeon. The Breast Cancer Patient Education Act of 2015 established an educational campaign to inform patients about breast reconstruction, and the WHCRA requires health plans that cover mastectomies to also pay for breast reconstruction. Breast reconstructive procedures have risen dramatically in the United States over the past two decades. This can be attributed to

- greater awareness of reconstruction
- more reconstructive options
- improved procedures that produce better results
- more surgeons who routinely perform breast reconstruction
- advancements that safely preserve most of the breast skin, including the nipple and areola
- enhanced protocols before, during, and after surgery that reduce pain and shorten recovery
- state and federal laws that require insurance companies that cover mastectomies to also pay for reconstruction

FIGURE 5.1 Traditional breast reconstruction involves at least two and sometimes three steps.

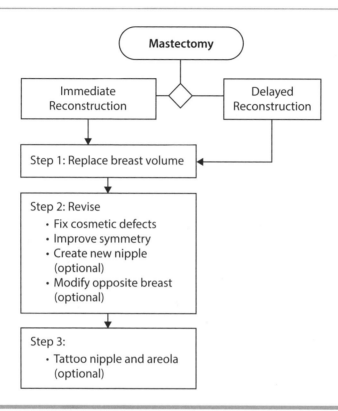

FIGURE 5.2 After mastectomy (*left*), the traditional approach to breast reconstruction first creates the breast mound to restore volume (*center*), and then later adds the nipple. Tattooing the nipple and areola completes the reconstructive process (*right*).

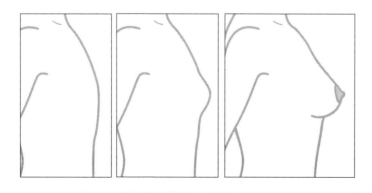

Reconstruction after Lumpectomy

Although lumpectomy preserves most of your breast tissue, in some cases, it may change the size or symmetry of your breast. Removing a small area of tissue may not cause more than a dent or a dimple along the incision line. When a larger mass is removed and creates a noticeable loss of volume or distorts the breast shape, *oncoplastic surgery*, a combination of lumpectomy and plastic surgery, may be performed. After removing the tumor, an experienced *surgical oncologist* can rearrange the remaining tissue to give you the best cosmetic appearance. If needed, your opposite breast—or both breasts—can be lifted or reduced for better symmetry. If you don't have access to an oncoplastic surgeon, a plastic surgeon can rearrange your remaining tissue after your breast surgeon removes the lump.

Timing Your Reconstruction

Your breasts can be rebuilt the same day as your mastectomy or anytime afterward, depending on your breast cancer treatment and personal preference.

Immediate Reconstruction

Immediate reconstruction occurs as soon as your mastectomy is complete and while you're still asleep on the operating table. The mastectomy and reconstruction are performed in a single visit to the operating room with one recovery. Your surgeon removes as much breast tissue as possible while leaving most

Reconstruction for Men

Men don't always need reconstruction after a mastectomy, because the amount of tissue removed isn't usually disfiguring. If a man's health insurance covers mastectomies, the WHCRA requires that it also pay for reconstruction—even though the name of the law implies that it's just for women. Depending on the extent of tissue removed and how much the chest contour needs to be improved, men may opt for one or more of the reconstructive options described in part II, "Rebuilding the Breasts," including

- fat grafting

- a customized silicone breast implant

- a small autologous flap (of their own tissue)

- optional nipple reconstruction and tattooing

of the breast skin intact. This often involves removing the nipple and areola as well. If you have a nipple-sparing mastectomy, your nipple and areola will be preserved. Once the mastectomy is completed and while you're still sedated, your plastic surgeon will replace your breast tissue with a temporary expandable implant, a full-sized implant, or a segment of your own tissue (figure 5.3). Although breast reconstruction can be performed any time after a mastectomy, immediate reconstruction offers several distinct benefits:

- Most of your breast skin is preserved.
- Your nipples and areolas may also be preserved.

FIGURE 5.3 After delayed reconstruction, the mastectomy scar remains on the new breast (*left*) but fades in time. Immediate reconstruction results in minimal visible scarring (*right*).

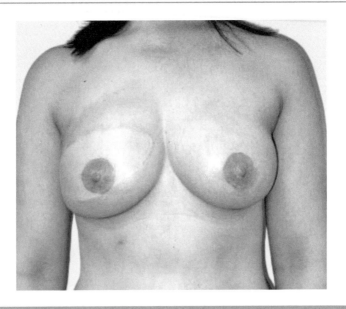

Image provided by PRMA Plastic Surgery, Center for Advanced Breast Reconstruction

- Your mastectomy incision is minimized and may be completely hidden on the new breast.
- Your mastectomy and reconstruction are completed in a single visit to the operating room.
- You wake up from surgery with a breast mound or a full-sized breast in place, so you never experience a flat chest.

Delayed Reconstruction

It's never too late to have breast reconstruction. A postponed or *delayed reconstruction* can be performed as a separate operation any time after your mastectomy has healed—20 days or 20 years later. In most cases when reconstruction is delayed, the "going flat" mastectomy procedure described in chapter 3 is performed (table 5.2). After your breast tissue is removed, just enough skin is left to pull the incision closed. If you have reconstruction at a

TABLE 5.2 Comparing Mastectomy with and without Reconstruction

MASTECTOMY WITH IMMEDIATE RECONSTRUCTION	MASTECTOMY WITHOUT RECONSTRUCTION
retains most breast skin	removes most breast skin
may retain nipple and areola	removes nipple and areola
two surgeries in one visit to the operating room	single surgery
incision is minimized and may be hidden	incision visibly spans the chest
new breast mound after mastectomy	flat chest after mastectomy
one or more days of hospital stay*	outpatient or overnight hospital stay
longer recovery period	shorter recovery period
higher chance of problems	lower chance of problems

*Some procedures may not require an overnight stay.

later date, your plastic surgeon will reopen your mastectomy scar to replace your missing breast tissue with a breast implant or an autologous flap. The scar will remain on your new breast, but it will fade considerably after a year or two (figure 5.3). Although delaying reconstruction may be disappointing, waiting has some advantages. You'll have more time to consider your reconstructive options, you'll have a shorter initial surgery for delayed reconstruction (because you've already had a mastectomy), and you'll have an opportunity to try breast prostheses. When immediate reconstruction isn't possible due to breast cancer treatment, a staged approach to reconstruction can be done instead (see "Delayed-Immediate Reconstruction" later in this chapter).

It may be best to delay breast reconstruction when

- you're unsure or undecided about reconstruction at the time of your mastectomy
- you want to focus on managing your diagnosis and treatment
- you want to try a prosthesis before committing to reconstructive surgery
- your doctor advises you to complete chemotherapy, radiation, or other cancer treatment before reconstruction

- you have a health condition that may increase your surgical risk or impede healing
- you're pregnant

My mastectomy was overwhelming. I just couldn't deal with reconstruction too. I changed my mind three years later when I still couldn't face myself in the mirror, and I was still uncomfortable being naked around my husband. For me, delaying reconstruction was the right decision.

—*Copper*

My oncologist suggested I wait a few months after my mastectomy to see how I felt about reconstruction. I so feared looking down and seeing only a flat, scarred chest. If I was going to lose my breast, I wanted to replace it as soon as possible.

—*Diana*

Health Matters

Breast reconstruction procedures are generally safe, but like any surgery, complications can occur. Mastectomy with immediate reconstruction involves two operations; it's more complex and more invasive than a mastectomy alone and carries a higher likelihood of postoperative issues. Certain health conditions can affect the timing of your reconstruction, how you withstand the surgery, your recovery, and your overall result.

Obesity

Carrying excess weight doesn't automatically limit your ability to have reconstruction (figure 5.4). Obese women are as likely to be satisfied with the results of their reconstruction as thinner women. Obese women are more susceptible to having postoperative infections, delayed wound healing, partial or total autologous flap loss, greater risks of blood clots, and longer hospital stays and readmission.[3] Having a plastic surgeon who is experienced in performing procedures for obese women can result in fewer problems and better manageability when problems do occur. Your surgeon may recommend that you reduce your weight before having reconstructive surgery.

FIGURE 5.4 Obese women can have successful breast reconstruction, although they may experience more complications from surgery.

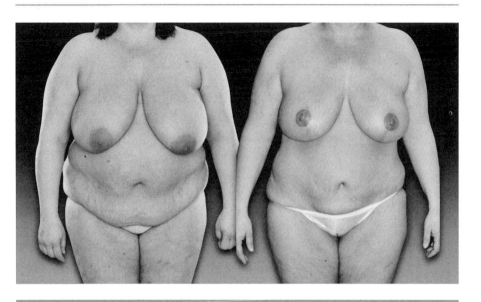

Images provided by Dr. Frank J. DellaCroce, Center for Restorative Breast Surgery, LLC

Underlying Conditions

Your doctor may advise against reconstructive surgery if your overall health is poor or if you have severe heart disease, lung disease, or chronic high blood pressure. Having lupus, scleroderma, rheumatoid arthritis, and other autoimmune diseases also increases the risk of slow-healing wounds and infection. Being diabetic significantly raises the chance of wound infection and complications.[4] Your overall health and fitness, rather than your age, influence how you weather the experience. Age doesn't necessarily mean more complications, although older women often have more health issues that may be problematic when combined with surgery. Women aged 65 or older who have autologous flap surgeries, which tend to last for several hours, have a significantly greater risk for *venous thromboembolism*, which is a blood clot that develops in a deep vein of the leg or lungs.[5] A clot that breaks away and blocks another blood vessel can be serious, so certain precautions, including the use of blood-thinning medications, may be needed.

Smoking, vaping, and/or using any type of tobacco product compromises your overall health. Carbon monoxide, nicotine, and other cancer-causing toxins from tobacco smoke can invade and affect most of the body's organs and raise the risk of numerous health issues, including breast cancer. These toxins greatly increase the chance of excessive scarring, infection, and other postoperative setbacks. They also delay healing by reducing respiratory capability and restricting blood flow to the skin and tissues of the reconstructed breast. Chemical substances in tobacco increase the body's need for oxygen but reduce its capacity to use oxygen. While this isn't optimal for reconstruction with breast implants, it can be disastrous for breasts created with your own tissue. You can greatly decrease your chance for complications if you stop smoking for four weeks or more before your procedure; every tobacco-free week after that improves blood flow and health outcomes by 19 percent.[6] You'll need to stop smoking several weeks before and after your surgery. You don't want to go to the trouble of having reconstruction only to potentially lose part or all of your new breasts.

Coordinating Reconstruction with Treatment

While breast reconstruction can restore your breasts and boost your self-image, treating your cancer is your medical team's priority. *Neoadjuvant therapy* (given before a mastectomy) generally doesn't affect the timing of when reconstruction can be performed. In some cases, however, *adjuvant therapy* (given after a mastectomy) may postpone reconstruction, depending on the stage of your cancer and recommendations for your treatment. If you're in good health, these treatments may not delay your reconstruction unless you have an underlying condition that increases the likelihood of postoperative problems. In that case, your doctor may recommend you postpone your reconstruction until your breast cancer treatment is completed. Alternatively, you might consider a staged approach to reconstruction (see "Delayed-Immediate Reconstruction" later in this chapter).

Reconstruction and Chemotherapy

While certain side effects from chemotherapy can be difficult to handle, chemotherapy is an essential part of treating many cancers. Erring on the side of caution, oncologists previously recommended delaying reconstruction for their chemotherapy patients to avoid potential postoperative problems that might interfere with or delay treatment. Research now supports the safety of immediate reconstruction, showing that it doesn't significantly interfere with or delay chemotherapy.[7] When postoperative complications occur, the resulting delay in chemotherapy isn't usually clinically significant.[8] For many women, having immediate reconstruction four weeks before a chemotherapy regimen begins is enough time to recover and heal sufficiently. If you need to begin chemotherapy without delay, a tissue expander can be placed in your chest at the time of your mastectomy and then inflated during your chemo treatment. If you don't feel up to the tissue expansion, it can be delayed until your chemotherapy is completed. Talk to your oncologist and plastic surgeon about the best timing for your reconstruction, given your treatment plan and overall health.

> I was disappointed when my oncologist said I should delay reconstruction for at least a year after my mastectomy. Intellectually, I knew chemo was more important, but emotionally, I didn't want to be without breasts. I'm glad I waited because it gave me time to think about my options.
>
> —*Kandy*

Reconstruction and Hormone Therapy

Anti-estrogen therapies—tamoxifen and aromatase inhibitors (Arimidex, Aromasin, and Femara)—reduce the risk of recurrence and improve survival for individuals with early-stage, hormone-receptor-positive breast cancers. But these medications also raise the risk of developing blood clots and may delay wound healing, so your surgeon may advise that you briefly discontinue taking them before and after autologous surgery.[9] (You should discuss this temporary "break" from your treatment with your oncologist.)

Reconstruction and Targeted Therapies

Treatment for breast cancers that overexpress the HER2 protein may include monoclonal antibodies, which are engineered molecules that mimic the body's antibodies to boost immune system response to cancer cells. Treatment with trastuzumab (Herceptin) combined with pertuzumab (Perjeta) may elevate the chance of wound complications after immediate breast reconstruction.[10]

Trastuzumab alone doesn't appear to have the same effect, although more study is needed.

Reconstruction and Radiation Therapy

The ideal reconstruction involves skin that hasn't been treated with radiation therapy. However, not all women who have reconstruction have skin that has not been irradiated. Radiation therapy usually follows lumpectomy and is often needed before or after a mastectomy to destroy any remaining cancer cells in the breast, lymph nodes, and chest wall. It's a highly effective treatment: radiation destroys cancer cells by damaging their DNA. Unfortunately, it affects neighboring healthy cells in the same way. Even improved radiation therapy that is more precise and causes fewer side effects can damage surrounding healthy tissue. This damage reduces blood flow and elasticity in the skin. Received before or after a mastectomy, radiation can affect the shape, volume, and position of a rebuilt breast, regardless of the reconstructive procedure. While radiation therapy often makes breast reconstruction more challenging and increases the potential for problems, reconstruction may still be successful, but the timing and type of procedure become more critical to the outcome. Delaying reconstruction for six months to a year after the last session is often advised to give the skin and tissues a chance to heal and settle before proceeding with additional surgery.

Radiation, Tissue Expanders, and Breast Implants

If asked which reconstruction procedure has the most complications, most surgeons would probably answer without hesitation: "Implant reconstruction after radiation." Radiation therapy given before or after reconstruction is tough on tissue expanders and implants. The results following this type of reconstruction are difficult to predict. Some women have satisfactory reconstructive outcomes, but the odds of having problems and needing to remove the implant are high. One exception that tends to have fewer complications after radiation is a breast implant that is covered with an autologous flap (chapter 8).[11] Irradiated skin can be difficult to expand and is more likely to develop an infection, heal slowly, harden scar tissue that naturally forms around the implant, or break down. Sometimes it works; frequently, it doesn't. Expanders and implants have a better chance of succeeding with fewer complications when they're placed before radiation; even then, radiation may compromise or sabotage the reconstruction. In some cases, exchanging a tissue expander for an implant may be problematic or impossible if irradiated skin doesn't sufficiently recover.

Radiation and Autologous Flaps

Radiation can also affect reconstruction with your own tissue. The new breast might contract, harden, or shrink as the irradiated tissue contracts, and the pigment of the skin may change. A portion of the flap may die, and in rare cases, the entire flap may fail. Because autologous flaps bring healthy tissue and new blood supply to the mastectomy site, they produce better cosmetic results when they're performed after radiation. Autologous reconstruction, whether immediate or delayed, tends to provide superior outcomes to implant reconstruction; the rate of complication is similar whether the chest is irradiated before or after autologous radiation.[12]

FIGURE 5.5 The decision-making process for delayed-immediate reconstruction.

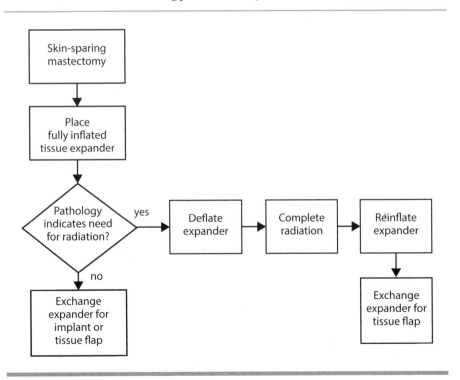

Delayed-Immediate Reconstruction

Knowing whether you need radiation after a mastectomy makes it easier to plan the timing of your reconstruction, but sometimes this isn't clear until the postmastectomy pathology results are available. If your oncologist suspects you may need radiation after a mastectomy, you'll probably be advised to delay your reconstruction. Delaying your reconstruction can be difficult to accept because it means you'll wake up from your mastectomy with a flat chest and miss the cosmetic benefits of immediate reconstruction. *Delayed-immediate reconstruction* is a staged approach to this issue. During the first stage, as soon as your breast tissue is removed, a tissue expander is placed under the chest muscle to preserve your breast shape and skin. If you then don't need radiation, you can proceed with the next reconstructive stage, which is swapping the expander for an implant or an autologous flap. If radiation is recommended, the expander can be deflated, left in place during your treatments, and then reinflated in a couple of weeks after your last session. (Deflating expanders addresses the concern that they may interfere with the precise delivery of radiation.) In three to six months when your skin has healed, the expander can be removed, and your breast can be reconstructed with an autologous flap. Implants aren't generally advised because of the high potential for complications following radiation therapy (figure 5.5). Having radiation therapy while you still have a tissue expander allows your surgeon to remove any radiation-related scar tissue before the final implant is put in.

Part II
Rebuilding the
Breasts

After a mastectomy, your breasts can be recreated with breast implants or with your own tissue. Within these two options are many different procedures and techniques. No single reconstructive procedure is right for everyone. Each alternative has different benefits and limitations, and a different length of surgery and recovery period. You may not be a candidate for every option, and some may not appeal to you. Because not all plastic surgeons perform all procedures, your choices may be limited by the reconstruction offered by your local surgeons or within your health-care network.

This central section of the book will equip you with a solid understanding of the many ways reconstruction of one or both breasts can be accomplished. Armed with this information, you'll have a good idea of which procedures appeal to you and which don't. You'll also be better prepared for effective conversations with plastic surgeons so you can make informed decisions about reconstruction.

Five key points in this section include

- traditional and advanced methods of reconstruction with breast implants
- the reason tissue expanders are used and what to expect from them
- traditional and advanced methods of reconstruction with your own tissue
- the difference between muscle-sparing and muscle-preserving procedures
- potential problems from reconstruction and how they can be resolved

Chapter 6

Reconstruction with Breast Implants

I don't mind if my implant must be exchanged in the future. I consider it required maintenance, like getting my car serviced. I can take the time to do that if I need to. Besides, it may be an opportunity to trade up to a newer, better model.

—BELLE

In the early days of modern breast reconstruction, implants were the only method of replacing breast tissue. Implants are still the simplest method. Compared to reconstruction with your own tissue, implants are less invasive, leave fewer scars, and do not require advanced surgical skills. Recovery is also faster. In most cases, the overall reconstruction process takes longer to complete.

Breast reconstruction with implants is a good option if you

- want the shortest surgery and the quickest recovery
- don't want to scar an additional area of your body
- don't have an active infection anywhere in your body
- are too thin for autologous flap reconstruction
- aren't healthy enough or don't want to endure a lengthier autologous reconstruction operation

- haven't previously had radiation therapy on your chest/breast and it won't be irradiated as part of your current treatment
- are willing to alter your healthy breast, if necessary, to achieve symmetry (if you have unilateral reconstruction)

Implants Inside and Out

Reconstruction with breast implants is the most common method of rebuilding breasts after a mastectomy. In the United States, implants from the following four manufacturers are approved by the FDA: Allergan, Ideal, Mentor, and Sientra. Decisions regarding reconstruction with implants are best made during a consultation with your plastic surgeon, who will describe where your incisions will be made, explain the different types of implants available, and discuss which device and procedure are best for you.

- Interior filling: saline or silicone
- Shape: round or teardrop
- Implant surface: smooth or textured
- Size: big or small
- Projection: low, moderate, high, or very high
- Placement: over or under your chest muscle
- Procedure: tissue expansion or direct-to-implant

Saline or Silicone

Breast implants used in the United States are medical-grade silicone shells filled with sterile *saline* (salt water) or *silicone gel*. A breast reconstructed with a saline implant feels like a filled water balloon. (Essentially, that's what it is.) A saline implant lacks the softness and bounce of silicone, which more closely mimics the feel of natural breast tissue. *Cohesive silicone gel* implants have a thick semi-solid interior with a consistency like Jell-O. They create a breast that is soft and feels natural. *Highly cohesive silicone gel implants*—often called "gummy bears"—are said to be "form stable." Like gummy bear candies, they maintain their teardrop shape even if the shell is cut or torn. Although not without potential issues, soft-but-sturdy highly cohesive gel implants are thought to have fewer complications, are less likely to rupture, and are likely to last longer than older types of breast implants. These improvements, combined with shorter

TABLE 6.1 Comparing Saline and Silicone Breast Implants

CHARACTERISTIC	SALINE IMPLANT	SILICONE IMPLANT
Components	silicone shell filled with salt water	silicone shell filled with silicone gel
Texture	firm, like a filled water balloon	soft, more like breast tissue
Interior	filled by surgeon during operation	prefilled by manufacturer
Incision required	shorter (implant is deflated when inserted)	longer (implant is full when inserted)
Rupture	obvious	may be undetected
Follow-up	annually with plastic surgeon	annually with plastic surgeon; periodic MRI or ultrasound recommended

surgery and recovery than autologous reconstruction, make silicone implants popular: About 93 percent of all breast reconstructions involving implants use silicone devices.[1]

During your consultation appointment, you can ask to see and hold saline and silicone implants to compare how they feel. (Some surgeons only use one kind or the other.) Speak with other women who have had implant reconstruction (your plastic surgeon can put you in touch), so you'll have the benefit of learning from their experience, as well. Consider the advantages and disadvantages of silicone and saline before you make your final decision about how your reconstruction will be done (table 6.1).

Shape and Surface

Breast implants are either round or shaped like a teardrop (also called anatomic) (figure 6.1). Round implants create more cleavage and fullness above the nipple. Teardrop-shaped implants are contoured more like a natural breast: longer and thinner at the top with more fullness at the bottom. All teardrop implants are filled with highly cohesive silicone gel. They're firmer than round implants and better maintain their shape and position. Teardrop implants have a rough, *textured exterior* that adheres to the surrounding scar

FIGURE 6.1 Breast implants are either round (*left*) or shaped like a teardrop (*right*).

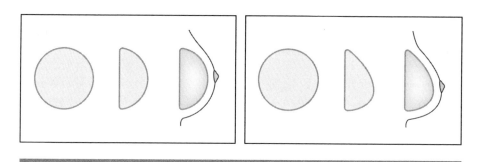

tissue, making them more likely to stay in place without shifting or rotating and distorting breast shape. Breast shape distortion is less of an issue with round devices, which generally retain their shape even when they move in the pocket: A round implant that rotates is still round. Texturing is also intended to reduce the likelihood of *capsular contracture*, which is the hardening of the scar tissue that forms around an implant. Round implants can have a textured exterior or have a *smooth exterior* that allows them to move under the skin or muscle, much like a natural breast does.

Size and Projection

If you have unilateral reconstruction, your surgeon will choose an implant that closely matches the size and shape of your opposite breast. (If you prefer your reconstructed breast to be smaller or larger, your healthy breast can be modified with one of the procedures described in chapter 10.) With bilateral reconstruction, you have a clean slate and can choose new breasts that are smaller than, bigger than, or similar to your natural breasts.

Communicating how big or how small you'd like your new breasts to be isn't as easy as saying "make me a 36C" because breast implant capacity is measured in cubic centimeters (cc): 30 cc equals about 1 ounce. Implant size doesn't readily translate to bra size. Although breast implants sold in the United States are available from 100 cc to 800 cc, the diameter and shape of your chest influence the size of your implant, with some variation in width, height, and projection. Your plastic surgeon will take careful measurements—nipple to nipple (cleavage), base width, and chest circumference—to determine which implants

FIGURE 6.2 Breast implants provide varying levels of projection.

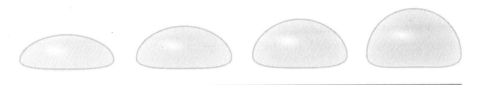

best fit while providing the volume and projection you want. Generally, a narrow chest requires a higher profile implant to look natural and achieve the desired breast size. High-profile implants provide more projection; low-profile implants have less projection. If you have a large body frame, low- or moderate-profile implants, which are wider at the base, may provide a better fit than high-profile implants. Although high-profile implants have more projection, they are designed to fit individuals with a smaller body frame and a narrow chest (figure 6.2).

Choosing an appropriately sized implant is important. Implants that are too small won't give you the volume you want. Implants that are too large might upset the aesthetic proportions of your body. The shape and profile of an implant, as well as your unique anatomy, can also affect how an implant looks in proportion to the rest of your body: A 480 cc implant will look larger on a 5′ 4″ woman who weighs 120 pounds than on a 5′ 9″ woman who weighs 160 pounds. Many women leave the choice to their surgeons. However, actively participating in the decision increases the likelihood that you'll be satisfied with the size of your reconstructed breasts and that you won't be surprised or disappointed with breasts you think are too big or too small. Be sure you and your surgeon are on the same page about what you want before you have surgery.

Prepectoral and Subpectoral Placement

Implants can be placed above or below the pectoralis major, the largest muscle on the chest wall. Each option has advantages and disadvantages that should be carefully discussed with your surgeon during your consultation appointment.

Prepectoral Placement

Prepectoral placement (above the chest muscle) is a minimally invasive procedure that positions the implant naturally—between the skin and muscle where the breast tissue was removed. It's the most anatomically correct way of rebuilding breasts with implants (table 6.2). Prepectoral placement requires *mastectomy flaps* (the breast skin and underlying fat that remain after a mastectomy) that are thick enough to supply the skin with a healthy blood supply. Thin mastectomy flaps increase the likelihood of visible *rippling* and *wrinkling* of the implant under the skin.

Implants above the muscle are wrapped in an *acellular dermal matrix (ADM)*, a sterilized, biodegradable tissue replacement mesh made from donated human or animal skin that retains collagen but has been stripped of its DNA and cells so that your body won't reject it (figure 6.3). ADMs are FDA-approved

FIGURE 6.3 For prepectoral implant placement, a layer of acellular dermal matrix or other surgical mesh provides a cushioning layer between the implant and the breast skin.

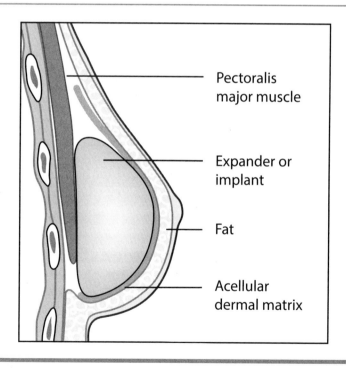

Pectoralis major muscle

Expander or implant

Fat

Acellular dermal matrix

for hernia surgery and to repair or replace large areas of skin that has been burned or otherwise injured. ADMs are also widely used to provide a supportive biological framework for implant-based breast reconstruction, although this use is off-label (it is not approved by the FDA). Your own blood vessels quickly integrate into the mesh. (Other surgical mesh products may also be used instead of ADM.) ADM smooths the breast contour and cushions the skin from direct contact with the implant. The muscle isn't cut, stretched, or disturbed, so recovery is quicker and less painful than subpectoral placement. You'll more quickly be able to return to routine activities and move with a full range of motion. Because some studies have found higher rates of seroma and infection when reconstruction involves ADM, one or two surgical drains may be inserted into the new breast for several days. (Some ADMs may also increase the chance of infection, reoperation, and removal of the implant.)[2]

Subpectoral Placement

Breast implants for reconstruction are often placed under the chest muscle. *Subpectoral placement* has traditionally been used to reduce the likelihood of the implants poking through skin that has been made thinner by a mastectomy. Improved mastectomy procedures that preserve more fat and skin and the increasing use of ADMs with breast implants make prepectoral placement possible and in most cases, preferred. However, most breast reconstruction with implants still involves the traditional subpectoral two-step process described in "Tissue Expander-to-Implant Reconstruction." Compared to prepectoral implant reconstruction, placing the breast implant beneath the muscle increases recovery time and related discomfort because the muscle is manipulated during surgery.

Tissue Expander-to-Implant Reconstruction

Most breast reconstruction with implants involves *tissue expansion*, a safe and effective way to replace large areas of severely burned skin, to repair other physical deformities, or to create a pocket to hold implants in a postmastectomy chest. Expansion slowly stretches tissues and creates new skin, similar to the way a woman's belly expands during pregnancy. In the first step, the lower edge of the pectoralis major muscle is cut away from the chest wall and lifted, and a tissue expander—a temporary, inflatable implant—is placed behind it (table 6.2). The expander will be round or teardrop-shaped to match the shape of your implants. The muscle is then pulled down over the expander. Because the muscle is only long enough to cover the top half of the expander, a patch of ADM is sewn to the lower edge of the muscle. This fully covers the expander and acts as a sling to support it (figure 6.4).

Initially, the expander is partially filled with saline or air. This pushes the muscle forward, creating a small bulge. When you wake up, you'll have starter breast mounds, and your chest won't be completely flat. During the second step, the expanders are gradually inflated in your surgeon's office, usually weekly for 6 to 8 weeks (or sometimes longer), until your skin and/or muscle stretch enough to accommodate your full-sized implants. (Expansion is described in more detail in chapter 7.) The expanders are then exchanged for implants in a short, outpatient operation. Shorter revision surgery to improve symmetry and contour can be performed in another three months when your implants have settled into place (chapter 9). New nipples—if you choose to have them—may be created during this operation or in a later, separate procedure. The final, optional step is tattooing the nipples and the areolas several weeks later.

TABLE 6.2 Comparing Prepectoral and Subpectoral Implant Placement

	PREPECTORAL	SUBPECTORAL
Expansion required?	less likely	more likely
Procedure	less invasive	more invasive
Recovery	shorter, less discomfort	longer, more discomfort
Chest muscle cut and lifted?	no	yes
Thins chest muscle?	no	yes
Capsular contracture	more likely	less likely
Animation deformity*	no	yes
Visible rippling/wrinkling	more likely	less likely

*Visible implant movement whenever the chest muscle contracts.

FIGURE 6.4 For subpectoral implant placement (*left*), adding ADM or another type of surgical mesh to the lower edge of the muscle extends coverage to the entire implant (*right*).

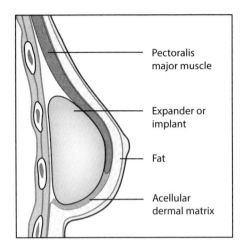
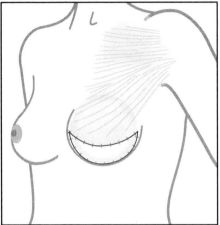

Pectoralis
major muscle

Expander or
implant

Fat

Acellular
dermal matrix

You might wonder why expansion is necessary, considering that women who have breast augmentation to enlarge their natural breasts don't typically need it. These women, however, have enough breast tissue and skin to accommodate an implant. After a mastectomy, that breast tissue is gone, and the remaining breast skin is thinner. If you had breast augmentation before your mastectomy, your new implant may be placed in the existing pocket.

Your plastic surgeon may recommend tissue expansion if

- your breast skin is thin or fragile, especially if you're a smoker or your breast has been irradiated
- you don't have enough breast skin to cover an implant
- you have delayed reconstruction with implants (a mastectomy removed most of your breast skin)
- the blood supply to your breast skin isn't healthy

Direct-to-Implant Reconstruction

Direct-to-implant (also called "one-step") *reconstruction* streamlines the reconstruction process. Unless complications occur or revisions are necessary, this

TABLE 6.3 Typical Timeline for Reconstruction with Breast Implants

PROCEDURE	FILLS	EXCHANGE FOR IMPLANT	REVISION SURGERY; NIPPLE RECONSTRUCTION	TATTOO NIPPLE AND AREOLA	TOTAL TIME
Direct-to-implant	not needed	not needed	not needed	not needed	initial surgery only
Tissue expander*	2–3 months	3 months	3 months	3 months	11–12 months

*Intervals may vary depending on how often you have fills, how much saline is added at each fill, and additional time needed for complications that may delay completion.

skip-a-step procedure completes reconstruction in a single procedure what tissue expansion achieves over several weeks (table 6.3). There's no need for expansion, exchange surgery, nipple reconstruction, or revision procedures with direct-to-implant reconstruction. You enter and leave the operating room with full-sized breasts (figure 6.5). For many women, a mastectomy and direct-to-implant reconstruction through a single, small incision below the breast creates an "invisible" reconstruction during a single visit to the operating room.

If direct-to-implant reconstruction appeals to you, consider the following:

- It's the quickest and least invasive method of breast reconstruction.
- Your breast skin must be healthy, with an adequate blood supply.
- It requires a nipple-sparing mastectomy.
- It may limit the size of the implant you can accommodate.
- Although more women are having direct-to-implant reconstruction, the tried-and-true expansion process is more appropriate for some women and preferred by most surgeons.
- Choose a plastic surgeon who is well experienced with the procedure.
- A "one-step" reconstruction may require additional procedures to improve symmetry, appearance, and resolve any problems that may develop.

FIGURE 6.5 Before (*left*) and after (*right*) bilateral nipple-sparing mastectomy with immediate direct-to-implant reconstruction.

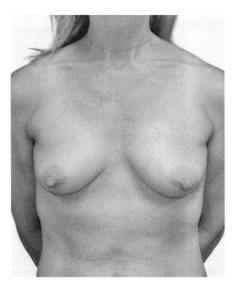 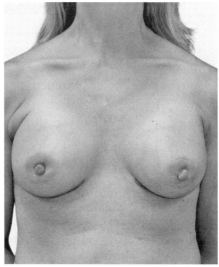

Images provided by PRMA Plastic Surgery, Center for Advanced Breast Reconstruction

— EXPERT INSIGHT —

Another Option with Implants

KAREN HORTON, MD, FACS

An alternative to tissue expansion and direct-to-implant reconstruction involves the placement of a smooth, round saline-filled implant that is permanent but postoperatively adjustable, giving patients control over their final results. Precisely matched to the dimensions of your breast, chest, and aesthetic goals, the implant can be placed prepectorally (on top of the muscle) in nearly every instance, allowing for a more natural look and shape. After surgery, just one or two saline fills, if any, are done in the office via an injection port that is left in place for three months after surgery. While an adjustable device gives you the option to keep the saline implant to avoid more surgery, most patients choose to switch to a more natural-feeling silicone implant after the swelling is gone and the port is removed.

When combined with a nipple-sparing mastectomy, this type of prepectoral breast reconstruction is completed within three months. The chronic tightness and pain that some patients experience is avoided, as is the animation deformity, which can be embarrassing for patients, that results from putting implants under the muscle. Submuscular implants tend to sit high and wide on the chest, as the implant follows the pull of the chest muscle in an up-and-out direction toward the shoulder. Women who initially have their implants placed under the muscle for reconstruction are candidates for conversion to a prepectoral reconstruction, even if years have passed since their reconstruction or radiation therapy.

I had risk-reducing, nipple-sparing mastectomies and reconstruction with prepectoral placement of breast implants. After much research, I chose the prepectoral approach because I felt it would give me the best option for continuing my occupations of yoga, acrobatics, and aerial arts. I did not want my pectoralis muscles moved as they are in subpectoral reconstruction. I am happy with my reconstruction. I am glad I do not have to do this again, but I would make the same choices. I was back at yoga, a bit wobbly, at seven weeks post initial surgery and three weeks after exchange and fat grafting. Are my reconstructed breasts perfect? No. There are some ripples when I bend over. Fat grafting has helped, but much of the fat has been resorbed. Is the appearance of my breasts better than the originals? Yes! Sensation is returning in my nipples, but they are always hard and the sensation is not pleasant. In a bra, bathing suit, and clothing, I look better than I did before surgery. More importantly, I can still do the things I love without pain, weakness, or animation deformity.

—*Amy*

I did not think I would be able to look in the mirror if I had no reconstruction, but I knew I did not want to have fat removed from other parts of my body and endure more scars and healing time. I wanted my reconstruction to be over and done; I did not want to have to go back for fills and more surgery. Then I discovered nipple-sparing mastectomy with direct-to-implant reconstruction. The surgery was minimal, and recovery was short. My procedure was a success; and three or four weeks later, I felt very good. I was an A-cup before my mastectomy; now I am a B-cup. I look so much better than before, and I have sensation in the outer parts of my breasts. My nipples react to cold, yet I have no feeling on or around them. I love the results.

—Leslie

Are They Safe?

Breast implants have been around in one form or another since the early 1960s. By the time the US Food and Drug Administration (FDA) began regulating implants in 1976, thousands of women already had them. Lawsuits filed by women in the 1990s claimed that silicone implants caused arthritis, immune system disorders, and a host of other health problems. Implant companies and plastic surgeons were caught between a rock and a hard place: though implants had been used for 30 years, their long-term safety had never been established. Although no scientific evidence has linked silicone breast implants to any significant health issues, in 1992 the FDA banned the use of the devices for cosmetic purposes, reclassified them as experimental, and approved their use only for breast reconstruction and clinical studies until manufacturers could prove the devices were safe. The Institute of Medicine studied the issue comprehensively, concluding in 1999 that although implants have inherent problems, "a review of toxicology studies of silicones and other substances known to be in breast implants does not provide a basis for health concerns."[3] Subsequent studies in the United States, Canada, and Europe concurred. With no evidence of a cause-and-effect relationship between silicone breast implants and health concerns, the FDA reversed the ban in 2006. Numerous studies since then have come to the same conclusion, finding no link between silicone implants and long-term health issues.

More recently, reports of illness, complications, and certain cancers in women who have implants have been reported (see "Breast Implant Illness," "Breast Implant–Associated Anaplastic Large Cell Lymphoma," and "Breast Implants and Other Cancers" later in this chapter). As a result, following the recommendations of an advisory panel that reviewed and revisited the issue of breast implant safety, the FDA issued this statement in 2020: "some patients may not be receiving or understanding important information regarding the benefits and risks of breast implants in a format that allows them to make a well-informed decision about whether or not to have a breast implantation."[4] So that everyone has the information they need to make decisions about breast implants, all implants now carry an FDA-mandated "black box" warning—information on the packaging of products with potentially serious safety risks.[5] Additionally, sales and distribution of implants in the United States are restricted to surgeons and other healthcare providers who must review a Patient Decision Checklist of potential risks and benefits of implants with patients before they have breast augmentation or reconstruction. Patients must also have the opportunity to initial and sign the document.

If you're considering breast implants for augmentation or breast reconstruction, or if you already have them, be sure to read "Things to Consider Before Getting Implants," which is the required labeling for all breast implants (https://www.fda.gov/medical-devices/breast-implants/things-consider -getting-breast-implants). Talk to your plastic surgeon about what is currently known about the risks associated with these issues and check for updates on the FDA website (www.fda.gov). If you develop a problem related to breast implants, the FDA encourages you to file a report through the MedWatch Safety Information and Adverse Event Reporting Program (https://www.accessdata .fda.gov/scripts/medwatch).

Breast Implant Illness

Silicone is manufactured by combining certain chemical substances with silicon, the second most common natural chemical element on the planet. We're all exposed to silicon as a part of modern life. It's ubiquitous in the environment, and it's used in thousands of everyday products, including cosmetics, nonstick cookware, and even antacids. It's also found in small amounts in the body, including breast milk, even in women who don't have silicone implants. Silicone breast implants are the most studied medical devices in the history of medicine; and, inherent problems aside, they're considered to be relatively safe. Medical-grade silicone is the most common material used in artificial joints, pacemakers, and other devices that are placed in the body. Some women with silicone breast implants develop characteristics of autoimmune conditions that are collectively known as *breast implant illness (BII)*, a term that encompasses a range of symptoms that some women experience immediately after they have augmentation or reconstruction with implants or years later. Women with saline implants have also reported symptoms of BII but to a lesser degree. Anyone in the United States who has a silicone implant becomes part of a national database that tracks and evaluates problems.

The most frequently reported BII symptoms include but aren't limited to

- unexplained fatigue
- chronic headaches
- persistent pain
- interrupted sleep
- decreased libido
- depression and anxiety
- joint and muscle pain
- issues with memory and concentration ("brain fog")
- hair loss
- heart palpitations
- psoriasis

Many of these symptoms are similar to what is experienced with lupus, rheumatoid arthritis, some autoimmune and connective tissue diseases, and other health conditions. BII isn't well understood; and without standard diagnostic screening or testing, it's difficult to say what the cause is or isn't or whether implants are somehow involved. Symptoms may be attributed to breast implants when no other cause can be identified. Despite decades of study, no undeniable evidence links silicone implants with connective tissue disease, breast cancer, or reproductive problems.[6] (Some textured breast implants are associated with a rare type of lymphoma. See "Breast Implant–Associated Anaplastic Large Cell Lymphoma" in this chapter.)

There are no identified risk factors for BII, so it's unclear why some women with breast implants develop symptoms and so many others don't. Health experts point out that these symptoms occur no more frequently in women who have silicone implants than in women who don't. Further, some people who are predisposed to having an immune reaction to materials in breast implants develop inflammation that causes these symptoms. Some healthcare professionals believe that silicone may be problematic for women whose immune systems are already weakened when they get implants.

Removing implants and the surrounding scar tissue seems to eliminate or improve symptoms for many women, while others report that their symptoms remain. Findings from a significant study of BII found that patients who self-report BII demonstrated a statistically significant improvement in their symptoms after *explantation* (removal of their implants) and that this improvement persisted for at least six months; improvement was less frequent in women with known autoimmune disorders.[7] BII will remain a mystery until larger clinical studies can shed light on what it is and what it isn't and whether it should be classified as a medical condition.

Breast Implant–Associated Anaplastic Large Cell Lymphoma

Women who have or previously had breast augmentation or reconstruction with textured tissue expanders or implants have a very low but increased risk of developing *breast implant–associated anaplastic large cell lymphoma (BIA-ALCL)*, a rare but treatable type of non-Hodgkin lymphoma (cancer of the immune system). Worldwide, the majority of individuals diagnosed with BIA-ALCL had Allergan's Biocell textured breast implants at the time of diagnosis.[8] Most cases of BIA-ALCL have been found in the capsule of scar tissue or fluid surrounding the implant. How or why BIA-ALCL develops is unclear. Some experts suspect that harmful bacteria may grow more easily on the dimpled surface of textured implants; and when the immune system responds by isolating bacteria with white blood cells, chronic inflammation may lead to lymphoma. Compared to the microtextured devices of other manufacturers, Biocell devices are macrotextured, with a larger and rougher surface that may harbor more bacteria. Biocell textured breast implants and tissue expanders were voluntarily recalled worldwide in 2019. Many surgeons now only use smooth round implants for breast reconstruction; others use textured implants from other manufacturers.

Most women with BIA-ALCL notice one or more changes: swelling or a lump in one or both breasts, fluid that collects in the breast, or pain near the implant. These symptoms may occur well after the surgical incision has healed, often years after implant placement. It's important to recognize the symptoms of BIA-ALCL and to take action early. The FDA recommends seeing a physician promptly if any of these symptoms or unexplained changes develop. Removing the implant and the surrounding capsule of scar tissue resolves most early-stage cases; undiagnosed or untreated, BIA-ALCL can spread throughout the body and become life-threatening. Chemotherapy, radiation therapy, or other treatment may also be needed for advanced cases. If you already have textured implants, experts say it isn't necessary to remove them, but you should be monitored annually.

Breast Implants and Other Cancers

Although there are few documented cases, squamous cell carcinoma (SCC)—a common type of skin cancer—and various lymphomas in the capsule of scar tissue surrounding the breast implant have been reported in medical literature and to the FDA. (These are not the same lymphomas involved in BIA-ALCL.) Implants that are smooth or textured, as well as saline and silicone devices, have been involved. While the connection between implants and these cancers is still unclear and these occurrences are believed to be very rare, a 2022 safety communication by the FDA advised healthcare providers and people who have implants to be aware of this issue. The agency doesn't recommend immediate removal of breast implants but does advise people to be aware of any changes that may develop (including swelling, pain, lumps, and skin changes) and to consult with a surgeon or other healthcare provider if any abnormal changes appear.

Recovery

The length and intensity of your recovery after implant reconstruction will depend on the procedure you had and your ability to heal (table 6.4). Initially, your chest will be numb and may feel heavy or ache for several days, but any discomfort will be controlled by pain medication. If lymph nodes were removed during your surgery, your underarms may also be numb or sore. You'll be encouraged to get up and begin walking the day after your surgery. You should take progressively longer walks each day, and perform the exercises recommended by your surgeon to gradually improve your range of motion. You'll be tired and sore for a couple of weeks, but your strength will slowly return. Each day, you'll spend more time awake and less time napping. You'll need to initially restrict upper body motion and should avoid strenuous activities and movements that pull excessively on the muscle until cleared by your surgeon.

Before reconstruction, you may wonder if you'll always be conscious of your implants. Will they ever feel a part of you, as your natural breasts did? They may feel heavy at first. If you had subpectoral placement, you'll feel the implants shift in the pocket when you stretch or lift and move when your chest muscles flex or contract. This recovery process shouldn't be painful, although it can feel odd until you become accustomed to it. After several months, your implants will become softer, feel better, and drop into a more natural position

Breast Implant Warranties

All four US implant manufacturers provide product warranties, each with its own coverage, benefits, and conditions. You'll be automatically enrolled once your implants are in place. It's a good idea to read the fine print to know when replacements will be covered and when they won't, because while the device may be warrantied for its lifetime, the cost of replacing it isn't usually covered after 10 years. (Some people choose to have their implants replaced before the 10-year period is up.) Guaranteed coverage typically includes "necessary" replacement as determined by your plastic surgeon. Usually, this means rupture or deflation due to a device failure; it doesn't cover the cost of replacement if you decide you'd like to upgrade to a different size, type, or style of implant. If you've had bilateral reconstruction and one implant ruptures, both implants may be replaced. Warranties usually provide a flat amount towards replacement surgery, which doesn't necessarily cover all related costs. Extended warranties at varying fees provide more coverage to defray the costs of additional replacement surgeries that may be needed.

Once your implants are in place, be sure you have your implant ID card, which lists your implant's manufacturer, type, size, and serial numbers, before you leave the hospital. You'll need this information to register your warranty. Then keep it in a safe place. Your doctor or a member of the office staff should provide you with a copy of the manufacturer's warranty for your device and explain its terms. (You can also read the warranty terms online at the manufacturer's website.)

TABLE 6.4 Typical Intervals for Implant Reconstruction and Recovery

PROCEDURE	SURGERY AND HOSPITAL STAY	MOST ROUTINE ACTIVITIES RESUMED
Direct-to-implant	about 2 hours per breast; outpatient or overnight hospital stay*	4–6 weeks
Tissue expansion	about 1 hour per breast; outpatient or overnight hospital stay*	4–6 weeks
Exchange surgery	up to 1 hour per breast; usually outpatient	2–4 weeks

Note: Surgical expertise and individual healing affect recovery times.

*Delayed reconstruction may be performed as an outpatient procedure.

on your chest. Women who have implant reconstruction say that you get used to them in time.

Bras are optional after implant reconstruction. Even though you won't need a bra, you might enjoy wearing lingerie after reconstruction. If you decide to shop for new bras, you may need a different size than the one you wore before your mastectomy because your new breasts may not have the same shape, size, or profile. You may be limited to wearing seamless stretch or lightly padded bras if your breasts don't project enough to fill a regular bra cup, particularly if your nipples were removed. After unilateral reconstruction, it may be difficult to find a bra that fits both breasts correctly unless your healthy breast was modified for better symmetry.

Potential Problems and Fixes

Though many women are happy with their breast implants, complications are not uncommon and can require revision surgery. You can find information online, including the type and frequency of complications, for each manufacturer's device. Search for "Labeling for Approved Breast Implants" at www.fda.gov/breastimplants or check the implant manufacturer's website. You can also ask your plastic surgeon for a copy of the implant packaging; either option will have the same information.

Your new breasts will continue to improve as they heal. Don't be disappointed if they're initially a bit too high, too low, too big (wait for the swelling to dissipate), or don't look quite right. These aesthetic issues can be corrected during your second-stage revision surgery. Other temporary issues that may develop will resolve as your new breasts continue to improve over several months to a year. Some problems, however, may occur over time and may make additional surgery necessary. Odds are that you'll need one or more re-operations for one reason or another at some point. Like all manufactured devices—washing machines, tires, and virtually all medical devices that are im-planted in the human body—breast implants don't last forever; they have no finite shelf life. There's no way to predict how long yours will last, although highly cohesive silicone gel implants are estimated to last 10 to 20 years. Some implants last longer, while others develop problems sooner. Even though some implants may endure for years without complication, the odds of needing a replacement procedure at least once during your lifetime are high. According to the FDA's patient information regarding breast implants, "The longer people have them, the greater the chances are that they will develop compli-cations, some of which will require more surgery."[9] While any reconstructive surgery has the potential for cosmetic shortcomings, many, including the fol-lowing, are unique to breast implants. Other potential problems from surgery that aren't inherent in implants are discussed in chapter 15.

- Placing breast implants under the chest muscle commonly causes *animation deformity*, meaning that the implant visibly moves upward when the chest muscle contracts, as it does during exer-cise, and then back down when the muscle relaxes.
- *Asymmetry* is a mismatch in size, shape, or position that may be unsatisfactory from the initial reconstruction or could change over time because your implanted breast doesn't droop or reflect weight changes as your natural breast does, particularly if skin was re-moved during a mastectomy or if radiation is required. Your reconstructed breasts may not look alike. After unilateral recon-struction, it can be difficult to match your natural breast without additional surgery because implants can't be shaped and sculpted like living tissue.
- Capsular contracture can be mild, moderate, or severe (see figure 6.6; sidebar on page 102).
- Some degree of rippling or wrinkling, indentations that look like small waves under the skin, can occur with any implant, especially

if your breast skin is thin. The cause may be from a too small subpectoral pocket or a prepectoral pocket that is larger than the implant. Scar tissue around the implant that sticks to the surface of a textured implant or saline implants that are underfilled or leak and lose volume can also be problematic. Rippling and wrinkling can also occur if your breast skin is thin, stretches, and/or becomes even thinner over the years or if you lose weight after your reconstruction. Some of the stiffer, highly cohesive silicone implants tend to ripple less. Saline implants more frequently show ripples and wrinkles and are routinely overfilled to decrease the likelihood of this occurring. Overfilling also increases the firmness of the implant. (Each implant has a range for overfilling set by the manufacturer; exceeding these limits can affect the implant durability and may also void the warranty.)

- A *rupture* is a tear in the outer shell of a saline or silicone implant that can result from injury to the breast or normal aging of the implant. Although ruptures and leaks are believed to be less frequent in newer, more durable implants, they can still occur. Tears or cuts in an implant shell are usually the cause of ruptures. A manufacturing defect, a weak point that develops as the implant ages, or a faulty valve that allows saline to leak may be the culprit. An accidental nick from a scalpel during surgery or from a needle during a biopsy can also lead to a rupture. Chronic contraction of the muscle over a subpectoral implant can create a "fold flaw," a weakness in the shell that continues to become thinner until it breaks.

  A silicone implant that ruptures may cause a hard knot, breast pain, swelling, numbness, or a change in breast size or shape. Cohesive silicone gel that retains its shape usually remains in the pocket or the scar capsule around it, so you may be unaware of a rupture. Because there are often no visual changes to indicate this *silent rupture*, the FDA recommends a breast MRI or high-resolution ultrasound five years after silicone implants are initially placed and every two to three years thereafter (your health insurance may not pay for these screenings). If an MRI or ultrasound shows that a rupture has occurred, the implant can be removed and replaced. This occurrence isn't an emergency because the scar tissue around the implant contains the gel. If a saline implant leaks, your reconstructed breast will deflate in a very obvious way (figure 6.7 on page 104).

- *Malposition* occurs when implants move too far up, too far down, or to the sides of the pocket. Your reconstructed breasts may droop more than you'd like if the weight of the implants pulls them down because your skin is too thin. This is less likely if your implants are supported by an ADM. *Bottoming out* occurs when the breast skin and underlying tissue can't hold the implant in place, and it drifts below the inframammary crease.

- The weight of a tissue expander or an implant under skin that was thinned during a mastectomy may cause *extrusion*, causing it to break through the skin, particularly in women who smoke or whose skin is thin or has been irradiated. When this occurs, the implant must be removed and the skin allowed to heal before a new implant can be placed.

- Repairing *symmastia* is one of the more difficult revision procedures. Sometimes called "uniboob," this issue occurs when the space between the breasts is eliminated, so they appear to be joined in the middle (figure 6.8 on page 104). This can happen when too much of the muscle is cut when the subpectoral pockets are formed or the implants are too big or too wide. The implants must be removed and the pocket revised or reinforced with ADM to create a more natural distance between the breasts before replacing the implants. Alternatively, the implants can be moved above the chest muscle. Prepectoral symmastia is sometimes improved by moving the implants beneath the muscles.

- Silicone *gel bleed* occurs when microscopic droplets of silicone leach through the outer shell of the implant into the surrounding capsule of scar tissue, despite the cohesiveness of silicone gel. (This is different than an implant rupture, where the shell develops a break or tear.) This "intracapsular rupture" is usually silent and harmless. Some data suggest that cohesive silicone implants bleed no more or no less than older types of silicone implants.[10] It's ordinarily identified when an implant is removed or by MRI imaging. FDA labeling guidelines for improving patient communication about silicone breast implants say, "The patient should also be informed

FIGURE 6.6 Capsular contracture can distort breast size, shape, and position (*left*). This reconstruction was salvaged by replacing the implant with an autologous flap from the abdomen and lifting the opposite breast for symmetry (*right*).

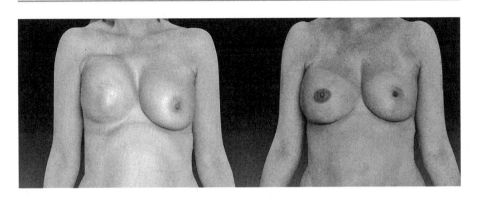

Images provided by Dr. Frank J. DellaCroce, Center for Restorative Breast Surgery, LLC

that most of these chemicals stay inside the shell of the implant but small quantities have been found to diffuse (gel bleed) through the implant shell of silicone gel-filled implants even if the implant is intact and not ruptured or leaking." Small amounts of platinum, which are used during the manufacture of silicone implants, may also bleed through the implant shell and move into the surrounding tissue. The FDA's position is that "the platinum contained in breast implants is in the zero oxidation state, which would pose the lowest risk, and thus that the small amounts of platinum that leak through the shell do not represent a significant risk to women with silicone breast implants."[11] The implant and the capsule of surrounding scar tissue can be removed and, if desired, the implant can be replaced.

Capsular Contracture

The body surrounds a breast implant with a thin capsule of scar tissue, similar to the way the membrane of an egg holds the yolk in place. A capsule that thickens, contracts, and squeezes the implant causes capsular contracture, the most common reason for reoperation after implant reconstruction. Capsular contracture is believed to be caused by inflammation from bacterial biofilm that forms around an implant within a few months of reconstruction, or even years later. This is why avoiding wound-healing problems is important and why surgical drains are used.

- Grade I is asymptomatic and doesn't affect any aspect of the reconstructed breast.

- Grade II may cause the breast to feel firmer without affecting its appearance.

- Grade III somewhat distorts the appearance of the breast and makes it abnormally firm.

- Grade IV severely distorts breast shape, hardens the breast, and is painful (figure 6.6).

Capsular contracture occurs more commonly after breast reconstruction than cosmetic breast augmentation because blood supply to the tissue surrounding the implant is decreased after a lumpectomy and radiation or a mastectomy. It also develops more frequently in smokers. It's a mystery why some individuals experience capsular contracture repeatedly or develop it in one breast and not the other, and others never experience it.

Your surgeon may recommend anti-inflammatory medication, vitamin E, muscle relaxants, ultrasound massage, or physical therapy for mild to moderate cases of capsular contracture. Two asthma medications, Accolate and Singulair, are sometimes prescribed off-label to reduce capsular contracture. However, these medications can have potentially serious side-effects. Standards haven't been established for dosage or when the drugs should be given, and long-term studies of their effectiveness for this purpose are lacking. Bacteria that contaminate the pocket can be difficult to clear without a *total capsulectomy* to remove the implant and the scar tissue around it. Recurrent contracture is often best treated by converting to an autologous reconstruction or staying flat for at least a year before trying implants again. Some people elect to remain flat after their breast implants are removed.

FIGURE 6.7 Although a silicone implant rupture may go unnoticed, a saline rupture is obvious.

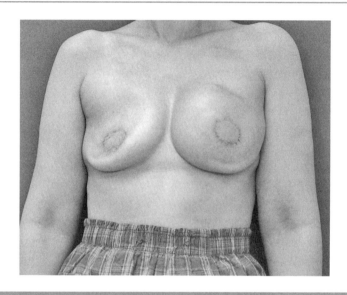

Image provided by Gail S. Lebovic, MA, MD, FACS

FIGURE 6.8 Symmastia occurs when the breasts appear to be joined in the middle (*left*). Revising the pockets and replacing the implants can resolve the problem. This patient chose to replace her implants with an autologous flap of fat from her buttocks (*right*).

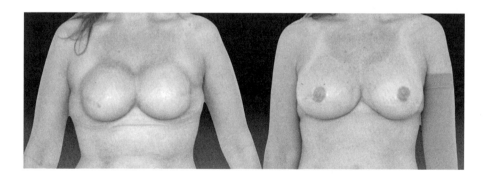

Images provided by Dr. Frank J. DellaCroce, Center for Restorative Breast Surgery, LLC

Questions for Your Plastic Surgeon

- Am I a candidate for reconstruction with breast implants?
- What shape, size, and exterior do you recommend for me?
- How much projection will I have after my reconstruction?
- Do you recommend saline or silicone implants for me? Why?
- Am I a candidate for direct-to-implant reconstruction?
- Do you recommend subpectoral or prepectoral placement? How will that affect my recovery?
- How many operations/procedures will I need?
- How many additional operations can I expect to need in the future?
- How long will it take to complete my entire reconstruction?
- How long will my recovery be and what should I expect?
- What kind of follow-up will I need and when?
- How long can I expect my implants to last?
- What results can I reasonably expect?
- What risks or complications may I experience? How will you address them?
- What changes can I expect in my reconstructed breasts over time?
- May I look at your before-and-after patient photos of the procedure you recommend?
- May I speak to other patients who have had the procedure you're recommending for me?
- Will my insurance cover my reconstruction with implants and any related problems that may occur later?

Chapter 7

The Expander Experience

Once I scheduled my mastectomy and tissue expander surgery, I had plenty of time
to worry. I spent hours on the internet reading about it. The first time I had a fill I
was nervous. I felt the first contact the needle had with my skin, almost like a bug
bite. After that, the only discomfort was when the muscle and skin stretched between fills. I took Tylenol before each one. That worked! Other than that, I went
about my day. By nighttime, the discomfort was gone, and I would forget all about
it until my next appointment.

—MICHELLE

M ost breast reconstruction with implants begins by placing tissue expanders under or over the pectoralis major muscle. Although tissue expansion
can be tedious and uncomfortable, it's a reliable and amazing process, and
it's the first reconstructive step for many people.

Traditional tissue expansion with subpectoral placement starts by inserting an expander into a pocket created under the chest muscle (as described in
chapter 6), reinforcing it with an ADM to secure it in place and partially filling it with a small amount of saline. The muscle acts as a barrier between the
expander and the breast skin, minimizes the chance of capsular contracture,
and reduces the risk of rippling and wrinkling. Your surgeon may recommend
subpectoral placement if your postmastectomy skin is thin, fragile, or weak,
especially if your breast was irradiated. Although under-the-muscle expanders are efficient, the process has downsides. Cutting the muscle and stretching
it causes temporary discomfort, tightness, and muscle weakness. Compared

to those who have expanders above the muscle, some women experience significantly more pain, tightness, and discomfort.[1] Animation deformity—noticeable movement of the expander when the chest muscle is flexed—is also likely when expanders are put under the muscle.

Tissue expanders may also be placed above the muscle. Wrapping the expander with a covering of ADM or other surgical mesh and then suturing it to the surrounding tissue supports it throughout the expansion process. In this prepectoral placement, the ADM rather than the muscle acts as the barrier between the skin and the expander. A small amount of saline or air, which puts less pressure on your skin as it heals, is introduced into the device when it's placed into the chest, forming a small bulge that will eventually become your breast mound. Prepectoral expanders gradually stretch the surrounding tissue to make space for your implant. The benefit of over-the-muscle expanders is less pain and discomfort because the muscle isn't cut or stretched. Compared to subpectoral placement, prepectoral expanders can also accommodate more saline, requiring fewer office visits to your surgeon. Placing the expander above the muscle slightly increases the risk of infection around the expander, as well as risk of rippling and wrinkling.

Getting Your Fill

In three or four weeks, when your mastectomy incision has healed sufficiently—or anytime thereafter if you have delayed reconstruction—you'll begin the process of having your expanders slowly inflated in your surgeon's office. Your surgeon will inject sterile saline through a needle fitted into a port on the surface of the expander or the top of your skin (figure 7.1); you may be able to feel the port under your breast skin. You probably won't feel the needle because your breast will be numb. Every week or two, you'll return to repeat the process, which takes only a few minutes.

The constant pressure created by adding more saline stretches the breast skin; if you have a subpectoral expander, it also enlarges the pocket as the muscle stretches. More saline is added at each office visit until the pocket is large enough to accommodate your breast implant. During your last appointment, your expander will be somewhat overfilled. This ensures that you'll have sufficient skin to cover your implant and enough space so that it will sit in a more natural position in the pocket, instead of unnaturally high on your chest.

FIGURE 7.1 Adding saline to the tissue expander (*left*) gradually stretches the muscle and surrounding skin until the flat mastectomy site slowly grows into a fully formed breast mound (*right*).

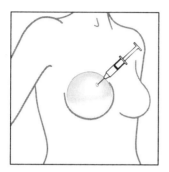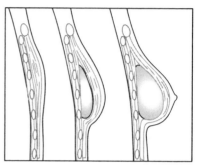

Traveling with Tissue Expanders

Airport security scanners can detect metal and may be set off by the metal ports on expanders. (You won't have the same issue when you have your implants, because they don't contain metal.) If you plan to fly with expanders, ask your surgeon for a letter explaining that you have a medical device in your chest. It's also helpful to have the Device Identification Card for the expander handy. You should receive this from your surgeon or before you're discharged from the hospital after your initial procedure. The card lists the manufacturer, type, size, and serial numbers of your expanders. If you're concerned about being in a pressurized cabin while you're being expanded, don't worry. Airplane pressurization doesn't affect expanders.

TABLE 7.1 Sample Intervals for Tissue Expansion

	INTERVALS TO 540 CC**			
VOLUME ADDED WEEKLY (CC)*	4 WEEKS	6 WEEKS	8 WEEKS	10 WEEKS
50	300	400	500	540
60	340	460	540	
100	500	540		

Note: Expanders are usually slightly overfilled once the desired volume is reached.

*Assumes 100 cc is added at initial surgery.

**Equivalent to about a C-cup size.

How Long Will It Take?

Expansion is often completed in six to eight weeks. Your interval may be different, depending on the elasticity and the fragility of your skin, how much your skin needs to stretch to accommodate the implant, how your skin reacts, and how well you tolerate the process. If your surgeon recommends a more conservative approach or you feel that you need to go more slowly, the process will take longer (table 7.1). Using an acellular dermal matrix to provide complete coverage of the expander allows for more saline to be added during the initial operation and in subsequent fills, thereby shortening the expansion interval. Expanding irradiated skin can be especially challenging; this must be performed cautiously and can add several weeks to the expansion timeline, especially when the skin is thin or damaged. Tissue expansion sometimes works on irradiated skin, and sometimes it doesn't. It helps to have a plastic surgeon who has a good deal of experience working with irradiated skin and tissue. If you have chemotherapy treatments during expansion, talk to your oncologist about the best time to have your fills. It may be helpful to have them a day or two before your chemo, when your resistance to infection is strongest.

Minimizing Discomfort

Expanders are built for function—to create room for your implants—and not so much for comfort or form. During subpectoral expansion, the lower portion of your chest where the muscles attach to the ribs may feel heavy or tender. It will feel fuller and tighter each time more saline is added; but, in many cases, this often subsides within a day or two. It's a bit like having dental braces. As soon as you get used to the braces, it's time to have them tightened, and they're uncomfortable all over again. Your pectoral muscles may contract or spasm as they stretch between fills. You can expect less discomfort with prepectoral expanders, which don't involve the muscle. Some women sail through the process with minimal discomfort, while others find it stressful and uncomfortable. One day, the muscles will relax, and you'll feel much better. In the meantime, if you experience discomfort, the following tips may provide relief:

- If the process is too uncomfortable, talk to your surgeon about taking an over-the-counter pain reliever 30 minutes before each fill. If that doesn't do the trick, ask for prescribed pain medication.
- Wrap a cold gel pack, ice cubes, or frozen peas in a towel and apply for up to 20 minutes at a time for temporary relief. You may not feel the chill, so be sure to move the pack frequently.
- Try gentle self-massage along the front and side of your rib cage to relax your muscles. Or ask your surgeon for a referral to a physical therapist who can massage and relax the connective tissues in your chest.
- Take a warm shower or two each day to relax your muscles.
- Exercise is beneficial during expansion, as long as it doesn't involve aerobics, jogging, swimming, or other strenuous, high-impact activities; wait until your surgeon gives you the okay to do these activities. Slowly and gently move your arms to stretch your pectoral muscles. Avoid lifting weights or doing other activities that increase or strengthen your pectoralis muscles before surgery so it won't become more difficult to stretch them. Perform the arm and shoulder exercises your nurse will show you. It may be easier to do these after a warm shower.
- Try deep breathing or meditation.
- If your expansion is unbearable, ask your surgeon to remove some saline from your expanders, allow more time between fills, or add smaller amounts of saline. You'll be eager to be done with the process, but take time to listen to your body. It will be worth it in the long run.

I had an amazing experience with subpectoral tissue expanders without any real complications. The pain was brutal at times, but staying on top of pain meds, resting when needed, and using muscle relaxants made it doable. I was excited to watch the "growing" process unfold each week. I was truly in awe after each fill, despite the tightness that occurred a few hours later and continued through the evening. However, the next day I felt well again. I returned to full-time work five weeks after my mastectomy. Tissue expanders are not for everyone, but they can be a positive experience for those who go into the procedure knowing what to expect.

—*Lenore*

My doctor filled my expanders with 120 cc every seven days. I was very uncomfortable for two or three days afterward. It felt like a metal band was crushing my ribs. I finally asked him to put in only 60 cc at a time. My expansion took longer, but it was more tolerable.

—*Lin*

Living in Limbo

After surgery to place your tissue expanders, you'll leave the hospital with a surgical bra. When your doctor clears you to wear a sports bra in two weeks or so, be sure that it supports you without compressing the expander. Avoid underwire bras, which can put too much pressure on the inframammary fold of your new breast, until your surgeon says you've healed sufficiently to wear them.

Dressing during expansion can be a challenge. During unilateral expansion, your growing breast mound may not be the same size or shape as your healthy breast, and it may sit higher on your chest, so finding a bra that fits both can be difficult. Placing a small prosthesis in your bra on the expanding side may help to correct an imbalance in your shape. Wearing a padded mastectomy bra while your new breast is being expanded is another option. As your breast mound grows, you can remove some of the stuffing from that side of the bra to give yourself a more symmetrical look. Sleeping comfortably may also require some trial and error. You'll need to sleep on your back for a while; many women find it helpful to sleep with a wedge pillow.

The expansion process may seem endless, and you may become impatient with the tightness and cosmetic flaws, but there is light at the end of the tunnel. Don't be disheartened with your asymmetry. Hang in there if you feel lopsided or misshapen or if your reconstructed breasts are flatter than you expected. Don't be overly concerned with incisions that seem uneven or puckered; they can be improved during your exchange surgery. Remember, you're a work in progress. Expanders are temporary. Your discomfort is temporary. And this isn't the way your finished breast will look or feel. Keep the end result in mind. In a few weeks, your expansion will be complete.

> Initially, it was difficult to look at the bruising and the flattened, mis-shapen appearance of my breasts, but my husband, the doctor, and his staff were very encouraging and gave me confidence and peace of mind that this phase was only temporary. Once my incisions were healed, I was fitted for breast forms and mastectomy bras by a certified fitter. The bras and forms were covered by my insurance, and I was able to wear them under my clothes while my expansion was being completed. I didn't need the forms for long, but it was a blessing to have the option of a formed breast silhouette on some occasions with certain clothes.
>
> —Cara

Exchange Surgery

Surgeons have different ideas about how long expanders should remain before replacing them with implants. Some like to rush the process along. Others prefer a more cautious approach, particularly when skin is fragile. You may need to wait a while longer if your surgeon wants to give your irradiated skin more time to heal or if your schedule causes a delay.

Exchange surgery is usually performed two to three months after the last fill when the pectoral muscles have stretched sufficiently and the expanders have settled into the pocket. When the pocket above or below your chest muscle is large enough to hold your implant, you'll have a short outpatient surgery to replace your expanders with softer, full-size, better-shaped saline or silicone implants. Once you're asleep in the operating room, the surgeon will reopen your mastectomy scar, remove the expander, and take out any scar tissue around the pocket, which will soften the overall appearance of your new breast. Your implant will then be inserted into the pocket and adjusted to match the position of your opposite breast. The incision will be closed, and a surgical bra will be put in place to discourage swelling. Your surgeon may perform fat grafting at the same time (chapter 9) to improve the shape or size of your new breast.

Compared with your mastectomy or your initial operation to place your tissue expanders, exchange surgery is a snap. The procedure takes about an

A Double-Duty Expander/Implant

With an outer layer of silicone and an inner chamber that is inflated with saline, the Spectrum implant does double duty as an expander and an implant. Saline can be added or removed to fine-tune your breast size during the six months after the implant is fully expanded. The fill valve is then removed, which triggers the expander to seal itself. The expander becomes the implant, eliminating the need for exchange surgery.

hour or so for each breast. You'll notice the difference as soon as you wake up: most, if not all of the tightness in your chest and ribs will be gone, and the implants will feel vastly more comfortable than the expanders. You should be back to your normal routine by the following week. At your post-op appointment in a week or two, your surgeon will remove the hospital dressing; and, for the first time, you'll get a look at your new breasts. They'll be a big improvement compared to the expanders, but they're still not the final product. Over the next few weeks, most of the swelling will subside and your implants will drop to a more normal position, although you may continue to have mild swelling for two to three months. Your reconstructed breasts will continue to settle and become softer over the next several months.

I was amazed to have hardly any swelling or bruising after my mastectomy, and I had cleavage from the expanders! At first, they gave me a flat bulk, like a bodybuilder. My new breasts looked okay when I looked down, but there wasn't much there from a side view. I was so upset. Even though the expanders were better than no breasts at all, they were nothing like the breasts I had seen in my surgeon's patient photos. In hindsight, I should have listened to my surgeon who said my implants would be very different. Of course she was right. My implants are so much better, and they continue to improve.

—Carole

Potential Problems and Fixes

Most women don't have serious problems with tissue expanders, but complications can occur. Expanders aren't recommended if you have a history of poor wound healing or infection anywhere in your body. Delayed healing after a mastectomy, poor circulation to the skin, or other problems may also postpone or preclude using expanders. If the breast skin dies, the expanders must be removed and the skin allowed to heal before another reconstructive procedure, if desired, can be tried. Problems that may occur include the following:

- An infection can develop around the expander. This can be treated with antibiotics; otherwise, the expander must be removed until the infection clears and reconstruction can then continue with a new expander. Diabetes, smoking, obesity, and previous radiation therapy to the chest increase the risk of infection.
- Expanders may rupture if they're damaged or compressed excessively. A nick from a scalpel during surgery or from a needle while the surgeon is filling the expander, a damaged port, or a blow to the chest can also cause a leak. Be protective of your chest during your expansion. It's a good idea to avoid strenuous exercises, gym machines, yoga positions that put pressure on your chest muscles, and any activities or sports with a high risk of falling. A fall against furniture or an accidental blow to your chest can cause a rupture; the expander may then leak saline and lose volume. The saline inside is harmlessly absorbed by the body, but the ruptured expander must be removed to prevent infection. It's a frustrating setback, but your reconstruction can be continued with a new expander.
- Capsular contracture can develop as scar tissue forms and tightens around the expander, especially with prepectoral expanders. The tissue expander must then be removed and/or replaced.

- Breast skin that doesn't get enough oxygen can weaken and die (necrosis). When this happens, the expander may push through to the surface of the skin (extrusion) and will need to be removed.
- Certain textured tissue expanders are linked to a very low but increased risk of developing breast implant–associated anaplastic large cell lymphoma (BIA-ALCL), an extremely rare and serious but treatable type of non-Hodgkin lymphoma (cancer of the immune system) (chapter 6). These expanders are no longer used; several other types of expanders that aren't linked to BIA-ALCL are available.

Questions for Your Plastic Surgeon

- Am I a candidate for direct-to-implant reconstruction?
- Will I need tissue expanders for my breast reconstruction with implants?
- Will you place expanders above or below my chest muscle?
- Will my expanders have a smooth exterior?
- How often will I need fills?
- How long will it take to achieve my desired breast size?
- What can I do to avoid excessive discomfort and pain while I have tissue expanders?
- Once my fills are completed, how long do I need to wait for exchange surgery?
- How long will my exchange surgery last?
- May I speak to other patients who have had tissue expanders?

Chapter 8

Autologous Tissue Flaps

The best thing about my gluteal scar is that I don't have to see it every time I look in the mirror.

—SONDRA

Autologous reconstruction (also called tissue flap reconstruction) uses your own living tissue to recreate durable breasts that look and feel natural. Compared to reconstruction with implants, autologous procedures require advanced surgical skills, a lengthy initial surgery, more time in the hospital, and a longer recovery that involves not only the chest, but also one or more donor sites. Breasts reconstructed with your own tissue will be warm and soft and move much like your natural breasts.

Reconstruction with your own tissue is a good option if

- you prefer the most natural reconstruction
- you want a reconstruction that will last your lifetime
- you want to avoid the inherent problems with breast implants
- your chest or breast has been or will be treated with radiation therapy
- you're healthy enough to undergo autologous surgery
- you have access to a surgeon who performs autologous breast reconstruction or you're willing to travel to one who does

Tissue Flap Basics

Autologous reconstruction forms full-size breasts during the initial operation by transferring a "flap" of fat, skin, blood vessels, nerves, and sometimes muscle to the chest, where it's then shaped into a breast. Excess tissue for autologous reconstruction can be removed only once from a particular *donor site*: your abdomen, thighs, hips, buttocks, or back. If one breast is reconstructed with your own tissue and you later need the opposite breast reconstructed, tissue must be taken from a different donor area. Autologous flaps are always placed above the muscle and below the skin in the space where the breast tissue has been removed (figure 8.1). The start-to-finish interval is longer than direct-to-implant reconstruction but shorter than reconstruction with tissue expansion (table 8.1).

Autologous reconstruction is often performed by two plastic surgeons at the same time: one prepares and places the flap on one side of the chest while

FIGURE 8.1 Autologous flaps are placed over the chest muscle.

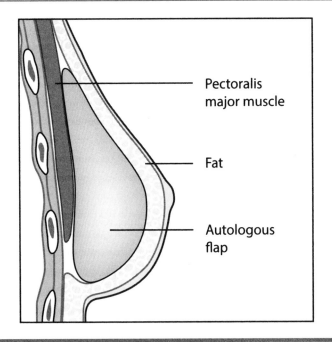

Should You Gain Weight before Autologous Reconstruction?

Unless you have an abundance of abdominal tissue, you might wonder whether you should try to gain weight before your reconstruction, especially if you don't have enough fatty tissue for the breast size you'd like. Considering the health problems associated with obesity, many experts consider deliberately adding weight to be inadvisable. Weight gain is usually distributed throughout the body, and it's difficult to target added weight to a specific donor site exclusively. On the contrary, you should strive to be in the best possible shape before your procedure to better facilitate your recovery. Even though a part of your tummy, thigh, or buttock will be your new breast, it will continue to respond to diet and exercise, reflecting overall weight losses and gains as though it were still in its original location.

TABLE 8.1 Typical Timeline for Reconstruction with Autologous Flaps

INITIAL PLACEMENT	REVISION SURGERY; NIPPLE RECONSTRUCTION	TATTOO NIPPLE AND AREOLA	TOTAL TIME
Tissue flap	3 months (outpatient)	3 months (outpatient)	6 months

Note: Intervals may vary depending on the preferences of you and your surgeon; additional time may be needed for complications, which may delay completion.

the other surgeon does the same on the opposite side. In three or four months when the new breast has settled into position, you return to the operating room for revision procedures to improve the size, fine-tune shape and symmetry, and create new nipples. If you had unilateral reconstruction, your opposite breast can be modified at this stage to better match the shape and position of your reconstructed breast.

Being thin or overweight shouldn't necessarily preclude you from having this type of reconstruction. Experienced surgeons routinely perform autologous reconstruction in both cases. A medical workup and a thorough evaluation will determine if you're healthy enough and which donor site will be best for you. You have a higher probability of problems if you're heavily overweight or obese, if you smoke, or if you have certain underlying health conditions. Careful planning before, during, and after your surgery can help manage most of these issues.

Advantages of Autologous Reconstruction

- It creates breasts with a natural feel, look, and movement.
- Some flaps preserve the donor site muscle.
- It continues to improve as scars fade and the tissue softens.
- It improves the chances of regaining sensation.
- It doesn't require tissue expansion.
- It avoids capsular contracture, rippling, and other inherent complications of implants.
- It may provide more volume than the largest breast implants.
- It is less likely than implants to be compromised by previous radiation.
- The tissue can be sculpted to match the natural shape and position of the opposite breast (if you're having unilateral reconstruction).
- It improves contour at the donor site, particularly the abdomen, hips, and thighs.
- It lasts a lifetime.

Disadvantages of Autologous Reconstruction

- Surgery and recovery involve two or more areas (the mastectomy and donor sites).

- It leaves a scar at the donor site.
- Some procedures sacrifice muscle and may affect long-term strength and functionality at the donor site.
- The area around the donor site incision may remain permanently numb.
- Fewer surgeons have the required qualifications, training, and experience.

Options for Reconstruction with Your Own Tissue

Decisions regarding autologous reconstruction are best made with your plastic surgeon, who will explain the different types of procedures, describe the benefits and risks of each procedure, and discuss which one is best for you:

- Donor site(s): abdomen, thighs, buttocks, back, or hip
- Procedure: muscle left in place or removed with the flap
- Incisions: number of incisions and their locations
- Size: whether multiple flaps or an implant will be needed to achieve the breast volume you want
- Symmetry: modifications to achieve better symmetry with your opposite, healthy breast (if you're having unilateral reconstruction)

Muscle-Sparing and Muscle-Sacrificing Flaps

Look at the human anatomy and you'll see three layers of tissue over the body's organs: skin on top, fat in the middle, and muscle underneath, with blood vessels running through all three layers. The distinction between different autologous procedures, aside from the donor site, is how blood vessels are included in the flap. Traditional autologous procedures remove some or all of the muscle surrounding the blood supply; advanced procedures preserve the entire muscle by carefully detaching blood vessels from the flap and then reconnecting them to blood vessels in the chest (table 8.2). Regardless of the procedure, the appearance of the reconstructed breasts is the same. The difference, which is significant, is on the inside: after reconstruction, the muscle is either missing or remains fully functioning at the donor site.

Perforator Flaps

Perforator flaps are named for the *perforating arteries* that run through ("perforate") muscle and supply blood to the overlying fat and skin. (Arteries move blood away from the heart; veins carry blood to the heart.) These are *muscle-sparing procedures*; they transfer an entire flap of fat, skin, nerves, and the supporting artery and vein to the mastectomy site while leaving the muscle fully functioning and in place at the donor site. Perforator flaps are the most advanced type of autologous breast reconstruction. They require the specialized training, experience, and meticulous skill of a *microsurgeon*, who identifies the best artery for the flap (sometimes more than one perforator runs through the tissue) and uses high-powered magnifying equipment to carefully separate the fat away from the muscle, spread the muscle fibers, and separate and detach the perforating artery (figure 8.2). Using sutures that are thinner than human hair, the blood vessels in the flap are reconnected to blood vessels in the chest. (A small piece of rib cartilage may be removed to gain better access to the internal artery in the chest, particularly in women with narrow or small chests.) Not all surgeons are microsurgeons. Many limit their practice to traditional autologous procedures that sacrifice muscle and don't require microsurgery. Perforator flap reconstruction is complex and lengthy; yet compared with flaps that include muscle, it's a less debilitating operation with a shortened hospital stay and recovery.

FIGURE 8.2 Perforator flaps involve lifting an island of skin and fat away from the muscle (*left*). The perforator artery and a vein from the muscle are detached (*center*) and reconnected to blood vessels in the chest (*right*).

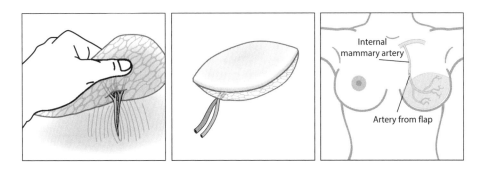

Preoperative Imaging

A preoperative *magnetic resonance angiogram (MRA)*, a *computed tomography angiogram (CTA)*, or a *handheld Doppler probe* (a small, portable ultrasound machine that detects blood flow) will provide your surgeon with a road map of your underlying blood vessels, showing whether the needed arteries are intact and undamaged. This is especially helpful if you have previously had abdominal surgery. Even with this advanced imaging, surgeons sometimes discover during the operation that the perforator artery they planned to use is damaged or too small to adequately supply the flap; they must then decide which procedure is the most advantageous.

When preoperative imaging identifies a less-than-adequate blood supply, performing a *surgical flap delay* (also called vascular delay) a week before an

Blood Supply to the Flap Is Critical

Without sufficient blood, part or all of a new breast can wither and die. Moving an autologous flap from a donor site to the chest with its blood supply intact is the most critical part of any flap reconstruction because, unlike breast implants, living tissue needs the essential nourishment blood provides:

- It brings nutrients and oxygen to all parts of the tissue.
- It circulates hormones.
- It carries infection-fighting antibodies.
- It transports carbon dioxide and other waste materials to the lungs, kidneys, and digestive system to be removed from the body.

autologous procedure can improve blood flow to the tissue that will become the flap. This preemptive preconditioning deliberately disrupts other nonessential blood vessels that feed the targeted tissue; the chosen perforator then dilates to become a single, more robust blood source that improves flap viability and accommodates a larger flap that provides more tissue for the breast.

Free Flaps

Free flaps also require microsurgery to disconnect tissue from its original blood supply, move it to another area, and then reconnect it to a blood supply there. Technically, all tissue flaps that involve disconnecting and reconnecting blood vessels are included in this category: the blood supply is "freed" from its source and reconnected in the chest. A free flap may remove some or all of the muscle that surrounds the necessary blood supply. Perforator flaps are free flaps, but not all free flaps are perforator flaps.

Pedicled Flaps

Pedicled flaps were developed before plastic surgeons began using microsurgery for breast reconstruction, when taking the muscle was the only way to include blood supply to the new breast. While some surgeons still perform pedicled flaps, most autologous breast reconstruction is now accomplished with perforator flaps. During pedicled flap surgery, one end of the muscle with the surrounding skin and fat is cut away from the donor site (most often from the abdomen or the back) and tunneled under the skin to the chest. The other end of the muscle remains attached to its original blood supply at the donor site. (The artery and vein form the "pedicle.") Microsurgical skills aren't required because the artery and veins aren't detached or reconnected. A pedicled flap creates a cosmetically fine breast, but it unnecessarily sacrifices a perfectly healthy muscle, which is taken only for the blood supply that runs through it. Compared to perforator flaps, pedicled flaps generally take longer to heal, make for a more uncomfortable recovery, and may reduce some functionality where the muscle is removed.

TABLE 8.2 Autologous Tissue Flaps

SOURCE	FLAP	TYPE
Abdomen	deep inferior epigastric perforator (DIEP)	preserves muscle
	superficial inferior epigastric artery (SIEA)	preserves muscle
	transverse rectus abdominis myocutaneous (TRAM)	removes muscle
Thighs	profunda artery perforator (PAP)	preserves muscle
	transverse upper gracilis (TUG)	removes muscle
Buttocks	gluteal artery perforator (GAP)	preserves muscle
Back	latissimus dorsi (LD)	removes muscle
	thoracodorsal artery perforator (TDAP) flap*	preserves muscle
	lateral intercostal artery perforator (LICAP) flap*	preserves muscle
Hips	lumbar artery perforator (LAP)	preserves muscle

*Primarily used for partial reconstruction after lumpectomy.

Borrowing from the Abdomen

Using skin and fat from the lower belly is the most common method of autologous breast reconstruction because that's where women often carry excess weight—and also where they would like to lose it. Abdominal tissue is a good choice for breast reconstruction. It's pliable and has the skin tone, texture, and thickness similar to breast tissue. Abdominal procedures provide a two-for-one benefit: the same tissue that is normally removed and discarded after a tummy tuck is used to create the new breast mound. You come out of reconstructive surgery with new breasts and a tighter belly.

Beneath the abdominal skin and fat are the long, flat rectus abdominis ("six-pack") muscles. You have two: one on the left and one on the right, extending from the fifth, sixth, and seventh ribs to the pubic bone. These are the sit-up muscles that support the abdominal wall, help you bend and flex at the waist, and keep your abdominal organs in place. Each muscle has two sources of blood: the superior artery and veins in the fatty tissue just beneath the skin, and the inferior artery and veins that run through the muscles near the groin (figure 8.3). One side of the abdomen is used for unilateral breast reconstruction; both sides are used for bilateral breast reconstruction.

FIGURE 8.3 DIEP flaps include fat, skin, and the deep inferior epigastric artery; SIEA flaps include skin, fat, and the superficial inferior epigastric artery. Both procedures preserve the abdominal muscles.

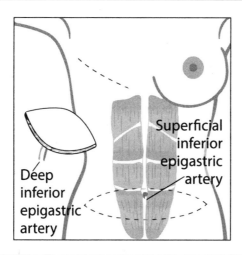

Reconstruction with an abdominal flap begins with a hip-to-hip elliptical incision above the navel and almost to the pubic bone, similar to the placement of a cesarean incision. (The resulting scar is covered by most bathing suits and underwear.) Your belly button may look different after your surgery. During the operation, it's freed from the surrounding skin but remains attached to the abdominal wall. When the flap has been removed and the edges of the incision are pulled together, a new hole is made, and the belly button is pulled through and sutured in place with tiny stitches.

DIEP Flaps

The *deep inferior epigastric perforator (DIEP) flap* is often referred to as a new method of breast reconstruction, but it's been performed since the early 1990s. DIEP flaps revolutionized breast reconstruction by providing an option for rebuilding breasts without breast implants and without sacrificing any muscle. They include only what is needed to reconstruct the breast: fat, skin, and blood vessels (figure 8.3). A small incision is made into the *fascia* (the fibrous tissue covering the muscles), and an artery and vein that run through the skin

FIGURE 8.4 After unilateral mastectomy (*left*), delayed DIEP flap reconstruction and mastectomy and immediate DIEP flap reconstruction of the opposite breast (*right*) with later nipple reconstruction and tattoos.

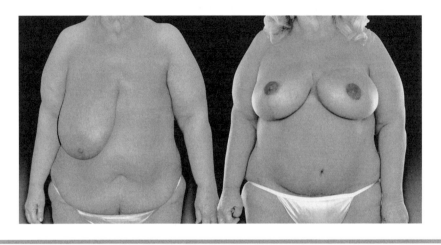

Images provided by Dr. Frank J. DellaCroce, Center for Restorative Breast Surgery, LLC

and fat are carefully teased away from the muscle fibers. If the perforator artery is tangled with scar tissue (perhaps from a previous cesarean section) or a cluster of muscle fibers, a very small incision in the muscle may be required. Generally, DIEP flaps don't involve cutting or relocating any part of the abdominal muscle, so it's not surprising that DIEP has a better rate of abdominal wall recovery and function, and a lower potential for causing abdominal bulging and hernia, compared to abdominal flaps that do sacrifice muscle.[1] A true DIEP flap preserves the entire muscle. The entire flap with its blood supply is cut away from the abdominal wall and moved to the mastectomy site, where the artery and vein are reconnected in the chest and the living tissue is shaped into a breast (figure 8.4). The incision is then closed. You leave the hospital with new breasts and fully functional abdominal muscles.

A prior cesarean delivery, hysterectomy, appendectomy, or hernia repair in the groin don't necessarily eliminate DIEP as a possible reconstructive method, as long as you have enough tissue and blood vessels that aren't damaged or missing. You aren't eligible for DIEP reconstruction if you've already had a cosmetic tummy tuck or you no longer have enough belly tissue after liposuction.

Is a DIEP Flap the Same as a Tummy Tuck?

Reconstruction with a DIEP flap is often said to be like a tummy tuck, and in some ways, it is—but it also has some differences. Both surgeries involve a hip-to-hip incision in the lower abdomen, remove an elliptical area of skin and fat, and improve the contour of the midsection. Abdominal tissue flaps are a reconstructive procedure, while tummy tucks are cosmetic. Unlike a tummy tuck, which removes excess fat to reduce the belly, an autologous reconstructive procedure focuses on preserving and relocating tissue and blood vessels to recreate a breast. Reconstructive procedures are more complex and require advanced surgical skills to relocate tissue that is otherwise discarded from a tummy tuck.

Variations of the DIEP flap

In a small percentage of women, the *superficial inferior epigastric artery (SIEA) flap* is a more accessible blood supply. Although the procedure and the cosmetic result of a SIEA flap are essentially the same as a DIEP flap, a different artery is used for the flap. SIEA blood vessels are found in the fatty tissue just beneath the skin and above the muscle (figure 8.3). The abdominal muscle and fascia are not only spared, but are also undisturbed, which reduces surgery time and improves recovery. Not all women have SIEAs. The superficial blood vessels are often too small to support the flap, or they've been cut during a previous abdominal surgery. When a SIEA can't be used, a DIEP flap is performed instead.

When a single perforator isn't adequate to nourish the entire flap or blood vessels are aligned in irregular locations in the abdominal muscles, the muscle structure between the required additional blood vessels may be cut to bring them closer. This causes muscle damage that can result in weakness and may elevate the chance of developing a *hernia* (a bulge under the skin caused when the intestines poke through the weakened muscle). In these cases, an *abdominal perforator exchange (APEX) flap*—a DIEP flap with a modified method of securing the blood supply—is an alternative for optimizing blood flow to the flap while fully preserving the muscles.[2] Blood vessels that run through the six-pack muscles divide into different branches, much like limbs from a tree trunk. During the APEX procedure, the "trunk" is disconnected between the branches; this allows the vessels to slip between the muscle fibers without cutting them. The entire flap—skin, fat, and the disassembled blood vessels—is then moved to the chest, where the separated vessels are reconnected, and the end of the main blood vessel is attached to a vessel in the chest; this restores blood flow to the flap through all of the additional branches. With this rearrangement of the blood supply, the flap is well-nourished, and the entire new breast remains soft and healthy. In addition, the muscles remain undamaged.

An *extended DIEP flap* lengthens the standard hip-to-hip incision to include abdominal and hip fat for additional volume. A *stacked DIEP flap* is a combination of two DIEP flaps, one from each side of the abdomen. For thin women with limited abdominal tissue, this produces a larger breast than what could be created with a single DIEP flap. The entire abdominal flap can be removed in one segment and folded, or both sides can be harvested separately and stacked to create the breast.

I met with several surgeons when I decided to have DIEP reconstruction. When my hometown doctors said I didn't have enough tissue, I traveled across the country to a DIEP specialist for my surgeries, and I have never looked back. I returned home with two beautiful D-cup breasts. I chose the most competent and caring doctors I have ever met. I now live in Israel; and when my doctors here see my results, they are blown away. My recovery was uneventful, with only some spitting stitches and hypertrophic scars. Five years later, I live a normal life. I see my scars, but I do not regret my surgery one bit.

—Debbie

TRAM Flaps

The *transverse rectus abdominis myocutaneous (TRAM) flap* was a major advancement when it was introduced in 1982 because it introduced a way to use a woman's soft belly tissue as a more natural alternative to breast implants. (The latissimus dorsi flap that uses a muscle from the back was the first autologous flap used for breast reconstruction.) A TRAM is a pedicled flap that uses the same fat and blood vessels from the lower abdomen as the DIEP flap; but, unlike the DIEP flap, it also includes the abdominal muscle. For many years, the TRAM flap was the most common method of autologous reconstruction. With DIEP and so many other muscle-sparing options now available, it's no longer necessary to sacrifice muscle; and less than 10 percent of all autologous breast reconstructions involve TRAM surgery.[3] In some areas, it might be the only available method of autologous breast reconstruction, however.

During a TRAM surgery, a segment of skin, fat, and the underlying six-pack muscle is cut away from the lower abdomen and tunneled under the skin to the opposite side of the chest. (The rectus abdominis muscle opposite the missing breast is used for unilateral reconstruction; both muscles are used for bilateral reconstruction.) The upper portion of the flap is sutured into position to provide fullness at the top of the new breast, while the lower edge is folded under, shaped to match the size and contour of the opposite breast, and stitched in place. The upper end of the muscle remains attached in its original position above the rib cage to maintain blood flow to the flap (figure 8.5).

FIGURE 8.5 A pedicled TRAM flap remains attached to one end of the rectus abdominis muscle and is tunneled under the skin to the chest. The opposite end of the muscle remains in its original location.

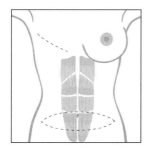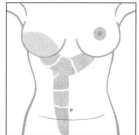

Synthetic mesh is placed in the abdomen to strengthen the abdominal wall, which is weakened when the muscle is removed. (Surgical mesh isn't required with a DIEP because the abdominal wall isn't cut or removed.) A bulge may develop five or six months after the operation as a result of tunneling tissue under the skin; this usually recedes as the muscle atrophies and thins.

Variations of the TRAM

A *free TRAM* procedure transplants the abdominal flap rather than tunneling it under the skin. The flap, along with the muscle that carries the necessary blood supply, is cut away from the abdominal wall and positioned in the chest. Compared to a pedicled TRAM, the blood supply of a free TRAM is more reliable, which allows for a larger breast that can be shaped more aggressively. During a *muscle-sparing TRAM* procedure, the muscle is cut across its width to remove a small portion that is included in the flap. The amount of muscle taken varies depending on your anatomy and your surgeon's skill. Leaving most of the muscle in place reduces postoperative pain and decreases the risk of abdominal wall weakness and hernia; surgical mesh isn't normally needed. If you're considering any type of TRAM procedure, it's important to understand how much of your abdominal muscle will be removed and the short-term and long-term potential for complications.

Recovery from Abdominal Flap Reconstruction

It's amazing how many movements involve the abdominal muscles. That's something you'll discover after a DIEP or TRAM surgery. Initially, it will be difficult to sit down, get up, or get in and out of bed; but you'll have medication to control your pain. With either procedure, your breasts and abdomen will at first be sore and tender. Within 24 hours of your operation, you'll be taking short walks, gradually increasing how far and how much you walk. Your flap will be closely monitored around the clock by nurses.

You'll need help during your first week home. You may have three incisions to care for: on your breast, on your abdomen, and around your belly button. If you had axillary lymph node dissection, you'll have another incision under your arm. You'll also need surgical drains for two weeks or more at your donor sites and chest. Lifting, bending, pulling, or pushing anything over 5 pounds may not be possible or advisable until your incisions heal. Avoiding motions or activities that strain your abdomen will encourage healing. Each day, you'll feel progressively better and less fatigued. Driving will have to wait until you no longer need narcotics.

Recovering from a DIEP flap

Because the chest muscle isn't cut or elevated and the abdominal muscle is undisturbed, DIEP recovery is significantly shorter and less painful than a pedicled TRAM, which removes one or both muscles. With the implementation of enhanced recovery protocols (chapter 13), many DIEP patients experience manageable discomfort after surgery; require few, if any, narcotics; and are discharged from the hospital in three days. Still, DIEP is major surgery and requires recuperation (table 8.3). Closing the incision after removing tissue considerably tightens the abdomen; for the first week or so, you'll need to walk hunched over at the waist. Some women need a bit longer before they can stand straight. By the second week, you should be able to gently increase your movement and range of motion. By the fourth week, you'll likely be able to return to many of your routine activities. Most women are back to normal without restriction by the fifth or sixth week. Swelling in your abdomen and new breasts may last for several months, and tightness in the abdomen should improve after three months or so. It may take up to a year for your tissues to heal completely.

Recovering from a TRAM flap

Pedicled TRAM surgery is the most difficult recovery of any breast reconstruction. You're recovering from not one but two significant operations and the loss of one or both major abdominal muscles. It's important to begin walking as soon as possible to reduce swelling and reduce the chance of blood clots. You may need four to six weeks until you can begin gentle stretching. You'll gradually begin more vigorous movement and should be back to most routine activities within two months; however, some women may require additional time to heal. You may feel tired for several more weeks as your energy level slowly returns and you can safely resume more strenuous movements and activities. Tightness in the abdomen should begin to soften and improve a few months after your procedure but may last longer. Wearing a compression girdle for several weeks will help to minimize swelling, which should gradually subside. The abdominal muscle (now part of your new breast) will slowly thin from lack of exercise, and your new breast will assume its final shape.

TABLE 8.3 Intervals for Autologous Reconstruction with Abdominal Flaps

FLAP TYPE	SURGERY; HOSPITAL STAY	MOST ROUTINE ACTIVITIES RESUMED*
DIEP	5–8 hours; 3–4 days	4–6 weeks
TRAM (pedicled)	4–5 hours; 4–5 days	6–8 weeks
TRAM (free)	6–8 hours; 4–5 days	6–8 weeks
TRAM (muscle-sparing)	6–8 hours; 4–5 days	6–8 weeks

Note: Reflects reconstruction without complications. Surgical expertise and individual healing affect recovery times.

*Additional time may be needed to regain full strength and mobility or return to strenuous activity.

Most women have no long-term ill effects from a pedicled TRAM, but removing the six-pack muscles and the fascia weakens the abdominal wall. Without the support of the rectus muscle(s), back pain may develop as other muscles work harder to support and stabilize the spine. Getting in and out of bed will be difficult without first rolling to your side, especially if both abdominal muscles were removed. You may need physical therapy to strengthen your back and core muscles, improve flexibility, and maintain proper posture.

Honestly, my TRAM hurt like hell. I spent a lot of the day crying and just stayed on medication until I got better. Now I'm just as excited about my flat stomach as I am about my new breast. For the first time in my life, I'm wearing clothes I never would have worn before my surgery.
—*Monique*

Other Donor Sites and Procedures

If you prefer reconstruction with your own tissue but an abdominal flap isn't right for you, then your thighs, buttocks, back, or hips may be a resource for your new breasts. You're a candidate for one of these flaps if you have enough fatty tissue and healthy blood vessels for the flap. These secondary autologous flaps can be used alone, stacked for more volume, or combined with a breast implant. These procedures aren't used as frequently as implants or abdominal flaps, but they produce very good reconstructive results. The length

Pregnancy after an Abdominal Flap

No large, long-term clinical studies have addressed pregnancy after DIEP or TRAM reconstruction, yet many people have delivered healthy babies after abdominal flap reconstruction with no significant complications. While this implies that pregnancy is safe after reconstruction with abdominal flaps, these are individual cases. They do not provide sufficient evidence to identify potential risks, suggest how long after surgery you should wait to become pregnant, or clarify who can expect to do so without problems. For some people, especially those who have bilateral pedicled TRAM, pregnancy could potentially place too much pressure on the abdominal wall and donor site scar. If you hope for a future pregnancy, speak with your obstetrician/gynecologist about this before deciding which reconstructive method is best for you.

Source: Fu A, Liu C. Is pregnancy following a TRAM or DIEP flap safe? A critical systematic review and meta-analysis. *Aesthetic Plastic Surgery,* 2021;45:2618–30; Moshrefi S, Kanchwala S, Momeni A. Should planned/desired pregnancy be considered an absolute contraindication to breast reconstruction with free abdominal flaps? A retrospective case series and systematic review. *Journal of Plastic Reconstruction,* 2018;71(9)1295–1300; Chai SC, Umayaal S, Saad AZ. Successful pregnancy during pedicled transverse rectus abdominis musculocutaneous flap for breast reconstruction with normal vaginal delivery. *Indian Journal of Plastic Surgery*, 2014;48(1):81–84.

TABLE 8.4 Intervals for Reconstruction with Other Autologous Flaps

FLAP	SURGERY; HOSPITAL STAY	RESUME MOST ROUTINE ACTIVITIES*
PAP	3–5 hours; 3–4 days	4–6 weeks
TUG	6–8 hours; 2–3 days	4–6 weeks
GAP	8–12 hours; 3–5 days	4–6 weeks
LD	3–6 hours; 3–4 days	4–6 weeks
TDAP or LICAP**	up to 3 hours; overnight	2–4 weeks

Note: Reflects bilateral reconstruction without complications. Surgical expertise and individual healing affect recovery times.

*Additional time needed to regain full strength and mobility or return to strenuous activity.

**Primarily used for partial reconstruction after lumpectomy.

of the surgery, hospital stay, and recovery vary depending on the procedure (table 8.4).

Flaps from the Thighs

When the belly isn't an available donor site, soft, pliable tissue from the thighs can be a source for reconstruction; the limited volume is usually enough to create only small- to moderate-sized breasts. Removing fat from this area slims the donor site, similar to a thigh lift. (After unilateral reconstruction, liposuction of the opposite thigh may be required for symmetry.) The crescent shape of thigh flaps offers a unique advantage over other autologous flaps: bringing the ends together creates a natural breast shape.

The point of the flap sometimes facilitates nipple reconstruction during the initial procedure (figure 8.6). Placing a few sutures around the tip of the flap refines the nipple and enhances projection, but some surgeons prefer to reconstruct a new nipple during later revision surgery. Because thigh skin tends to be slightly darker than breast skin, later tattooing of the nipple and areola after a skin-sparing mastectomy may be unnecessary unless you want a deeper pigment.

The scar that remains on the upper thigh is sometimes well disguised. Depending on the location of the blood vessels included in the flap, sometimes it may be visible in underwear and swimsuits. While there is no risk of a hernia, the chance of delayed wound healing is greater than with other types of autologous flaps.

PAP and TUG Flaps

The muscle-sparing *profunda artery perforator (PAP) flap* uses skin and fat from the upper thigh just below the buttock, leaving an acceptable overall contour and, in many cases, an inconspicuous scar in the buttock crease (figure 8.7). The exact placement of the incision depends on the anatomy of the blood vessels, which tend to vary among individuals. A segment of skin, fat, and blood vessels is removed and relocated to the chest where the blood vessels are reattached. This flap may be an option even if you've had liposuction on your thighs. The *vertical profunda artery perforator (VPAP) flap*, which uses the same tissue with a vertical incision on the inner thigh, produces a longer flap of tissue that creates a larger breast.

The *transverse upper gracilis (TUG) flap* includes skin and fat from the upper inner thigh; but, unlike the PAP flap, it also uses some or all of the gracilis muscle. Losing this muscle doesn't affect long-term functionality because other muscles pick up the slack. A TUG flap leaves a scar that may be tucked into the crease of the thigh, but sometimes it's necessary to make an incision lower on the thigh that results in a more visible scar. The TUG flap has a greater risk of donor-site wound healing issues and lower extremity lymphedema.

FIGURE 8.6 The PAP flap (*left*) uses tissue from the back of the thigh. The TUG flap (*center*) uses tissue from the inner thigh. In both procedures, the elliptical flaps are folded over (*center*) and moved to the chest (*right*).

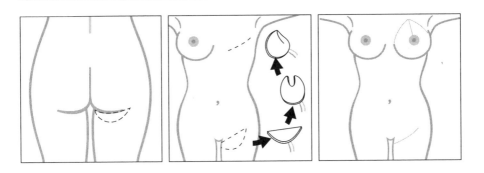

FIGURE 8.7 Expanders removed due to infection after bilateral nipple-sparing mastectomy (*left*), followed by delayed PAP flap reconstruction (*center and right*).

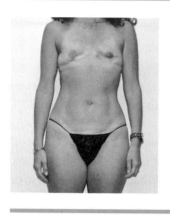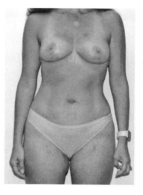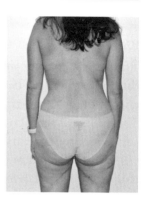

Images provided by Joshua Levine, MD, Center for Breast Reconstruction

Variations of Thigh Flaps

Additional volume can be accessed with a *vertical upper gracilis (VUG) flap*, which leaves a more noticeable incision on the inner thigh. A *diagonal upper gracilis (DUG) flap* is a TUG with a diagonal incision. The *lateral transverse thigh (LTP) flap* is uncommon, but it can serve as an alternative if you have excess skin and fat in your upper outer thigh. Although it improves the thigh-hip contour, it leaves an obvious scar; and, when used for unilateral reconstruction, it causes visible asymmetry with the opposite thigh.

Recovery

Thigh incisions make for a somewhat awkward and restrictive recovery because you'll need to refrain from flexing your hips or spreading your legs for a couple of weeks to avoid putting tension on the incision. Your soreness should begin to recede within two or three weeks. You'll need four to six weeks before resuming most normal activities. During that time, your surgeon will advise when to begin stretching and strengthening exercises for the donor site. The tightness you feel where the tissue was removed will gradually improve over several weeks. You may also experience some early weakness in the thigh muscles before strength eventually returns. A compression garment worn for about eight weeks will minimize swelling. Depending on the location of your incision, a later *scar revision* may be needed to achieve an acceptable result (chapter 9).

Flaps from the Buttocks

Posterior, derriere, backside, rump, tush, gluteus maximus. Popular jargon aside, a well-padded bottom can be a prime source of tissue for breast reconstruction. The tissue that provides a *gluteal artery perforator (GAP) flap* has a high fat-to-skin ratio and a robust blood supply, producing excellent reconstructive results without needing the muscle. Buttock fat is firm, which makes it more difficult to shape than fat from the abdomen or thighs, yet it creates soft, natural-feeling breasts. You probably have enough gluteal tissue to recreate one or both full, round breasts, even if you're slender and lack sufficient fat for an abdominal flap. You might not be a candidate for GAP reconstruction if you've already had gluteal liposuction. A unilateral flap causes buttock asymmetry, which can be improved with liposuction of the opposite buttock.

The *superior gluteal artery perforator (SGAP) procedure* creates a slanted elliptical incision on the upper buttock from the outer hip to the intergluteal cleft between the cheeks (figure 8.8). The resulting scar runs across the top of the buttock below the panty line (figure 8.9). A flap of skin and fat is carefully removed where the upper buttock meets the hip. Excess fat in the "love handles," the fatty area just below the waist or the lower back, can be incorporated into the flap if extra tissue is required. The gluteal artery feeding the tissue is separated from the muscle, reattached in the chest, and the flap is sculpted to form the new breast.

An SGAP flap tends to flatten the natural curve of the buttock. This can be somewhat offset by removing the fascia over the muscle, allowing the muscle to protrude into the space created by the flap, and restoring some of the natural contour.[4] Otherwise, symmetry can be achieved during a later revision surgery by rounding out the donor site with fat that is removed with liposuction from your hips or thighs or lifting the opposite buttock after unilateral reconstruction. The less common *inferior gluteal artery perforator (IGAP) flap* removes skin and fat from the lower part of the buttock (figure 8.8). Although the incision is hidden in the natural crease beneath the bottom, removing fat this low on the buttock can make sitting uncomfortable.

GAP flap surgery is meticulous and lengthy, requiring 8 to 12 hours under anesthesia, even when two surgeons work as a team. Bilateral GAP requires

FIGURE 8.8 SGAP reconstruction uses an elliptical flap on the upper buttock. An IGAP incision follows the natural crease below the buttock.

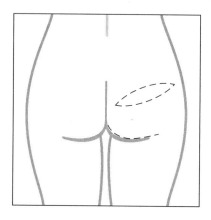

that you be turned twice during the procedure. During immediate reconstruction, you're first positioned on your back. Once the mastectomy is completed, you're gently turned onto your stomach so that fat and skin can be harvested from your backside. You're then returned to your back to complete the reconstruction. Delayed GAP flap reconstruction is somewhat shorter because the mastectomy has already been done. Few surgeons perform GAP reconstruction; even fewer surgeons perform bilateral GAP reconstruction, which requires two operations and two recoveries. If you're interested in this procedure, it's worth your time to consider surgeons who build both breasts in a single operation.

I had a bilateral prophylactic mastectomy with SGAP flap reconstruction using tissue from my upper bottom to rebuild my breasts. Initially, I had very limited sensation in my reconstructed breasts. For the first few months after surgery, I was very cautious and nervous about anything bumping into my chest. Gradually, some sensation returned to my breasts. Seven years later, I can feel pressure and warmth, but I have limited local sensation. I don't have any feeling in my nipples, which is unfortunate since I used to experience sexual pleasure from nipple stimulation. In the first year or two after surgery, I occasionally

FIGURE 8.9 Before (*upper and lower left*) and after (*upper and lower right*) bilateral SGAP flap reconstruction following removal of a failed implant after radiation to the right breast (*upper left*) and nipple-sparing mastectomy of the left breast (*upper left and right*).

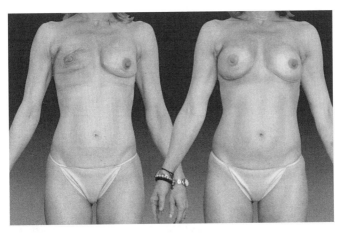

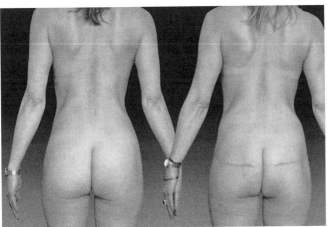

Images provided by Dr. Frank J. DellaCroce, Center for Restorative Breast Surgery, LLC

felt numbness, tingling, and short, shooting pain at the donor site. I'm still relatively numb along the donor site scars, but I don't feel any pain or tingling. While I was initially very aware of the changing feelings in my breasts and donor sites, now I mostly don't think about it, and overall I'm very satisfied with the results.

—*Ann*

Recovery

Recuperating from GAP reconstruction is generally less painful and quicker than recovery from reconstruction involving the abdomen or the thighs. Pain and tenderness around the gluteal incisions often subside during the first week. Surgical drains at the chest often remain for seven to ten days; donor site drains may be needed for a few more days. Wearing a compression bra around the clock for two weeks and a compression girdle for six to eight weeks discourages seroma and reduces post-op pain by supporting your incisions. Initially, it may be difficult to sit comfortably or lie on your back. You'll discover which positions are more comfortable as you heal. You may need to avoid heavy lifting, as well as strenuous sports and activities, for six to eight weeks.

Flaps from the Back

The *latissimus dorsi myocutaneous (LD) flap* is the original procedure for autologous breast reconstruction. It recreates the breast using the flat, triangular back muscle that runs from the shoulder to the hip. (When you stand facing a wall and push against it, the latissimus dorsi muscle enables that movement and facilitates twisting the body.) Although the LD flap is still used for head, neck, and shoulder repair, it's now performed less often for breast reconstruction. It's an alternative if you don't have enough donor tissue elsewhere and you've previously had radiation therapy to the chest wall or if you don't have access to a microsurgeon who performs autologous reconstruction.

An LD procedure is a pedicled flap. When the mastectomy has been completed, you're turned to rest on your stomach or side. An oval of skin, fat, and part or all of the latissimus dorsi muscle is lifted away from the back and tunneled under the skin and across the armpit to the mastectomy site (figure 8.10). The opposite end of the muscle remains connected to the artery in the back. You're then turned to your back, and the flap is placed over your chest muscle. Because the muscle is thin and the back typically provides less fat than other donor sites, this flap creates only small- to moderate-sized breasts and is usually combined with a tissue expander or an implant. (Covering the implant with the muscle reduces the risk of capsular contracture.) A vertical or horizontal incision on the back is easily covered by bras. A diagonal incision isn't hidden as easily, so if you choose this procedure, talk to your surgeon about the placement of your incision.

FIGURE 8.10 Removing a latissimus dorsi flap from the back (*left*) leaves a scar beneath the shoulder blade (*center*). The flap is then tunneled under the skin to the chest (*right*). An expander or implant is often used for added volume.

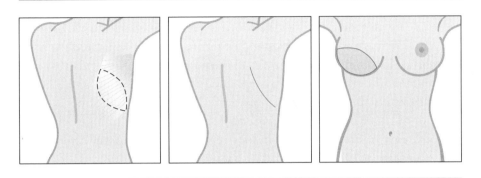

LD flaps generally produce good results with few problems. Because it's less likely to develop delayed wound healing, it's a reliable alternative for smokers and women who have diabetes or health issues that preclude having longer, more invasive surgeries. It isn't a preferred option if you have circulatory problems, persistent pain, or weakness in your back or shoulder. Other reconstructive methods may be better if you've had previous surgery in or near your armpit or near your lungs or heart, which can affect the blood supply to the back.

> As an aerobics instructor, I didn't want to risk reduced abdominal strength, even though my doctor said I'd be okay after TRAM reconstruction. I read about the back flap in a magazine. I'm glad I did because my surgery went very well.
>
> —*Dee Dee*

Variations of the LD Flap

When the back (especially the lower back) has a generous excess of skin and fat, an *extended latissimus dorsi flap* can create a larger breast, eliminating the need for an implant but also leaving a longer scar. During a *muscle-sparing latissimus dorsi flap* procedure, an incision is made lower on the back, and the muscle is divided vertically: a small portion is used to create the breast, while the rest remains functional in the back. An *endoscopic latissimus dorsi flap* procedure transfers the muscle through the mastectomy incision or a small incision under the arm, leaving an unscarred back and a shorter recovery. Other muscle-sparing flaps can be taken from the side of the chest under the arm. The *thoracodorsal artery perforator (TDAP) flap* uses a perforator and vein that run through the latissimus dorsi muscle; the *lateral intercostal artery perforator (LICAP) flap* includes blood vessels that run through the muscle between the ribs. The perforating arteries and veins are carefully separated from the latissimus dorsi muscle, and the tissue is rotated to the chest under the skin or removed from the back and transplanted to the mastectomy site. The entire latissimus dorsi muscle is preserved. These flaps yield only a small amount of tissue but can be combined with another flap or an implant for added breast volume. Most often, they're used to replace tissue removed on the outer portion of the breast during a lumpectomy.

Recovery

Recovery from LD flap reconstruction is generally shorter and less painful than reconstruction with other autologous flaps, especially from the abdomen or thigh. Your upper back may be sore for four or six weeks after LD flap reconstruction and will be numb until the nerves regenerate. Your underarm will be sore from tunneling the flap around to the chest. For a few months, you may experience tightness and limited movement and strength in your back. An LD procedure doesn't cause significant long-term weakness or interfere with day-to-day activities for most women. Physical therapy may be needed to regain strength and range of motion. Removing the muscle limits the ability to lift and twist, so your ability to swim, golf, play tennis, and do certain other athletic activities could be impacted, especially after bilateral LD reconstruction.[5] Drains normally stay in place for about two weeks because this flap tends to form a seroma, particularly in overweight and obese individuals. Because the blood supply is reliable, necrosis rarely occurs. A bulge that may develop under the arm from tunneling the flap to the chest will likely shrink as the muscle atrophies over time, although it may never disappear completely.

Flaps from the Hips
The *lumbar artery perforator (LAP) flap* is an uncommon procedure that uses the "love handles" to reconstruct the breasts. Removing tissue in this area leaves a horizontal scar where the waist meets the upper buttock that is usually hidden

by most bathing suits or underwear. A LAP flap preserves muscle, so recovery is shortened and less uncomfortable compared to other procedures that sacrifice muscle. Hip flaps can be stacked with flaps from other areas to create the desired breast volume. Few surgeons offer this type of reconstruction.

Hybrid Reconstruction

Plastic surgeons are always looking for new ways to exceed women's expectations and give them better results. One innovative example is *hybrid breast reconstruction*, a combination of breast implants and autologous reconstruction. This mix-and-match method is particularly advantageous for thin women who prefer autologous reconstruction but lack sufficient fatty tissue from a single donor site to create the breast volume they want.[6] Hybrid procedures provide the best of both reconstructive worlds, especially for bilateral reconstruction: the volume of full-sized implants with the softness of living fat.

Advantages of Hybrid Breast Reconstruction

- It provides the natural look and warmth of autologous reconstruction.
- It generally results in fewer complications and better aesthetics after radiation therapy.
- It facilitates prepectoral placement of an implant.
- It camouflages the breast implant and reduces rippling, wrinkling, and capsular contracture.
- Because the flap provides much of the breast volume, a smaller implant is often sufficient and is usually smaller than what it would be with implant reconstruction alone.
- It eliminates the need for tissue expansion in most cases; when needed, missing breast skin can be replaced with the autologous flap.
- It reduces the donor site incision/scar because implants supply a portion of the breast volume.
- It results in a scar that is lower and less visible than the typical scar from DIEP, SIEA, or TRAM flaps because tissue can be removed from the lower abdomen (which usually has less fat).
- It enhances projection of the breast and reconstructed nipples as the implant pushes the tissue forward.

Disadvantages of Hybrid Breast Reconstruction
- There is some chance of problems associated with breast implants.
- Routine screening of silicone implants is recommended (chapter 6).

Stacked Flaps

For women who lack sufficient fat in a single donor site but prefer not to have a breast implant, *stacked flaps* provide a purely autologous reconstruction with more volume. Two flaps—one placed on top of the other—can be used for unilateral reconstruction. Four flaps can be combined for bilateral reconstruction. Stacked flaps can provide exceptional aesthetics, with one flap adding fullness to the top of the breast, while the other provides fullness at the bottom. They usually involve a DIEP flap that is supplemented with another flap from the buttocks, thighs, or hips (figure 8.11). While the thought of having a procedure involving two or four flaps may seem overwhelming, an experienced two-surgeon microsurgical team can safely and efficiently harvest these flaps simultaneously with little added risk. Technically demanding, stacked flaps are recognized as a safe and effective method for reconstruction in women who don't otherwise have enough fat in one area to accommodate their reconstruction.

Potential Problems and Fixes

Complications can develop from any kind of surgery, and autologous reconstruction is no exception (chapter 15). Having a lengthier, more complex surgery increases the chance of problems. Compared to reconstruction with breast implants, autologous reconstruction involves a longer initial surgery and recovery from two, rather than one, area of the body. But it also produces a breast that looks and feels more natural, without implant-related problems. Complications that develop generally show up early on and resolve in time or can be remedied during revision surgery.

Uneven or Poorly Healed Scars

Your scars won't disappear, but your plastic surgeon can make them look more even and possibly less visible. Scars that don't heal well, are discolored, or are

FIGURE 8.11 Before (*upper and lower left*) and after (*upper and lower right*) nipple-sparing mastectomies with immediate stacked bilateral DIEP and SGAP flaps.

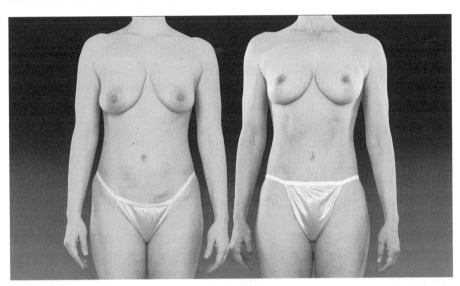

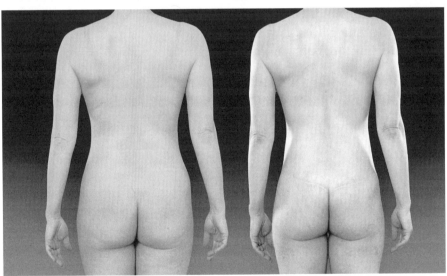

exceptionally wide can be improved (chapter 15). "Dog ears" can also be re-fined; these small puckered folds of skin often form at the end of round or elliptical incisions. (It's easier to avoid this issue with straight incisions because the edges can be evenly matched.) Dog ears are common after a mastectomy without reconstruction and autologous flaps, especially in individuals who are overweight or obese.

Hernia

A hernia can develop after any abdominal surgery, but it's more likely to oc-cur when part or all of the abdominal muscle is removed and weakens the ab-dominal wall. Hernias are less likely to develop after a DIEP procedure than a pedicled TRAM, which removes one or both abdominal muscles. In rare instances, a hernia or unusual bulge may appear after a DIEP flap, but these often disappear when the internal incision in the fascia heals. Repairing her-nias is important because they can be painful, and they can cause nausea, cramping, and bloating. If a hernia is left untreated, symptoms can worsen, and surgery is the only solution. Minor hernias can sometimes be repaired by tightening the abdominal fascia. Larger hernias are resolved by carefully push-ing any bulging organs back where they belong, closing the hernia opening, and reinforcing the abdomen with mesh to reduce the odds of recurrence.

Necrosis

When blood doesn't flow evenly throughout the flap, small areas of scar tis-sue may harden and feel like lumps in the breast. If the blood supply fails, the entire flap dies. This can be a devastating turn of events because instead of be-ing done with reconstruction, the entire breast needs to be removed. It's like a mastectomy all over again. If you want to try another reconstruction, you can have a different autologous procedure or implant reconstruction in a few months when your chest has had a chance to heal. Fortunately, complete flap failure rarely happens. Smoking or using other tobacco products raises sus-ceptibility to infection, seroma, hernia, and necrosis at the mastectomy and donor sites.[7] The likelihood of these problems is significantly reduced if you stop smoking for a month or more before your surgery. Being obese or dia-betic (or both) also raises the chance of complications after flap surgery, includ-ing seroma, infection, hernia, and partial or total flap loss.[8]

Questions for Your Plastic Surgeon

- Am I a candidate for autologous muscle-sparing reconstruction?
- Is a hybrid reconstruction a better option for me?
- Which procedure do you recommend for me? Why?
- How often do you perform this procedure?
- Do I have enough fat to achieve the size breasts I want?
- Where will my incisions/scars be?
- How many donor sites/incisions will I need?
- How many operations/procedures will I need?
- How long will it take to complete my entire reconstruction?
- What results can I reasonably expect?
- What should I expect from recovery?
- What problems might I experience? How will you address them?
- What changes can I expect in my reconstructed breasts over time?
- May I look at your before-and-after patient photos of this procedure?
- May I speak to other patients who have had the procedure you recommend for me?

Part III
Procedures to
Improve Symmetry,
Shape, and
Appearance

With little exception, most breast reconstruction involves a secondary surgery, called a revision surgery, to fine-tune the cosmetic appearance of the new breasts and improve or resolve any postoperative problems. Revision surgery is a planned opportunity to improve the size, shape, symmetry, or position of the breasts. Compared to the initial reconstructive procedure, this secondary operation is usually shorter and involves less recovery time.

This section describes five key concepts of revisions:

- common reconstruction revisions that use breast implants or your own tissue
- surgical procedures that use your own, excess, fat as a filler to improve the aesthetics of your new breasts
- surgical procedures to modify your opposite breast for better symmetry after unilateral reconstruction
- surgical procedures to create new nipples and areolas
- nonsurgical methods of adding nipples and areolas

Chapter 9

Revision Procedures

During my second stage revision, I had fat grafting to help fill in the areas of one breast that was smaller. I'm very thin, so the doctor had to be careful. He did a great job. I have a fuller reconstructed breast, and no one but me would know I used to have slightly larger thighs.

—KELSEY

It would be wonderful if every patient emerged from a single visit to the operating room with flawless results. The reality is that most breast reconstruction procedures require a second surgery to improve position, size, or cosmetic appearance of breasts, and to repair minor defects. Unless you have direct-to-implant reconstruction, you can expect revision surgery as a part of your overall reconstructive process. Sometimes even a direct-to-implant procedure results in a less-than-stellar reconstruction and needs a bit of professional tweaking. Revisions are part and parcel of the reconstruction process. They can be performed three to four months after your initial reconstruction, once the swelling has reduced, the tissue has healed and settled into position, and the scar tissue has relaxed. Your surgeon may suggest waiting a bit longer to see if other problems disappear without intervention. Revisions might also be delayed if you're being treated with chemotherapy or radiation therapy. If you're not ready for cosmetic revisions, they can be performed at a later date. A minor outpatient procedure may be all that is needed to correct a crooked scar, shift an implant into a better position, or improve other cosmetic flaws in an otherwise well-crafted breast. For people who are unhappy with their reconstruction and want a second chance at being satisfied, revision surgery may involve starting over and rebuilding the breast again (chapter 16).

Revision surgery addresses five areas of improvement:

- shaping and refining the overall appearance of the breasts
- revising mastectomy or donor site scars
- removing overly firm lumps or areas of dead tissue
- creating new nipples (if this is something that you want)
- improving or eliminating a source of pain, discomfort, or tightness

Making a Good Reconstruction Better

Not all complications require surgery, and, given time, some resolve on their own. Some remedies can be done quickly, under local anesthesia in your surgeon's office; most require general anesthesia in a hospital or surgery center. When possible, incisions are made along existing scars. Your surgeon will evaluate your issues and discuss how they can be improved or eliminated to give your breasts the best possible appearance, whether the issues are related to implants (chapter 6); autologous flaps (chapter 8); or infection, seroma, hematoma, or other problems that may develop from surgery (chapter 15). If your new breast isn't quite as full as you had hoped, this can be improved. A breast can be lifted if it's too low or dropped if it's too high. Displeased with the shape of your belly button after your abdominal flap? Your surgeon can improve this, too.

The length of recovery depends on the complexity of your revisions and how many procedures you need. In most cases, revision surgery and recovery take less time than the initial reconstructive procedure. Your breasts may be bruised for a couple of weeks and swollen for a bit longer. Initially, you'll need at least a week off from work and exercise, and one to two additional weeks off from strenuous activity to give yourself a chance to rest and heal. If your job is physically demanding, you may need a while longer. It might take several months for you to see the full benefits of your revisions.

Revisions for Reconstruction with Implants

Revisions for implant reconstruction may address symmetry, rippling, wrinkling, malposition, capsular contracture, or any of the other problems

Time to Speak Up!

Revision surgery is an opportunity to fine-tune your reconstructed breasts and take care of any other issues that you're unhappy about. Chances are your surgeon will know exactly what needs to be done to finesse your reconstruction so you can have the best possible results. Now is the time to speak out about your concerns, your dissatisfaction, and the improvements you'd like to see. You don't have to live with misshapen breasts, poorly formed scars, or lingering discomfort. Be candid about your concerns. Describe what you'd like changed. Ask what can be done to get the results you want, the advantages and disadvantages of each alternative, and what you can realistically expect. Also, ask to see before-and-after photos of patients who have had the same or similar revisions. The surgeon who performed your initial reconstruction doesn't necessarily need to be the one to revise your results. Get a second opinion if you're unhappy with what your surgeon proposes, or if your surgeon says that your problems can't be remedied or improved.

described in chapter 6. Implants that are too close together or too far apart can be repositioned. If you're dissatisfied with the size of your new breasts, your implants can be changed. If you lose weight, you might want to have smaller implants that fit better on your now-smaller shape. If you gain weight, you may decide that larger implants fit more proportionately to the rest of your body than the ones you currently have.

Animation Deformity

Placing breast implants under the chest muscle commonly causes animation deformity, meaning that the implant visibly shifts and may change shape when the pectoralis muscle contracts, as it does during exercise; when the muscle relaxes, the implant returns to its original position. Correction usually involves removing the implant and placing a new one above the muscle. If the animation is minimal, another fix can be used: the implant can be wrapped with an ADM or other biologic mesh to reduce the space between the implant and the pocket.

A few years after my initial reconstruction with silicone implants under the muscle, my cosmetic results weren't ideal. My breasts didn't sit naturally, and there was noticeable animation deformity when I moved (for example, when exercising or washing my hands). My plastic surgeon thought I would get a better result by changing to over-the-muscle saline implants. In a three-hour surgery, he removed my old implants, sutured my pectoral muscles back together, and inserted saline implants over the muscle. This gave my breasts a much more natural appearance with no animation deformity. The recovery process was doable, with some pain, and I needed surgical drains for about a week. I'm happy I moved forward with the revision. Even though the most important goal is to prevent or remove cancer, we live in our bodies 24/7, and it matters that we're comfortable in our skin.

—*Krystin*

My surgery was planned as a two-stage process, beginning with bilateral mastectomy and reconstruction, followed three months later with revision surgery. After SGAP flap reconstruction, using tissue from my upper bottom to reconstruct my breasts, I was left with indentations at the donor site and outer thighs. During my revision procedure, my surgeon used liposuction and fat grafting to smooth out these imperfections, reshape my breast mounds, and flatten my incision scars. The results are beautiful! My breasts are perky and round, and the scars have largely faded. The donor site area is also smooth, well-shaped, and fits better in clothing than before surgery. I often don't wear a bra. My donor site scars, while noticeable, are flat, faded, and easily hidden by underwear or bikini bottoms.

—Angela

Asymmetry

Asymmetry is a mismatch in size, shape, or position of the breasts that can often be corrected by adjusting the subpectoral pocket, performing *fat grafting* (see "Fixes with Fat" in this chapter), or replacing the implant with one of a different size. After unilateral reconstruction, your opposite breast can be augmented, lifted, or reduced to better match your reconstructed breast (chapter 10).

Capsular Contracture

Unless capsular contracture distorts the breast or causes pain, it doesn't necessarily need to be corrected. The fix for more severe cases may involve *capsulectomy*, which is removing the scar capsule. (Capsulotomy, cutting into the capsule to release the scar formation, is controversial and its success is often temporary. The FDA doesn't recommend closed capsulotomy—manually applying pressure to the outside of the breast in an attempt to break up the scar tissue.) Replacing the implant with a new one that is wrapped in an ADM may help to reduce inflammation and decrease the risk of capsular contracture, but capsular contracture may reoccur.

Poor Cleavage

Creating or improving cleavage—the gap between the breasts—can be included in revision surgery. If your implants are too far apart, they can be moved somewhat closer together or replaced with wider, low-profile implants. Breasts that are too close together can be moved farther apart or swapped for narrower, higher-profile implants. Adjusting the size of the pocket (if you have subpectoral implants) or shifting from subpectoral to prepectoral placement may also help. Regardless of the reconstruction method, the cleavage between the breasts and in the upper pole can be plumped with fat grafting to better define the natural inner curve of the breasts.

Extrusion

The weight of an implant may cause extrusion—the implant breaks through the skin—particularly in people who smoke or whose skin is thin or has been irradiated. When this occurs, the implant must be removed and the skin allowed to heal before a new implant can be placed.

Gel Bleed

Treatment isn't usually required when droplets of silicone gel leak through the implant shell and into the surrounding scar tissue, unless a specific complication is diagnosed or treatable symptoms develop. Droplets that migrate to the tissue and beyond are more concerning because they may incite an inflammatory response in the scar capsule around the implant, which can lead to capsular contracture. If this occurs, surgical excision of the scar tissue (capsulectomy) and implant exchange can usually be performed as an outpatient procedure. Gel bleed that migrates and causes swelling in the lymph nodes or hard lumps in other areas of the body requires evaluation by a physician.

Malposition

Breast implants that shift too far up, down, or to the side of a subpectoral pocket can often be repositioned by reducing the size of the pocket. Bottoming out (when implants drop below the inframammary fold) is corrected by reinforcing the inframammary fold with sutures or surgical mesh to keep the implant where it belongs. The size of the pocket can be reduced, the breast can be lifted, or the implant can be replaced with a smaller device.

Rippling and Wrinkling

Visible rippling or wrinkling of an implant can be improved in several ways. Prepectoral implants can be moved under the muscle or a layer of ADM can be added between the implant and the skin. Textured implants can be swapped for smooth implants. Tightening the breast skin around the implant may also help. Highly cohesive implants that are stiffer but ripple less may also provide a solution.

Ruptures and Leaks

A ruptured implant, whether saline or silicone, must be removed, and can be replaced with a new implant. If you have no symptoms (a silent rupture), your surgeon may suggest taking a wait-and-see approach or may recommend removing and replacing the implant. Your surgeon can explain the pros and cons of leaving the implant in place or removing and replacing it. In either case, the capsule of scar tissue that naturally forms around it is also removed. In some cases, the implant may be withdrawn through small incisions made in the capsule. Silicone that may have leaked into the surrounding tissue is also removed. When a saline breast implant ruptures, the breast deflates and the body safely absorbs the liquid, but the implant must then be removed, and, if desired, replaced with a new implant.

Symmastia

Repairing symmastia is one of the more difficult revision procedures. Once the implants are removed, the subpectoral pocket must be revised to create a more natural distance between the breasts before inserting narrower implants. The skin is then reattached to the sternum with internal stitches and the pocket can be strengthened with an ADM. Prepectoral symmastia is sometimes improved by moving the implants beneath the muscles, while subpectoral symmastia is sometimes rectified by placing implants over the muscle.

Wrong Size

If you're unhappy with the size of your implants and it's something you'd rather not live with, they can be replaced with a different size. Health insurance providers typically must cover the replacement cost if the initial implant doesn't fit the chest or causes problems; they don't typically pay for replacement because you changed your mind about the size you want. The insurance codes submitted by your surgeon's office make all the difference. It's a good idea to make sure that you and your surgeon are on the same page regarding the size of your implants before your reconstruction and talk about whether a replacement procedure will be covered by your insurance.

Removing Your Implants

Complications with implants are often remedied with minor procedures, but in many cases, *explant surgery*—removing the implant—is necessary. There's no reason to replace an implant if it doesn't cause problems, and some people have their implants for 10 to 15 years, or more. Some implants, however, need to be explanted to remedy painful capsular contracture, a leak or rupture, an infection in the breast that can't be treated with antibiotics, or some other issue. Replacing an implant isn't particularly lengthy or difficult, but it does require another visit to the OR. If you have subpectoral implants, the pocket is already under the muscle, so most of the work is done. (Positioning your new implant over the muscle instead may be advantageous.) It's even easier to replace prepectoral breast implants. In either case, explant procedures are usually performed by reopening the mastectomy scar, removing excess scar tissue, and swapping the existing implant for a newer model. If you decide not to replace your implants, you may choose to have another reconstruction with your own tissue or go flat.

No matter how simple it may be to replace an implant, it can be emotionally disruptive: You're happily living your postmastectomy life when you find that you need more visits to the doctor and additional surgery to correct a problem with your new breast. Some people say it's like reliving their reconstruction all over again. Other people view replacement surgery as a price they're willing to pay. Either way, it's an important consideration when deciding whether breast implants are right for you.

Revisions for Autologous Reconstruction

Revision surgery after autologous reconstruction might be done to improve breast contour, refine shape, create deeper cleavage, improve the appearance of the donor site, or remedy other issues. If your new breasts are smaller than you'd hoped they would be, your surgeon can add fullness and volume. After unilateral breast reconstruction, your opposite breast can be modified if needed—lifted, augmented, or reduced—to better match your reconstructed breast (chapter 10).

Dog Ears

Closing a circular or elliptical incision in a straight line often creates dog ears, puckers of skin at the ends of the incision. Dog ear scars may improve over time, but they often require a short surgical procedure to improve their appearance or get rid of them. Correction is usually straightforward: a portion of the scar is reopened, excess skin is removed, and the incision is reclosed, resulting in a somewhat longer, but flatter, scar. Unless other revisions are needed, this is done in the surgeon's office with local anesthesia. (Read more about improving scars in chapter 15.)

Hernia

Repairing hernias is important because they can be painful and cause nausea, cramping, and bloating. Left untreated, symptoms worsen. Surgery is the only solution. Minor hernias can sometimes be repaired by reopening the incision and tightening the abdominal fascia. Larger hernias are resolved by carefully pushing any bulging organs (usually part of the intestines) back where they belong, closing the hernia opening, and reinforcing the abdomen with surgical mesh to reduce the odds of recurrence.

Necrosis

Small areas of necrosis that don't resolve on their own need to be trimmed away. If the blood supply is inadequate or fails and most or all of the flap dies, the new breast must be removed. Fortunately, this rarely occurs. Reconstruction can then be repeated after a period of healing. If you want to try another reconstruction, a different autologous procedure or implant reconstruction can be performed after a few months, once your chest has had a chance to heal. (Read more about necrosis in chapter 15.)

Fixes with Fat

Performed as a separate procedure or in combination with other revisions, fat grafting (also called *lipofilling*) is an integral part of many breast reconstruction procedures. It's also the primary method of breast reconstruction in men. Surgeons have used it for years to contour sunken facial areas, correct cosmetic hand defects, and plump buttocks and other parts of the body. It's also used to increase the volume of a healthy breast without an implant (chapter 10). Fat transferred from your belly, thighs, buttocks, "love handles," or behind the knees—anywhere you have it but don't want it—can improve the appearance of your reconstructed breast. The "from" area becomes slimmer, while the breast takes on soft fullness. (Although fat from the lower abdomen and thigh is sometimes touted as having more stem cells and therefore a higher likelihood of being retained in the breast, multiple studies show that fat retention is pretty much the same regardless of the donor site.)[1]

Fat is an ideal "filler" for breast defects because it's readily available and biocompatible; it's your own living tissue, after all. It's a versatile tool for improving and enhancing almost any reconstruction: replacing tissue that was removed during a lumpectomy, improving not-so-good reconstruction results, and making a good reconstruction even better (figure 9.1). Fat grafting also appears to rejuvenate irradiated tissue on the chest wall, which reduces capsular contracture and other common complications with breast implants after radiation therapy.[2] With earlier fat grafting methods, much of the repositioned fat was *resorbed* (assimilated back into the body). Newer procedures are vastly improved, making fat grafting more effective and more reliable. Your surgeon transfers fat from a single area—your abdomen or thighs, for example—or from multiple sites.

Fat transferred to your new breast can

- add volume up to an additional cup size
- smooth contour irregularities and fill in dimples and dents
- create or improve cleavage
- further define the inframammary fold

- fill in flat or sunken areas in the upper breast
- hide the edges of implants and camouflage rippling and wrinkling
- soften and improve the texture of previously irradiated tissue
- refine the appearance of scars
- improve postmastectomy pain

The Three-Step Process

Removing and transferring fat is a relatively simple procedure, but fat grafting involves more than just scooping fat from your hips, plopping it directly onto your breast, and hoping for the best. Performed as an outpatient procedure under local or general anesthesia, fat grafting involves three distinct stages: (1) harvesting the fat, (2) purifying the fat, and (3) injecting the remaining living fat cells into the breast. (Standard protocols haven't been established for any of

FIGURE 9.1 Reconstructed breasts after nipple-sparing mastectomy with DIEP flap reconstruction (*left*) are fuller and rounder with improved cleavage after fat grafting (*right*).

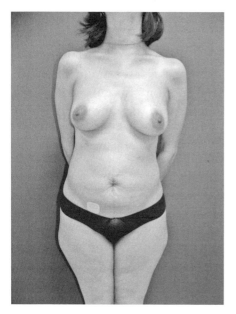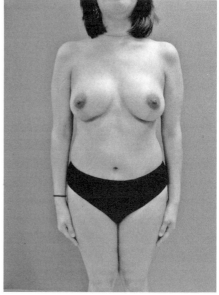

Images provided by PRMA Plastic Surgery, Center for Advanced Breast Reconstruction

these stages, and techniques vary widely among surgeons.) Before the fat is harvested, the donor site is infused with a combination of lidocaine (a local anesthetic) and epinephrine (adrenaline) to minimize bleeding. A small puncture, usually a quarter of an inch or less, is made in an existing scar, a fold of skin, the top of the belly button, or another inconspicuous spot. A thin cannula (a hollow surgical tube) is then inserted through the puncture, and fat is removed via liposuction with a vacuum or retrieved manually. (Using small cannulas allows reduced points of entry and results in minimal scarring, but somewhat larger cannulas gather more fat. Ask your surgeon which will be used for your procedure.) The extracted fat is then either processed in a centrifuge machine or rinsed with sterile saline. Cleansed of cellular debris, blood, and excess fluids (which can promote inflammation), the remaining healthy fat is loaded into syringes and injected in minuscule amounts precisely where it's needed in the new breast. Injection points are chosen to be as inconspicuous as possible, often in the inframammary fold or along the edge of the areola.

Unlike autologous flaps, which are large areas of fat with or without muscle that are transferred to the chest with their blood supply intact, fat grafts consist of much smaller fat particles that must connect to blood vessels in the reconstructed breast to survive. Layering small amounts of fat into different areas of the breast increases the odds that the grafts will successfully latch onto small blood vessels. It's difficult to predict how much fat will take hold and remain in the breast. A general rule of thumb is about 50 percent of the fat harvested will be injected, and 50 to 70 percent of that will remain in the breast; the body will likely resorb the rest. So, if your surgeon determines that a graft of about 150 to 200 cc is about right, your liposuction procedure might remove about 600 cc of fat, which should yield about 300 cc to be injected, of which 150 to 210 cc may remain in your breast. Two or more sessions, at least three months apart, are usually needed for optimal results.

The living cells in fatty tissue are fragile and must be handled gently. Unlike cosmetic liposuction, after which removed fat is tossed away, a surgeon's expertise, skill, and method of introducing the fat into the reconstructed breast affect the outcome, and careful handling and processing of the fat are absolute requirements. Your overall health, your hormone levels, and the levels of fluid in your fat also influence how much stays in the breast. While the fat that remains becomes a permanent part of your breast, it continues to function as it would in its original location: increasing or decreasing in volume with weight fluctuation.

Recovery

Recovery largely depends on how much fat is harvested and how many donor sites you have. Downtime is generally short, with minimal discomfort in the breast and some swelling, bruising, and tenderness at the liposuction area or areas for a week or two. Most people are up and about the next day and resume work and other normal activities by the second week. Recovery may take longer and be more uncomfortable when more fat or additional donor sites are involved.

You'll need to wear a compression garment at the liposuction site or sites for at least two or more weeks to minimize swelling and accumulation of fluids. You'll also need to avoid compressing your breasts for any reason, including wearing a bra or sleeping on your stomach; you can go back to wearing regular bras when your bruising resolves. Soreness, particularly at the donor site, may last longer, depending on the amount of fat removed. It may take several weeks before the swelling completely subsides. In about three to four months, your breasts will show their final shape and size.

Aside from injected fat not staying in the breast, complications related to fat grafting are generally few. They may include bleeding; fat necrosis, which is less likely when small amounts of fat are applied to the breast over multiple sessions; and infection. Firm lumps that may develop can be anxiety-provoking and should be brought to your surgeon's attention. An MRI or ultrasound may be necessary to determine whether they are fatty cysts, calcifications, or something else.

Is It Safe?

Fat grafting for reconstruction has gone mainstream. Initially, experts questioned whether stem cells and growth factors in transferred fat might elevate the risk of breast cancer recurrence, particularly in high-risk individuals. Studies at MD Anderson Cancer Center, the Mayo Clinic, Cleveland Clinic, and elsewhere have found similar rates of recurrence among women who had postreconstruction fat grafting and those who didn't, although no long-term, controlled studies with standard criteria, validated measurements, and appropriate follow-up have been conducted.[3]

Advantages of Fat Grafting

- Your body won't reject the fat, because it's your own tissue.
- Transferred fat feels similar to breast tissue.
- Transferred fat improves the overall shape and fullness of the breast.
- It may somewhat slim the donor area.
- It is minimally invasive.
- It has a low risk of complications.
- The procedure and recovery are shorter and less invasive than the surgery for an initial breast reconstruction.

Disadvantages of Fat Grafting

- There are no established procedural standards.
- Multiple sessions are usually required for the best results.
- Fat retention is influenced by the surgeon's experience and technique.
- No long-term (10 to 20 years) clinical studies have been conducted.
- Harmless cysts or areas of fat that die can feel like a hard lump, requiring ultrasound or other imaging.

Questions for Your Plastic Surgeon

- How long do I need to wait before having revision surgery?
- What revisions do you recommend to improve my reconstruction?
- What will be included in my revision surgery?
- How many of these procedures have you done?
- May I see your before-and-after photos of patients who had the same type of revisions?
- How long will I be in surgery?
- What should I expect from recovery?
- How long after my surgery will I see improvements?
- Will my insurance cover the full cost of these revisions?

Additional questions regarding fat grafting:

- How much fat will you remove and from where?
- What size cannula will you use?
- Will I have visible scarring?
- How do you process the fat?
- Where on my breast will you inject the fat?
- How much fat can I expect to remain in my breast?
- How many fat grafting sessions will I need to obtain the results I want?
- How will my donor site look afterward?
- What complications might occur and how will you address them?

Chapter 10

Modifying Your Opposite Breast

At first, I didn't want to have any more operations beyond my initial reconstruction, but my surgeon suggested a breast lift for better symmetry. I'm glad I did because both breasts now closely match.

—MANDA

W hen both breasts are reconstructed at the same time, plastic surgeons can usually ensure they're of similar size, shape, and position and have well-placed nipples. Unilateral reconstruction presents a different problem: how to achieve a balance between your reconstructed breast and your natural breast. An optional cosmetic procedure on your healthy breast can help you obtain the best possible symmetry. Your reconstructed breast may not be an exact match, but even natural breasts aren't usually identical. Often, however, reconstructing one breast and altering the other minimizes the differences between them. Performed during revision surgery or as a separate procedure, this opportunity for a breast makeover is something many people may have considered before a mastectomy, yet never pursued. (Health insurance companies that cover mastectomies are required by the WHCRA to pay for modifications to your remaining breast to achieve symmetry as part of your overall reconstruction.)

After unilateral reconstruction, you have three alternatives for your opposite breast:

- Leave it as it is. If you prefer not to alter your healthy breast, symmetry with your reconstructed breast will depend on the reconstruction method you choose. Generally, it's easier to match the shape and position of a natural breast with autologous reconstruction than a breast implant. Implants come in a variety of sizes and shapes and can often closely match the opposite breast, but they cannot be shaped and sculpted like living tissue can.
- Surgically modify it. Your healthy breast can be augmented, lifted, or reduced to match your reconstructed breast. Generally, these procedures are done under general anesthesia in a hospital or surgical center. Your natural breast may age differently than your reconstructed breast, depending on time, gravity, and weight changes (especially if you had reconstruction with a breast implant).
- Remove and reconstruct it. If you have a high risk of contralateral breast cancer, you may want to consider prophylactic removal of your healthy breast. In that case, you'll have both breasts removed with immediate reconstruction, which is the optimal way to obtain breasts that match.

Breast Augmentation

Augmentation mammoplasty to enlarge the breast with an implant or with your own fat is the most common cosmetic procedure in the United States. You may need a baseline mammogram of the breast before either procedure. Afterward, you should continue with routine self-exams and mammography. (Let the technician know that you have implants or fat grafts.)

Augmentation with a Breast Implant

If your breast was reconstructed with an implant, your opposite breast will be enhanced in the same way, with an implant placed under or over your pectoral muscle. (Tissue expansion isn't needed.) A saline or silicone implant is inserted through an incision made under the breast, along the bottom of the areola, or in the underarm; the underarm procedure doesn't scar the breast, but it makes for a more difficult placement of the implant and leaves a small scar that may show when you raise your arm (figure 10.1). A *transumbilical breast augmentation* is a less common option that has a higher risk of complications.

FIGURE 10.1 Breast augmentation incisions can be made around the bottom of the areola, under the breast, or in the underarm.

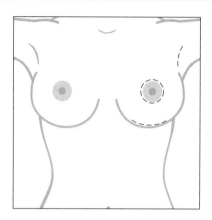

A deflated saline implant is inserted through a small incision made at the top of the belly button, tunneled under the skin to the chest between the breast tissue and muscle, and then fully inflated. No incision on the breast means no additional scarring.

Recovery

Your first week after augmentation will be the most uncomfortable. You'll have pain medication, but you should take it easy, limiting your activity to short, slow walks. Bruising and swelling are to be expected; these should begin to gradually dissipate a week or two after your surgery. Your surgeon will recommend a bra that supports your breast and discourages swelling. You may be able to return to light exercise and work that isn't physically demanding after a week or so (table 10.1). Still, you should refrain from lifting heavy objects, lifting your arms over your head, and doing strenuous activities until your tissues have healed. Be patient if your augmented breast seems excessively tight, firm, or flat. It will drop and soften over the next several weeks as your skin stretches to accommodate the new fullness; the bottom of your breast will become rounder and your nipple will become better positioned. If your breast appears to be too high on your chest, your surgeon may place an elastic bandage above it to force it down.

TABLE 10.1 Average Intervals for Breast Modification Procedures

PROCEDURE	SURGERY; HOSPITAL STAY	RETURN TO NON-STRENUOUS ACTIVITIES; ALL ACTIVITIES
Augmentation with implant	1–2 hours; outpatient	1 week; 4–6 weeks
Augmentation with fat grafting	2–4 hours; outpatient	7–10 days; 6 weeks
Reduction	2–3 hours; outpatient	1–2 weeks; 4–6 weeks
Lift	2–3 hours; outpatient	1–2 weeks; 4–6 weeks

Note: Individual recovery times may be somewhat shorter or longer depending on how the procedure is done and individual healing.

Aside from the potential risks of surgery and implants, breast augmentation causes few problems. Because fine nerves in the breast can be irritated during surgery or compressed by swollen tissues, you may initially experience numbness or reduced sensation; these should gradually improve as the swelling subsides and your breast heals. You can also expect to experience changed or reduced sensation in your nipple, which should resolve within six months. Some people experience a temporary hypersensitivity after augmentation, including tingling, burning, or sharp pain.

Augmentation with Fat Transfer

Your healthy breast can be increased by up to a full cup size with autologous fat transfer (the same fat grafting procedure described in chapter 9). A single session might yield enough to make you half a cup to a whole cup size fuller; additional sessions—opportunities to slightly reduce areas where you have excess fat—or an implant would be needed to achieve a greater increase in size. Breast augmentation with fat doesn't visibly scar the breast, and because it doesn't require an implant, it avoids the risk of capsular contracture and other implant-related problems.

Fat transfer is versatile. Fat can be added to the upper pole, cleavage, or wherever else it's needed to improve the size or shape of the breast. Breast augmentation with your own fat looks and feels natural—it's your tissue, after all—but the breast will droop more quickly and noticeably than if it was an implant. This is because implants lift and support breast tissue, while fat adds weight. If your healthy breast already has an implant, fat grafting can improve rippling, wrinkling, and other contour defects you may have. You're a candidate if you're in good health and you have enough fat deposits (almost everyone does) to accomplish augmentation in this way.

Recovery

Augmentation with fat transfer is less invasive than augmentation with implants, which shortens recovery. You'll feel more discomfort than pain for the first few days after your augmentation. Most bruising recedes by about three weeks after surgery, and your breast may be swollen for several months. Until the swelling resolves, you'll need to wear a surgical bra and a compression garment at the donor site. Excessive lifting and movements that strain or put direct pressure on your chest should be avoided until your tissues heal; this applies to all breast surgeries. Complications are rare, but bleeding, infection, and necrosis are possible. The amount of fat that stays in the breast depends on many variables, including your surgeon's technique and experience.

Breast Lift

All-natural breasts head south over time. As gravity takes its toll, tissue loses elasticity, breasts hang lower on the chest, and areolas may become larger. A *breast lift* (mastopexy) raises and reshapes a breast that sags due to age, excessive weight, pregnancy, hormones, or genetics. If your nipple points downward, a breast lift will reposition it so that it matches the nipple on your reconstructed breast. Small, sagging breasts can be lifted and augmented; overly large breasts can be lifted and reduced. Incision placement depends on your breast size and shape, the amount of skin to be removed, the position of your nipple and areola, and how much your breast sags (figure 10.2). Making an incision, removing excess skin, and then suturing the wound closed tightens and reshapes the breast tissue. A breast lift doesn't reduce or enlarge the breast. The same amount of tissue is now held together by less skin, so your breast is firmer and sits higher on your chest (figure 10.3). Cutting sensory nerves during the procedure may lead to changed feelings or a temporary loss of sensation in the nipple that lasts for several months. In some cases, sensation may be permanently lost. It may take six to twelve weeks for your breast to settle into its final shape.

Breast Screening after Augmentation with Fat Transfer

Although the popularity of no-implant augmentation has skyrocketed, some experts worry that lumps, cysts, or calcifications that form in the breast when fat grafts don't survive might interfere with mammography or cause unnecessary biopsies if they appear to be suspicious. The other side of this argument is that calcifications are known to occur in the breast after just about any other breast surgery, including biopsy, reduction, and reconstruction, without worry; radiologists know how to read these changes and know when to recommend an additional MRI or ultrasound. Even though newer, more sophisticated mammography equipment, particularly digital mammography, can better distinguish between benign and cancerous cells, a biopsy may be needed to determine whether a suspicious area is cancerous. Well-controlled, long-term studies are needed to settle the issue. Although hardened lumps of dead fat aren't cancerous or harmful, they sometimes become painful and should be checked and removed.

FIGURE 10.2 A small breast with minimal sagging can be lifted by removing a small segment of skin through an incision around the areola—the scar will be hidden in the border (*left*). A lollipop incision (*center left*) is often used to lift and reshape a moderately sagging breast, while a very large or heavily sagging breast may require an anchor incision (*center right*). A crescent incision may also be used (*right*).

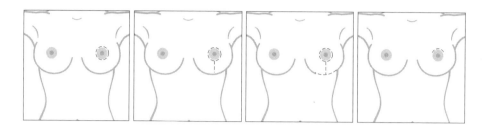

FIGURE 10.3 Before (*upper left*) and after (*upper right*) delayed DIEP flap reconstruction of the left breast and lift of the right breast. Before (*lower left*) and after (*lower right*) unilateral mastectomy and stacked DIEP flap reconstruction of right breast and lift of the left breast for symmetry.

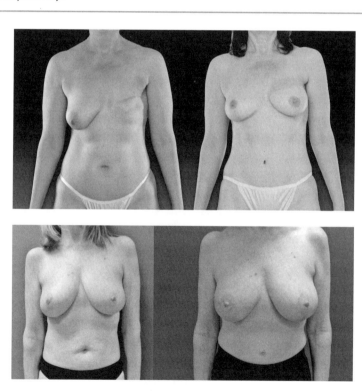

Upper images provided by Dr. Frank J. DellaCroce, Center for Restorative Breast Surgery, LLC. Lower images provided by PRMA Plastic Surgery, Center for Advanced Breast Reconstruction

Recovery

After a breast lift, you'll need to wear a support bra or bandage for about a month before progressing to a non-underwire athletic bra, which you will need to wear around the clock for several weeks. Bruising and swelling will last for up to a month or more. As with other breast surgeries, you'll need to protect your chest until it heals. Avoid straining, lifting, or exerting pressure on your chest, which can increase swelling; and avoid sleeping on your stomach until your surgeon says it's okay to do so. Scars from this procedure tend to be red and lumpy for several months before they fade and become smoother.

Breast Reduction

If you have back and shoulder pain, deep indentations from your bra straps, or other complications from heavy, oversized breasts, you may have wondered whether *breast reduction* (reduction mammoplasty) might relieve your discomfort. This surgical procedure removes excess breast tissue, fat, and skin to reduce the size and weight of overly large breasts. It can also resize your natural breast so it's in better proportion with your reconstructed breast and in a position that matches it. Making the breast smaller is a more complex procedure than augmentation and breast lift and involves more recovery. It can be performed in different ways, depending on your surgeon's preferred technique, where the incisions are made, and the amount of tissue removed (figure 10.4).

During the procedure, the nipple usually remains attached to its nerves and blood vessels on an island of skin that is pulled up and out of the way until the excess tissue is removed. If the breasts are overly large, the nipple may be removed and temporarily grafted to a higher position; this may cause permanent loss of some or all nipple sensation. Once the excess tissue is removed, the remaining tissue is shaped, and the nipple is recentered on the now smaller breast. (If your areola is too large for your now smaller breast, it, too, can be reduced.) The sides of the incision are pulled together, creating a firmer, tighter contour. Breast reduction may also be performed before a nipple-sparing mastectomy and immediate reconstruction for people with ptotic breasts (figure 10.5).

If your breast has a large proportion of fat but isn't particularly droopy, overly dense, or excessively large, you may be a candidate for liposuction-only

FIGURE 10.4 Excess tissue, fat, and skin can be removed through a circular incision around the areola (*left*) or a lollipop incision (*center*). The anchor incision (*right*), also known as the Wise Pattern, is most commonly used for breast reduction. It produces the most scarring, but it's often the best for large and saggy breasts and when more tissue and skin are removed.

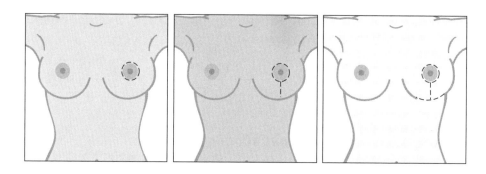

FIGURE 10.5 Before surgery (*left*), incisions are marked for breast reduction (*center*). After breast reduction followed by bilateral mastectomy and immediate implant reconstruction (*right*). Reducing ptotic breasts before reconstruction ensures that the nipples are properly centered on the new breasts.

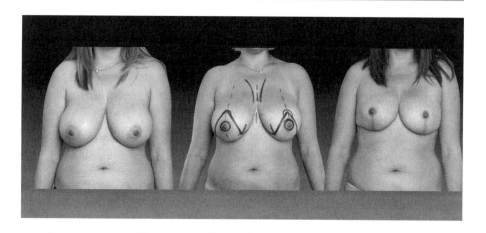

Images provided by Dr. Frank J. DellaCroce, Center for Restorative Breast Surgery, LLC

breast reduction. Fat is removed through two small, well-hidden incisions made under the breast. Liposuction can be used alone or in combination with other reduction methods. It's less invasive, has fewer complications, and requires a somewhat shorter recovery time. A surgical drain is placed at the site, and either the resized breast is wrapped in an elastic bandage or a compression bra is worn.

> For as long as I can remember, my breasts have been much too large for my frame. I always wanted to have them reduced, but I never seemed to have the time; and, frankly, I was afraid to have it done. When my plastic surgeon suggested doing a reduction before my breast reconstruction, I thought the timing couldn't be better, and I had to take advantage of the opportunity. The recovery was a bit tough, but it was well worth it.
>
> —*Veryl*

Recovery

Breast reduction is a significant procedure and recovery can be uncomfortable, especially for the first few days after surgery. After that, you'll be up and about, but you'll need plenty of rest and will be restricted from lifting or exerting too much. Bruising and soreness are routine side effects of reduction and may last two to three weeks, but they will dissipate as you heal. Bandages are usually removed a few days after the operation, although you'll need to wear a compression bra around the clock for several weeks. Depending on how you heal and the nature of your job, you may be able to return to nonstrenuous work after two to three weeks, but you'll need to refrain from lifting and straining for at least a month. Your breast, including the nipple, will likely be numb for up to eight weeks. Feeling gradually returns over a time period of several months to a year. Disturbing or damaging sensory nerves during surgery can cause a temporary or long-term loss of sensation in the breast or nipple. In rare cases, the nipple and areola may die from inadequate blood flow. (This is more likely to happen if you're a smoker or have diabetes.) An area of partial necrosis may heal in time or may need to be trimmed away. If the entire nipple dies, a new nipple can be reconstructed, but it won't have sensation.

Breastfeeding after Breast Augmentation, Lift, or Reduction

Augmentation, lift, and reduction surgeries can affect nerves and ducts in the breast and impact lactation. You should be able to breastfeed after any of these surgeries, but you may be unable to produce a full milk supply for your baby. If you have difficulty expressing milk, a lactation consultant can help you. Your ability to nurse your baby is more likely to be preserved when your nipple remains attached to the skin and the milk ducts are left intact. That's because nearby nerves send signals to the brain to begin milk production and flow. Incisions that encircle the areola and procedures that separate the nipple and areola from the breast are more likely to affect milk production; damage to the ducts is less likely with an incision in the armpit or below the breast. Repositioning the nipple during breast reduction may disrupt the lobules that make milk and the ducts that deliver it. It's a good idea to discuss your procedure with your surgeon if you're concerned about the ability to breastfeed in the future.

Questions for Your Plastic Surgeon

- How closely will my reconstructed breast match my healthy breast?
- Will I need to alter my natural breast for symmetry?
- If so, which procedure do you recommend?
- When would this procedure be performed?
- Where will the incisions be made?
- May I see your before-and-after photos of patients who had unilateral breast reconstruction and the cosmetic procedure you recommend for me?
- Will sensation in my breast or nipple be affected?
- Will this procedure affect my ability to breastfeed?
- What are the best and worst results I can expect?
- What should I expect from recovery?
- When can I resume normal activity and exercise?
- What problems may occur and how will they be resolved?
- When should I schedule a follow-up appointment?

Final Touches: Recreating Your Nipple and Areola

My new nipple is amazing!

—KARLA

You've made it through a mastectomy. You have new breast mounds, and unless you've had a nipple-sparing mastectomy, you're now ready for the final reconstructive step: creating new nipples and areolas. Nipple reconstruction is simple and minimally invasive. It does involve a bit more surgery, but it's minor compared with what you've already been through. Optional tattooing is the last step in the reconstructive process. You're in the reconstructive home stretch.

The Icing on the Cake

Nipple reconstruction is a physical and psychological milestone. It completes the restoration of your missing breasts, and, for most people, it's the end of the breast cancer experience. Creating a nipple is the icing on the reconstruction cake, although not everyone likes icing. Reconstructed nipples are purely cosmetic. They add a finished, more natural look to breast mounds, but they have physical limitations. They're permanent bumps that don't react to temperature or touch and don't change from flat to erect and back to flat again (as natural nipples do) because they lack the infrastructure of nerves and small muscles that makes that happen. After a unilateral reconstruction, your new nipple will be flat or standing at attention when your natural nipple isn't. This is something to keep in mind when you're deciding how small or large you'd like your nipple to be.

Nipples can be created during revision surgery under general anesthesia, or in a later outpatient procedure under local anesthesia. After bilateral reconstruction, your new nipples will be positioned at the point of most projection on your breasts. The goal of unilateral nipple reconstruction is to match the position, size, shape, and projection of your opposite, natural nipple. The WHCRA requires group health plans and individual health policies that cover a mastectomy to also pay for all stages of reconstruction surgery, including nipple reconstruction and tattooing (chapter 18).

You may prefer to forego nipple reconstruction if you

- don't consider having nipples to be important
- feel as though you can't face another procedure
- don't want nipples without sensation
- prefer to wait and see how you feel in the future about having your nipples created
- have breast skin that is damaged or unhealthy

My surgeon tried to convince me to "finish the job," but nipples didn't seem important. That was four years ago, and I still don't regret my decision. If I change my mind, I can always have them added.

—*Karola*

Advantages of Nipple Reconstruction and Tattooing
- creates realistic-looking nipples that project from the breast
- adds a finishing touch to reconstructed breasts
- simple procedures with little to no downtime

Disadvantages of Nipple Reconstruction and Tattooing
- Nipples lack sensation and don't react as natural nipples do.
- Nipples may always be in the "up" position.

- Nipples eventually flatten unless they're filled.
- Tattoo pigment eventually fades.

Building the Nipple

Reconstructed nipples are fashioned from a small flap of skin on the front of the breast. Various patterns and techniques can be used, depending on the surgeon's preference. To begin, careful measurements are made to determine the center of the reconstructed breast. The flap pattern for the nipple is then marked on the breast skin. Incisions are made along the pattern lines, free small flaps of skin, and underlying fat. The sides of the nipple flap are folded to meet in the center, the top part is folded down, and the edges are stitched closed to support the new elevated nipple until it heals (figure 11.1). The entire process takes less than an hour for each nipple (table 11.1). Your surgeon can describe a preferred method and show you before-and-after photos of patients who have had the same procedure.

Antibiotic ointment is applied to the new nipples, which are then covered with a plastic protector or several layers of gauze with a hole surrounding the nipple. You'll need to wear this protective covering for a week or two or until your stitches are removed. No surgical drains are required. Try not to put any direct pressure on your delicate new nipples for a few weeks until they heal, because this might squash them. You can immediately resume your normal activities, but don't let the shower directly hit your new nipples or involve your nipples in sexual activity until your surgeon gives you the okay. Reconstructed nipples lack nerves; any discomfort should be mild and can be managed with over-the-counter analgesics. Your nipple needs a healthy blood supply to survive, so avoid smoking, caffeine, and aspirin or other blood-thinning medications (with your doctor's okay) for a few weeks before and after your nipple procedure, as directed by your surgeon.

Initially, you may be unimpressed with your new nipples. For the first week or two, they'll be red, swollen, crisscrossed with dark stitches, and covered with scabs. It can be a shock when you first see them; they'll be much larger than you expect them to be. Supersizing them is deliberate: nipples are made 50 percent larger than the desired size because they shrink considerably as they heal. When the stitches are removed, your new nipple will begin to flatten and shrink so that it is in better proportion to your breast. In about three to four weeks, soft, natural-looking nipples emerge from the scabby cocoons.

FIGURE 11.1 The bowtie (*above*) and star (*below*) flaps are common patterns for nipple reconstruction. In both cases, a small flap of skin and underlying fat is lifted from the breast, leaving one edge attached to provide blood supply to the new nipple (1). The side arms of the flap are joined in the front and stitched together (2), and the top is tucked down and sutured in place (3).

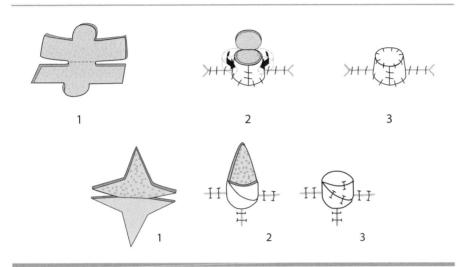

TABLE 11.1 Typical Intervals for Nipple Reconstruction and Tattooing

	TIMING*	PROCEDURE; HOSPITAL STAY	FINAL APPEARANCE
Nipple reconstruction	3–6 months after initial reconstruction surgery or anytime later	30–60 minutes; outpatient	3–4 months
Nipple and areola tattooing	3–4 months after nipple reconstruction or anytime later	30–60 minutes; outpatient	2–3 weeks

*May be longer if the breast needs more time to heal.

Skin Grafts

If you don't have enough breast skin to create your new nipple, your surgeon might transfer a *skin graft*, a small area of skin from your inner thigh, abdomen, or groin, to your breast. The grafting process creates an additional scar, and the donor site remains sore for a week or two. This method isn't necessary for most people, but some surgeons still prefer to use grafts, so it's worth asking how your nipples will be created before you have the procedure done.

Nipple Banking

Nipple banking is uncommon in the United States, considering the availability of nipple-sparing mastectomies, nipple reconstruction, and advanced tattooing techniques. In this procedure, the nipples are removed during a mastectomy. If they're clear of cancer cells, they're connected to a blood supply in the groin for several months until they're transferred to the newly reconstructed and healed breast mounds. Banked nipples have little or no sensation.

Nipple Sharing

Nipple sharing uses a portion of a person's healthy nipple to create a new nipple after unilateral reconstruction. Even though this ensures that the coloring of both nipples is perfectly matched, it can reduce or eliminate sensation and may affect your ability to breastfeed with your only fully functional nipple. If you're considering nipple sharing, ask your surgeon about the process and how your healthy nipple will be affected.

A Colorful Finish

When your new nipples heal in three to four months, they're ready for cosmetic tattooing, the final step in the reconstructive process (figure 11.2). Even though tattooing doesn't create texture or projection, it darkens the nipple and the skin around it to simulate an areola, adding a realistic finish to your reconstructed breast. (Before tattooing, a reconstructed nipple is the same color as the surrounding breast skin and doesn't have an areola.) If you're not ready for tattoos at this point, or you're happy with the way your unpigmented nipples and areolas look, you can forgo this optional step or have it done at any time in the future.

Tattooing is often done as an in-office procedure performed by the plastic surgeon or a member of their office staff. Many surgeons outsource nipple tattooing to professional tattoo artists, who are more likely to have a background in art and understand the subtle nuances of blending colors and shading for the most realistic effect. (Some people take this opportunity to have

FIGURE 11.2 Before (*left*) and after (*right*) nipple reconstruction and tattooing of nipples and areolas on reconstructed breast mounds.

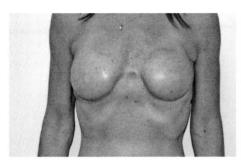 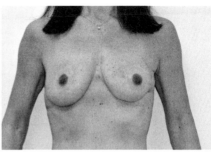

Images provided by Joshua Levine, MD, Center for Breast Reconstruction

flowers, vines, or other decorative patterns tattooed instead of conventional nipple coloring.) Your health insurance may reimburse part or all of the cost of having a professional tattoo artist color your areola and nipple, especially if you're referred by your plastic surgeon, but it's a good idea to check first. (Some tattoo artists who specialize in nipple tattoos provide no-cost services to mastectomy patients.) If you're going to the trouble of having tattoos, you want them to be as good as possible. No matter who applies the pigment, ask about the individual's specific experience coloring reconstructed nipples and review before-and-after photos of past work. Speak with some of the artist's previous reconstruction patients, if possible, to see whether the patients are happy with the results.

Choosing Your Colors

Whoever applies your tattoos should select the colors with your input. Review color samples together to decide which combination of pigments best matches your skin tone. After a unilateral mastectomy, you may want to match the color of your natural nipple. If you have bilateral reconstruction, some professionals recommend matching the natural color of your lips. Blending two or more shades of beige, brown, tan, or pink sometimes produces the most natural result. You may want to choose a hue that is somewhat darker than your final color because nipple tattoos fade considerably over time.

Before the ink is applied, your breast is swabbed with alcohol, and the circular outline of your new areola is marked on your breast skin. Check the markings in a mirror to be sure you approve of the position, shape, and size before any ink as applied. If you had unilateral nipple reconstruction, the outlined area should match your opposite areola. If both breasts are to be colored, the markings should be evenly centered. If you don't like what you see, it's easy to change the markings. If you're dissatisfied with the final tattoo, it's fairly simple to enlarge it or make it darker. It's not as easy to make it smaller or lighter. Once you've approved the outline, the color is loaded into an electric tattoo gun that holds sterilized needles. A series of short bursts inject the ink under the skin. The color is a bit shocking when you first see it: it looks like thick, shiny paint. It will fade under the skin to a more subtle shade in a few weeks. Because of reduced sensation in your breast, you'll probably feel more pressure, tingling, or slight stinging than pain. Local anesthesia isn't usually necessary; however, it can be applied if tattooing is too uncomfortable. Feeling a sting or a small amount of pain is actually good news; it means you've regained feeling in the front of your breast.

It takes about 30 to 40 minutes to ink each breast. Your newly tattooed nipples will appear brighter, darker, and redder than they'll be when they're healed. (The red is from blood mingling with tattoo color.) You might need two or three sessions to fill in any uneven spots and apply the full color; layering pigment can help your tattoo last longer. There's no downtime from tattooing, so you should be fine to return to work or home, or go off to lunch or a meeting. In four to five days, a scab will form over the tattooed area; it may take up to 10 days for it to fully heal. Take care not to rub, scrub, or pick at it before it falls off on its own, because that can create splotchy, uneven color.

Three-Dimensional Tattoos

More people are choosing three-dimensional (3-D) nipple and areola tattoos as an alternative to surgical nipple reconstruction. Traditional medical tattooing adds color to the breast in one or more sessions to make a small dark circle in the center that simulates a nipple and areola. 3-D tattooing is a more sophisticated combination of tattooing skills and artistry. It includes a broader selection of pigments and color that is less likely to fade. 3-D tattooing is detailed work that uses subtle shading and highlighting to create the illusion of

FIGURE 11.3 The subtle shading and highlighting of 3-D tattooing creates realistic-looking nipples.

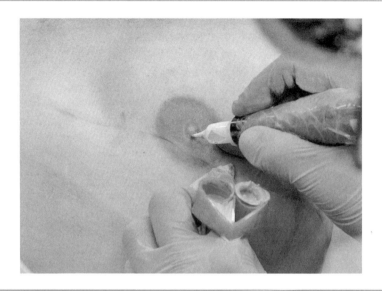

Image provided by Rose Marie Beauchemin-Verzella, Founder and President, Beau Institute of Permanent & Corrective Cosmetics, LLC

protrusion, so it looks as though you have nipples even though you don't (figure 11.3). Many surgeons have tattoo specialists on their office teams or outsource to local professionals who specialize in 3-D nipple tattooing.

The procedure is usually completed in an initial visit, to place the color, and a secondary visit (six to eight weeks later), to touch up as needed. Before you schedule an appointment, call the studio or check the tattoo artist's website to be sure the artist has experience in 3-D nipple tattooing, which requires special skill and experience. Set up a consultation appointment, then visit the studio to ensure that it's a meticulously clean environment. Explain what you have in mind, ask how many of these 3-D procedures the artist has done, and review photos of past work. You may also want to ask for a list of ingredients for the tattoo pigments, to be sure that you're not allergic to anything in the ink. One other option, 4-D nipple reconstruction, combines a surgically created nipple with 3-D tattooing.

— EXPERT INSIGHT —

What to Expect from Nipple Tattooing

ROSE MARIE BEAUCHEMIN-VERZELLA, FOUNDER,
THE BEAU INSTITUTE OF PERMANENT AND
CORRECTIVE COSMETICS, LLC

If you hope to have tattoos that are similar to your natural nipples and areolas, consider taking a photo of your breasts before your mastectomy and bringing it to your tattoo appointment. If you don't have a photo, answering simple questions like "Were your areolas light or dark? Pink or peachy?" helps the professional appreciate what you want while giving you the opportunity to understand your options and participate in color selection. Placing temporary dabs of pigment in different hues on your chest before the tattooing begins will give you a preview of how the different colors would appear. Once you agree on the color, the area to be tattooed is cleansed and carefully measured. A straight line is marked from the clavicle to the center of the breast mound and then repeated on the opposite side. A third line is then made across the bottom to join the two markings, forming a triangle; all three lines should be the same length. The triangle method may not always provide optimal symmetry; radiation and post-surgery complications can cause contractures (deep scarring) that pull the breast mound upward or sideways. The position of the areola may need to be higher, lower, closer to the center, or to the side to appear more symmetrical. For breast mounds that are very asymmetrical, a visual measurement is often more effective than the triangle technique.

Making the areolas a lighter color and the nipples a darker shade creates a contrast that shifts the light to the nipples. For a 3-D effect, leaving the top of the nipples without color creates the illusion of light from above, while using a darker color for the perimeter of the nipples creates both contrast and the illusion of protrusion. Tattooing a soft edge on the areola results in the most natural look. Simulating Montgomery tubercles with white pigment surrounded on three sides with the contrasting nipple color creates convincing realism.

Nonsurgical Alternatives

If you decide not to have nipple reconstruction, you might prefer adhesive semi-erect nipples, putting them on and taking them off whenever the mood strikes you. Rub-On Nipples (www.breasthealing .com) are one way to have nipples when you want them and forgo them when you don't. If you have one healthy breast and one reconstructed breast, using these products will give you an even appearance. Several companies customize prosthetic nipples in different sizes and skin tones. Feeling Whole Again (www.feelingwholeagain .com), Reforma (www.myreforma.com), and New Attitude (www .newattitudebreasts.com) provide customized nipples.

Problems and Fixes

Nipple reconstruction and tattooing are safe procedures, and when the breast skin is healthy, serious problems are few and far between. Complications that occur usually involve cosmetic issues that are easily corrected; but some issues, including the following, may develop, especially in irradiated or very thin skin.

Nipple Collapse

Reconstructed nipples are initially firm but eventually flatten, especially with skin that is thin, scarred, or has been irradiated. The solution is to plump the nipple with an ADM or your own fat or scar tissue. Doing this when the nipple is created maintains the rigidity of the nipple, but it also keeps it in the "up" position. Repeating the nipple reconstruction is another option, although there's no guarantee that the new nipple won't also eventually flatten unless it is filled to maintain its shape.

Poor Positioning

If your reconstructed nipple is off-center, your surgeon may be able to reposition it by tightening the surrounding skin. The best way to avoid nipples and areolas that are too high, too low, or off to the side is to wait until your reconstructed breast is fully healed before having nipple reconstruction and approve the positional markings before tattooing is applied.

Unsatisfactory Pigmentation or Fading

Nipple tattoos are generally made with semi-permanent pigments, and they eventually fade; some are only slightly visible after four to five years. Poorly distributed color can create a splotchy, uneven appearance that can be corrected by repeating the tattoo. While this is a common problem, certain conditions accelerate fading. Nipple tattoos are typically a combination of red and brown, colors that diminish more noticeably than the blues, greens, and blacks used in many body tattoos made with permanent inks. The type of pigment and the tool used to implant the color can also make a difference, and applying a local anesthetic may also inhibit color saturation. The quality of your skin may also affect the longevity of your tattoo: skin that has been irradiated or scarred often doesn't hold color as well. Exposing your tattoos to chlorine before they've healed can prematurely fade the color. Sun exposure also accelerates fading.

Necrosis

All or part of a reconstructed nipple may fail if the blood supply is inadequate. A small area of necrosis might be left to heal. If a larger area of the nipple or the entire nipple fails, it needs to be removed. Nipple reconstruction with or without tattooing can be retried when the skin has fully healed. Alternatively, a 3-D tattoo without nipple reconstruction is also an option.

> When I first saw my new nipples, I thought my plastic surgeon had made a mistake. They seemed huge in proportion to my breasts. But they kept shrinking as they healed, and after a few weeks they were the small nipples I had hoped for. When I later had them tattooed, I

thought the tattoo artist had applied too much color. They were several shades darker than I had imagined. Once again, they faded as they healed. Unfortunately, they kept fading, and four years later, they're barely visible. The only thing I can do is have them retattooed, but I just don't want to bother.

—*Kim*

Nipples in the Works

Nipple tattooing can produce lifelike nipples and areolas, but even the most realistically crafted nipples won't have sensation or react to touch. Researchers are looking for ways to restore these essential characteristics to individuals who have breast reconstruction. One possibility being studied is *nipple grafts*. Skin grafts have been used for years to replace skin that is damaged from burns or other injuries or removed during surgery. Nipple grafts may one day do the same to replace nipples and areolas that are lost to mastectomy. Like ADM, which has revolutionized breast reconstruction with implants, nipple grafts are made from donor nipple and areolar tissue. Because individual cells and DNA are removed from the graft, they won't be rejected by the patient's body, but proteins and collagen remain. Researchers hope that a patient's own cells will repopulate the grafted nipple-areolar scaffolding to regenerate a nipple and areola of their own cells. Just how much sensation might be restored remains to be seen.

Questions for Your Plastic Surgeon

- How will you recreate my nipple?
- How many of these procedures have you done?
- Where will the procedure be performed and how long will it take?
- How closely will my new nipple and areola match my healthy breast (after unilateral reconstruction)?
- What are my options to ensure my nipple doesn't flatten?
- Will tattooing completely hide my nipple scars?
- Will I have any downtime from building or tattooing my nipple?
- Who will tattoo my nipple and areola? What is their experience with breast reconstruction tattooing?
- What if I'm not satisfied?
- May I see your before-and-after photos of patients who had nipple reconstruction and tattooing?
- Will my insurance cover the cost of nipple reconstruction and tattooing?

Part IV
What to Expect from Prep, Post-op, Recovery, and Beyond

Contemplating reconstruction can be daunting. It's normal to fear or dread the unknown, especially when one or more operations are involved. Knowing what to expect and how to prepare for it can help you feel more confident and in control so that the anxiety you feel about what's ahead is minimized and less disruptive to your life. This section is an overview of what to expect before, during, and after your time in the hospital. Your surgeon will provide specific instructions before and after your surgery to ensure that your operation and recovery proceed as well as possible. Always follow your surgeon's instructions to the letter, and keep all of your scheduled follow-up appointments.

Five important takeaways from this section include:

- how to prepare during the four weeks before your surgery date

- what to expect in the hospital, from admission to surgery, the recovery room, and discharge

- managing medication, surgical drains, and other postoperative issues when you return home

- how to resolve physical and emotional complications that may develop as you recover

- how to navigate dating, intimacy, sex, and getting back to work

Chapter 12

Preparing for Surgery

Alone in my house, I cried all day. I was thankful for reconstruction, but I just couldn't come to grips with the reality of losing my breasts. My husband became so frustrated when he couldn't comfort me, he broke down and cried, too. That was the day I decided I was done crying.

—KATHY

By now, you've done all your research and seen all the photos. You've talked to your surgeon about your reconstruction, and you know what to expect. Your surgery date is circled in red on the kitchen calendar. There's a lot to be done before then. Improving your health now decreases your chances of complications and helps you recover faster. The more energy you invest in your overall well-being before surgery, the healthier your outcome will be. In all cases, follow your surgeon's instructions to the letter when you're preparing for surgery or recovering.

Countdown: Four Weeks to Surgery

Before scheduling your surgery, you should have a consultation with your surgeons about all of your mastectomy and reconstructive options, the benefits and limitations of each choice, and what to expect from each procedure. If you're being treated for breast cancer with radiation and/or chemotherapy, you should also understand how your surgeries will be coordinated with those treatments. Your surgeon will provide a list of pre-op instructions; generally, here's what you can expect within a month of your reconstruction surgery.

Finalize Insurance Coverage or Payment Arrangements

Ideally, you should have your health insurer's payment authorization or have a payment plan in place. Contact your insurance company to verify that the hospital or medical center, procedure(s), *and* your anesthesiologist and surgeon(s) are in-network or otherwise covered. Avoid "surprise medical bills" by knowing in advance how much your out-of-pocket cost will be. If you've requested pre-approval by your insurance company well in advance, this shouldn't be an issue.

Create Advance Directives

If you haven't already made an *advance directive*, now is a good time to do so to ensure that your preferences for healthcare will be carried out if you're unable to speak for yourself. There are two types of advance directives. A *living will* states your preference for treatment and resuscitation if you're unable to do so. A *durable power of attorney for healthcare* provides the name of the person you designate to make decisions for you if you can't. This is mostly a formality with a mastectomy and reconstruction, but it's always a good idea to have this on file.

Make Travel Plans

If you're traveling out of town for your surgery, make hotel, airline, or other needed arrangements. (See "Tips for Traveling to have Reconstruction" in Chapter 17.) Your surgeon's patient relations staff can provide information and assistance.

Have a Pre-op Evaluation

Within a month of your surgery date, you'll need to have routine pre-op testing to make sure you're healthy enough for surgery. Your surgeon will specify when these tests should be done. Pre-op testing may include a physical exam, routine blood tests, a chest x-ray, and an echocardiogram to check your heart rhythm. You may have additional tests, depending on your overall health, age, and the reconstructive procedure you're having.

Preoperative Mapping

If you're having a DIEP or other autologous muscle-sparing procedure, your surgeon may want you to have preoperative imaging that
provides a detailed map of blood vessels involved in your surgery.
This pre-op mapping identifies the strongest perforator artery that
feeds the flap of skin and fat that will become your new breast and
helps the surgeon plan the operation accordingly. (Everyone's
vascular anatomy is a bit different, and the location, quantity, and
quality of the perforators vary.) Many facilities use computed tomography angiography (CTA) for preoperative mapping. This is a CT
scan performed with *indocyanine green–based fluorescence*, a special
intravenous medical contrast dye that produces clear images of the
blood vessels at the donor site. Your surgeon may instead order a
magnetic resonance angiography (MRA). This is also used with
contrast dye, but the scan is performed with an MRI. Another type of
fluorescent imaging system, called SPY Elite, allows microsurgeons
to assess the strength of perforator arteries during the operation.

Let Others Help

Never underestimate the power and support of those who care about you. Recruit loved ones to pay bills and care for your children, pets, and home during
your hospital stay and recovery. When friends ask how they can help, suggest
they babysit your kids, grocery shop, mow the lawn, run other errands, schedule a meal brigade, or drive you to doctor appointments. Schedule a cleaning

service, if you need to. Arrange for someone to drive you to the hospital and take you home. Once home, you'll need someone to stay with you for at least the first 48 hours and longer if you have autologous (flap) surgery.

Fuel Your Body

Surgery is an assault on the body and its defenses, and fatigue is one of the most common side effects of general anesthesia. Up to this point, you've had to deal with many stressful decisions and issues, which take a toll on your mental and physical strength. If you've also undergone chemotherapy, it may have further weakened your resiliency. Now more than ever, your body needs special care to prepare for surgery and improve your ability to recover. This is no time to try a new diet. Eat nutritionally balanced meals with plenty of lean protein, whole grains, and plant-based foods. Stay well hydrated. Limit or avoid processed and sugary foods, which may be tasty but are short on nutrition. Your surgeon may recommend certain supplements to reduce inflammation and boost your immune system. Try for seven to eight hours of quality sleep each night.

Mind Your Weight

Carrying excess weight, especially if you're obese (a BMI of 30 or greater), makes surgery more difficult and increases the risk of complications. This can complicate anesthesia and raises the likelihood of problems. Diabetes, high blood pressure, and other weight-related health conditions may also increase your risk during surgery. Being significantly overweight raises the risk of breathing problems during surgery and increases the time it takes to regain consciousness. Being very underweight can be a risk factor for decreased wound healing while increasing the risk of infection and prolonged recovery. Talk to your doctor if you need help reaching and maintaining a healthy weight.

Boost Your Fitness

Just as you might prepare for an athletic event, increasing your fitness will help your body weather the stress of surgery. If you're used to being active, continue to do so up until your surgery. The sooner you begin, the better you'll fare. If you tend to be sedentary, try to increase your level of activity. Exercise vigorously for at least 30 minutes a day (45 minutes to an hour is even better):

- Enjoy a brisk walk each morning or evening.
- Walk, swim, dance, try a new exercise video, or engage in other cardiovascular activities to boost your immune system and strengthen your lungs and heart.
- Give yoga a try. Yoga is a particularly effective way to improve the mind-body connection. Regularly stretching the muscles increases flexibility, resilience, and range of motion and is beneficial before and after surgery. Yoga also calms anxiety. It can help to relieve the stress you feel before and after surgery.

Stop Smoking

Aside from raising the risk for several cancers, the 70 carcinogenic chemicals in tobacco products promote infections, delay healing, decrease the body's ability to use oxygen, and reduce survival; however, research shows that quitting four weeks or more before an operation lowers the risk of complications.[1] You must be free of nicotine several weeks before and after your surgery; if you aren't, your surgery will likely be postponed. That means no cigarettes, e-cigarettes, cigars, vaping, chewing tobacco, nicotine patches, nicotine gum, or other nicotine products. It's also important to avoid exposure to secondhand smoke. Ask your primary physician for helpful medication if you need it and check out the information at www.smokefree.gov. This could be the push you need to quit for good.

Avoid Alcohol

Drinking any kind of alcohol within 24 hours before surgery is a bad idea, and it can be dangerous. Abstaining for a week or two (or longer) before your procedure will help you get through surgery and help you heal. Drinking close to your surgery date creates the potential for a long list of problems: it weakens the immune system, thins the blood so that excessive bleeding may occur, may interfere with anesthesia, and can cause harmful interactions with pre-op and post-op medications. It also increases the likelihood of infection, delayed wound healing, and other post-op problems. If you're a consistent or heavy drinker or you're dependent on alcohol, speak honestly to your doctor as soon as you know you'll have surgery, so that you have time to seek treatment or gradually wean yourself from alcohol. The more you drink, the longer you need to refrain from drinking to give your body time to recover from the effects of alcohol.

Refrain from Recreational Drugs

Let your surgeon know if you use marijuana, narcotics, or any other stimulants. These substances can affect the type and amount of anesthesia you need and how you'll react to it.

Have a Recliner Ready

Finding a comfortable position to rest and sleep can be tricky after surgery. Sleeping in a recliner provides good support, making it easier to sleep comfortably. If you don't already have a recliner, consider buying or borrowing one.

Schedule Time Off from Work

Notify your workplace of your upcoming absence and when you think you might return. You don't need to reveal the exact nature of your surgery if you don't feel comfortable doing so, but you'll need to advise your supervisor or boss that you'll be gone and may need to work partial days when you return, particularly if your job is stressful or physically demanding.

Two Weeks before Surgery

With just 14 days before you head for the hospital, there's plenty to coordinate and accomplish.

Understand Your Pre-op Instructions

Your surgeon (or nurse) will explain preoperative do's and don'ts. Ask any questions you need to so that you're clear about how long your surgery will last and the length of your hospital stay.

Discontinue Certain Medications and Supplements

Your surgeon will advise which medications, vitamins, herbs, and supplements might interfere with anesthesia or increase bleeding and should be stopped weeks before and after your surgery. Taking aspirin, ibuprofen, or naproxen, which can thin the blood and inhibit clotting, is a definite no-no for at least two weeks and maybe more before and after surgery. You'll also need to stay away from medications that contain these ingredients, including many common non-prescription painkillers and anti-inflammatories such as Advil (ibuprofen), Aleve (naproxen), Motrin (ibuprofen), and others. When in doubt, read the label. Tylenol (acetaminophen) is usually okay for headaches, sore muscles, or other minor to moderate pains. If you take a blood thinner, your doctor may request a blood test just before your surgery to make sure your blood clots sufficiently. If you're taking tamoxifen to reduce your risk of breast cancer or recurrence, your doctor might advise you to temporarily stop for two to three weeks before and after autologous flap reconstruction, as both medications increase the risk of blood clots.[2] In all cases, your surgeon will advise what you may take safely and what you should avoid.

Prepare Emotionally

Well-documented studies show that people who are emotionally prepared for surgery have less pain and heal sooner. Try to deal with stress and anxiety proactively. Consider deep breathing, meditation, or exercise. Relaxation tapes and positive visualization are also helpful. *Prepare for Surgery, Heal Faster: A Guide of Mind-Body Techniques* by Peggy Huddleston is a classic resource. Or try journaling. Sometimes it's easier to express your feelings on a nonjudgmental piece of paper or a computer screen. It's also satisfying. You might be surprised at the depth of perspective it provides.

Breathe Deeply

Our bodies breathe reflexively. We don't have to think about breathing for it to occur. When you inhale, blood cells receive oxygen and release carbon dioxide, a waste product that is then exhaled. Deep breathing—consciously inhaling and exhaling to expand the lungs—brings more oxygen into the body, clears

Seven Tips for Maintaining Your Emotional Health

1. Create a support circle of a few trusted individuals who will support you without judgment, act as your safety net, and inspire you when you need an emotional boost.

2. Prioritize what you want to accomplish each day; you don't have to address everything at once.

3. Differentiate between things you can control and those you cannot.

4. Use positive self-talk to mentor yourself through difficult moments or days.

5. Do something enjoyable every day to lift your spirits.

6. Eat well and exercise regularly to maintain strength, boost your energy, and stabilize your mood.

7. Remember to breathe. No matter where you are or what you're doing, you always have time to pause for a few deep, calming breaths.

the mind, and offers a new perspective. It can improve concentration, and it's a potent anxiety reliever. It's an effective way to restore calm after a stressful day or to counter pre-surgery jitters, and you don't need any special equipment. Several methods of deep breathing trigger a relaxation response in the brain and body. Here's an easy one to try:

- Sitting or lying comfortably, place a hand on your stomach.
- Inhale deeply through your nose as you slowly count to four, feeling your stomach as it expands with air.
- Exhale fully as you slowly count to four.
- Repeat this sequence four or five times.

Go Shopping

If you'd like to wear something more personal than a generic hospital garment, one option is to buy an Annie and Isabel hospital gown (www.annieandisabel .com). Designed by two nurses, the gowns have an inside pocket, snap at the shoulders for easy access to surgery sites, and conform to hospital standards. Other options are available on the internet. Most hospitals provide surgical bras. However, if your surgeon recommends a different type, consider one (or two) that accommodates surgical drains, like the Elizabeth Pink Surgical Bra (www.mastheadpink.com). You can also order a special belt or camisole designed to hold your drains (described in chapter 14).

This is also a good time to shop for comfy, loose-fitting, and front-closing camisoles, pajamas, and other garments. If your reconstruction includes a flap from your abdomen, hip, thigh, or buttock, consider buying underwear and sweatpants a size or two larger than you normally wear to accommodate swelling and the compression girdle that you'll need to wear for several weeks. You'll also need lots of pillows to help you sleep and for placing under your knees and elevating your arms. Here's a checklist of things you might want to have on hand.

A Checklist of Things to Have on Hand
- ☐ soft cotton or silk camisoles
- ☐ front-zippered or buttoned tops and pajamas
- ☐ loose-fitting pull-on pants or pajama pants
- ☐ belt or camisole designed to hold surgical drains
- ☐ comfy, non-skid slip-on shoes or slippers
- ☐ large safety pins (for pinning surgical drains out of the way)
- ☐ front-closing bra (the type your surgeon recommends)
- ☐ shower chair and detachable showerhead
- ☐ a lanyard to hold your surgical drains and prevent them from dangling (shoestrings also work well)

- ☐ dry shampoo
- ☐ baby wipes (until you can shower)
- ☐ gauze (for changing dressings if necessary)
- ☐ drainage cups for measuring drain output (if your surgeon or hospital doesn't supply them)
- ☐ thermometer
- ☐ wedge, mastectomy, or other comfy supportive pillows
- ☐ recliner
- ☐ pen and notebook (if you want to journal)
- ☐ good stuff to read (e-reader, books, magazines) or audiobooks
- ☐ eye mask
- ☐ electric toothbrush

One Week to Go

As your surgery date draws closer, take time to get your house in order and prepare for your return from the hospital.

Fill Post-op Prescriptions

It's a good idea to have prescriptions for post-op pain medication and antibiotics filled now so that you'll have them when you get home. After your surgery, it may be difficult to press down sufficiently to open childproof lids, which puts pressure on your chest muscles, so ask your pharmacist to use a different type of lid.

Pamper Yourself

Now is a great time to get your hair cut and colored, have a facial, or engage in your favorite self-indulgent behavior. Enjoy lunch with friends. Finish that big project at home or work. Spend special time with your kids. Have fun. Shave your underarms or legs with an electric razor or consider waxing. Avoid razors that could cause nicks in the skin and encourage infection.

Notify Your Surgeon of Any Health Changes

Between now and your surgery date, notify your surgeon's office if you develop a cough, cold, infection, fever, or other health problem, no matter how minor it may seem. Your surgery may have to be rescheduled if there's a risk of infection—it's always better to be safe than sorry.

Talk to Your Kids

Many women feel better telling their children about reconstruction instead of keeping it a secret. Children know when something is wrong, even if they don't know what it is, and they want to be reassured that their world will remain unchanged. Kids process information differently. Some ask lots of questions, while others aren't interested, so it's a good idea to tailor your explanations to each child's personality and level of understanding. Your demeanor influences their reaction: if they see you're okay, they'll likely be okay. Keep it simple for little ones, giving them only the details they need to understand about why you'll be gone for a few days, and letting them know that you'll be all right. If they don't already know about your breast cancer and treatment, reassure them you're not ill because of anything they did. Some women prefer to avoid using the word "sick," which may frighten children. If you're emotional around your children, explain that Mommy is sad or angry or afraid but not because of them.

Older children and teens might want to know more. They may feel frightened or threatened if they sense that reconstruction is a taboo topic. Reassure them that you'll be fine and that your reconstruction is a way to help restore your breast after a mastectomy. Let them know how they can help during your recovery. Arrange to keep your kids' routines as normal as possible.

My four-year-old had already seen me bald and sick after chemotherapy, so when I told him I was going back to the hospital for a few days to get better, he didn't even blink.

—*Christine*

Our puppy had to have surgery after he swallowed pillow stuffing. When I scheduled my mastectomy, I explained that Mommy's boobs had a type of stuffing that could make me sick, so a nice doctor was going to replace the bad stuffing with good stuffing. I would be in the hospital, as our puppy had, and then I would come home and soon be all better. I gave each of my children a teddy bear I said was filled with "Mommy love" that would never run out. Whenever I couldn't hug them, they could cuddle the bears and it would be like me giving them a big squeeze.

—Cathy

Catch Up, Stock Up

A little preparation now will make things easier on you and your family when you come home from the hospital. You'll want to

- Stock up on groceries, particularly nutritious items that are easily prepared. Consider buying smaller quantities that will be lighter and easier to use: quarts of milk rather than gallons. If you have pets, be sure to have plenty of food (and treats) for them as well.
- Stash a batch of meals that can be reheated in the freezer, especially if you don't have someone who can deliver meals or shop and cook for you during your recovery. Have small bags of ice, frozen peas, or ice packs on hand to reduce swelling.
- Buy a thermometer if you don't already have one. It will come in handy if you think you might have a fever.

Prepare for Recovery

Do as much as possible now to prepare for when you get home from the hospital. This will be especially helpful if you are on your own or your caregivers' schedule is spaced out.

- Make a contact list of telephone numbers or e-mail addresses of friends and family who should be notified after your surgery and updated on your recovery. Consider appointing someone as a single point of contact for updates and information.
- Consider asking friends not to call for a few days after you come home from the hospital; having the phone ring just when you drop off to sleep can be disrupting. (Or silence your phone.) You can

always initiate calls when you feel up to it or ask a family member to call on your behalf.

- Arrange your nightstand with all the things you'll need at home, including pain medication, TV and DVD remote controls, books, audiobooks, e-readers, magazines, tissues, lotion, lip emollient, and phone. Baby wipes are handy for times when you just won't feel like getting up—although periodically getting up and walking around will be good for you.
- Have water and saltines or graham crackers handy for taking pain medication during the night. Keep a journal and pen, a digital tablet, or a mobile device with a recorder handy if you're inclined to document your thoughts.
- Clean your house or have it cleaned before you go into the hospital. You won't be able to sweep or push a vacuum for a few weeks.
- Change your sheets and pillowcases. You'll appreciate cool, clean linens during your recovery.
- Reposition bathroom and kitchen counter items so you can get to them without reaching. You'll need to avoid lifting or stretching your arms over your head for a while. If you're having an abdominal flap, reposition items that are under cabinets and on low shelves so that you can get to them without bending.

The Day before Surgery

With just one day to go before you head to the hospital, there are still a few last-minute details to take care of.

Remove Your Nail Polish

Your fingernails should be *au naturel* when you go into surgery (some surgeons say that light color is fine). Nail polish and acrylic nails can reduce the effectiveness of the fingertip sensor that your anesthesiologist will use to monitor your oxygen levels. If your oxygen dropped, your fingernails would turn blue, but this could be hidden by your polish or acrylics. Toe polish is probably okay because you'll be wearing socks in the operating room but ask your surgeon to be sure.

Take Some "You" Time

See a movie with friends, have dinner with your family or your favorite person, get a massage, or put on some music and stretch out in a warm bath. Engage in your favorite stress-reducing activity.

Don't Shave or Wax

Don't shave or wax your underarms or donor site because even small nicks invite infection. Bacteria in hair follicles can cause a skin infection if you happen to nick your skin with a razor (shaving with razor blades can cause microscopic skin breaks). You can shave or wax a few days ahead of your surgery; ask your surgeon about this.

Pack a Small Overnight Bag

Select a loose-fitting top that doesn't need to be pulled over your head and loose, comfy sweatpants or pajama bottoms, especially if you're having a tissue flap that involves your thighs, abdomen, or buttocks. Wear slippers or flat-heeled shoes. Take moisturizer, lip gloss or balm, floss, hairbrush or comb, and any other essential toiletries. If you're staying overnight, the hospital will supply a toothbrush, toothpaste, non-skid slippers, and a robe; but you can bring your own if you prefer. It's also nice to pack your favorite music, iPad or e-reader, audiobook, or magazines, particularly if you'll be in the hospital for more than one day. Remember your health insurance card and personal identification. Pack a special bag for whoever will stay in the waiting room during your surgery. Include water, snacks, something to read, and a list of family and friends to notify after your surgery. Bring loose clothing for discharge.

Hydrate

Drink plenty of water and clear, non-alcoholic liquids throughout the day. Avoid alcohol; it dries the tissues, and you need to be as hydrated as possible for your surgery. Clear fluids include water, juice, Gatorade and other sports drinks, tea, and coffee. (Tea or coffee should be taken without milk, which has a high protein and fat content and takes longer to digest.) Because patients who drink clear fluids are well-hydrated, they experience less anxiety, require fewer IV fluids during and after surgery, and recover better after the procedure.[3]

Eat a Light Dinner

New guidelines recommend refraining from eating eight hours before surgery, while drinking clear fluids up to two hours before an operation is encouraged. Your pre-op instructions may suggest avoiding dairy products and high-fiber, starchy, or fatty foods the evening before your surgery. Don't eat or drink anything beyond the cutoff time advised by your surgeon's office or the hospital.

Cuddle Up, If You Feel Like It

If you're so inclined, there's no medical reason to avoid sexual activity the night before your surgery. It may even help calm your nerves.

Scrub Up

Shower or bathe with the antiseptic soap your surgeon recommends. Apply gently, carefully cleanse the areas around the surgical sites, and rinse well. Generally, antiseptic skin cleansers are safe for everyday use, so you can use the remaining amount after your surgery as well; doublecheck with your surgeon before doing so.

Try for Eight Hours of Sleep

With your surgery looming, you'll have a lot on your mind. Try to get a good night's rest. If that's not going to be possible on your own, ask your doctor to prescribe a mild sleep aid. Don't take an over-the-counter sleep aid unless you have the doctor's okay.

Plant Positive Thoughts

Mental self-talk is powerful. Before you drift off to sleep, tell yourself that your surgery will be successful, you'll come through it beautifully, and you'll be just fine. Then believe it.

Follow Directions

Be sure to follow all of the preoperative instructions from your doctor and the hospital.

Reconstruction Day

Finally, the day of your surgery has arrived. You still have a few things to do before you head for the hospital.

Take Your Regular Medication

If your surgeon approved you to do so, take your regular medication with just a sip of water.

Take Another Shower

Even though you showered or bathed last night, doing so again will reduce bacteria on your skin and lower your risk of infection. Wash with Hibiclens, Dial, or other antibacterial soap recommended by your surgeon, paying special attention to the areas where incisions will be made. (Don't use antibacterial soap on your head or face.) This is the last chance to wash your hair for several days. Use only shampoo and conditioner; don't use any other hair products.

Leave It Off

Don't apply wigs, hairpieces, perfume, creams, lotions, or makeup (your natural skin tone is an indication of adequate circulation). Bring eyeglasses (and a case) if you need them; you can't wear contact lenses during surgery, and you probably won't feel like putting them in and taking them out (or getting up to rinse them) during your time in the hospital.

Leave Valuables at Home

Don't take anything you don't need. Leave cash, credit cards, your purse, your wallet, your watch, and all jewelry (including wedding rings, earrings, and body jewelry) at home.

Talk to Someone

Chat with your kids, your spouse, your significant other, or your best friend. It will help to quiet any concerns they're having. It will help you, too.

Leave Little Notes

If you have kids, tuck a note under their pillow or somewhere they'll be sure to find it, so they'll have a message from you even when you're not there. (Your partner or spouse would probably appreciate a note, too.)

Continue to Hydrate

Generally, you can continue to drink clear liquids up to two hours before your surgery, but your plastic surgeon may request that you refrain for a longer period. Drink water, plain tea, black coffee, or pulp-free juice; or eat Jell-O or popsicles. Avoid alcohol. Your nurse may give you a carb-loaded nutritional drink.

Try to Relax

It's natural to be nervous before surgery. But you can take steps to calm your thoughts and fears. Plant positive thoughts about your surgery, recovery, and outcome. Take a few moments for deep breathing. Focus on the most positive, beautiful thoughts you can: a happy time, a romantic vacation, or giggling with your children. Visualize a peaceful, happy postoperative you.

Chapter 13

What to Expect in the Hospital

Each time I enter a hospital, my hands shake and a feeling of dread comes over me. I had to find a more positive perspective to get through my reconstruction. I began to consider hospitals and doctors as places and people who did things for me rather than to me. I started to think of reconstruction as the process that would put me back on the road to wholeness.

—DORENE

Who doesn't get the jitters just walking into a hospital? It's a place we associate with the sick and ailing. Knowing what to expect once you're within those sanitized walls can help calm your fear of the unknown.

Admitting and Pre-op

The hospital will want you to arrive a few hours before your surgery. Once there, you'll be asked to review and sign pre-admission paperwork, including an informed consent form identifying the procedure to be performed—its purpose, risks, and expected outcome—and documents concerning your privacy and patient's rights. A nurse will show you to your room, where you'll be weighed, change into a hospital gown, and have your temperature and blood pressure taken. You'll also be asked to remove any jewelry, hairpins, hearing aids, dentures, and contact lenses. You may feel a tiny sting as a nurse inserts a thin needle into a vein on your hand or arm that is then connected to an *intravenous (IV) line*, through which you'll be given fluids and anesthesia during your operation. While you're waiting, your breast surgeon and plastic surgeon will come by for a brief visit before you enter the operating room. If incision lines haven't already been marked on your chest—and donor site if you're having a flap reconstruction—they'll be drawn now. The anesthesiologist will stop by to review your overall health, allergies, and experience with anesthesia, and explain the type of sedation you'll receive. If you have questions about your procedure, now is the time to ask.

There's always a lot of waiting around before surgery. Free to wander, your mind may go directly to uneasy. Try reading or watching TV. Breathe deeply. Concentrate on the positive aspects of your surgery. A mastectomy will remove your cancer (or reduce the threat of it), and reconstruction will restore your breasts. If it will make you feel better, discuss your fears with your nurse, spouse or partner, family members, or others who are with you or are just a telephone call away.

> I was so nervous the day of my surgery, I broke into a cold sweat. I remember wondering if I would be admitted for heart problems instead of reconstruction because I was sure I could feel my heart hammering beneath my shirt.
>
> —*Jasmine*

In the Operating Room

When it's time for your surgery, friends and family will be shown to the waiting room, and you'll be wheeled into the operating room. The first thing you'll notice is the temperature, which is kept low for the surgical staff. Their gowns are made of tightly woven material that protects against bacteria but doesn't breathe, and the room lights generate plenty of heat. A nurse will cover you with heated blankets and pre-surgery preparations begin. Small sensors will be taped to your arms and legs to monitor your blood pressure and heart rate. The pulse oximeter clipped onto your finger will measure the level of oxygen in your blood. It's natural to feel anxious at this point, but it won't last long; you'll soon be fast asleep. Your anesthesiologist will administer a customized anesthesia cocktail based on your weight and the length of your surgery through your IV and directly into your bloodstream. You'll be asleep before you can count to 10 . . . and maybe before you get to 5.

Modern anesthesia is precise and sophisticated. Your anesthesiologist will closely monitor your vital signs and adjust your sedation throughout your surgery, carefully controlling your level of consciousness to keep you in a deep sleep. Not too much, not too little—just enough. You'll also receive pain medication during your surgery, so you won't feel a thing. A surgical tube in your throat will help you to breathe, and a catheter inserted into your bladder will drain any urine. A nurse will cleanse your chest and donor site with surgical disinfectant. The rest of your body will be draped with sterile sheets, leaving only the surgical areas uncovered. The breast surgeon then begins your mastectomy. When that is done, if you're also having immediate reconstruction, your plastic surgeon begins recreating your breasts.

A Peek into Post-op

When your surgery is over, you'll be moved to the recovery room, and your surgeon will let your loved ones know your operation has been completed. You'll slowly wake up as the effects of anesthesia wear off, but you'll be drowsy and may continue to fall in and out of sleep. You'll be thirsty and your throat may be sore from the breathing tube. Ask your nurse for ice chips, water, juice, or throat lozenges. You'll have an automatic blood pressure cuff, and you may also have an oxygen tube in your nose. An IV that drips saline and antibiotics into your bloodstream will remain until you can take in fluids on your own. A nurse will frequently check your vital signs and closely monitor blood flow to your new breast if you've had autologous reconstruction. Your nurse may use a handheld Doppler probe, a small, portable ultrasound machine that detects blood flow.

Sequential compression devices sound ominous but these inflatable sleeves that are placed on your lower legs after surgery prevent blood clots from forming until you're able to move around on your own. You'll feel a gentle pressure and hear a soft whooshing sound as the pumping machine periodically inflates and deflates the sleeves to mimic normal circulation. If you had autologous surgery, you'll also have a compression garment at your donor site.

Your new breasts will be covered with gauze bandages under a surgical bra to hold them close to your chest. You may be curious and anxious to see what they look like, but unless you get a quick, upside-down peek while a nurse is checking your incisions, you won't see under the dressings until they're removed in your doctor's office in a few days. You'll also have surgical drains at your incision sites; these will be monitored by your nurses while you're in the hospital. Before you're discharged, you'll be given instructions on how to manage them at home (chapter 14).

Anesthesia suppresses the body's ability to function normally. You'll feel weak and tired and your head may feel fuzzy for the next 24 hours until its effects wear off. The longer you're under its influence, the harder your body works to recover. After surgery, it's important to restore your full lung capacity. You'll be given a *spirometer* to help expand your lungs, strengthen your breathing, and prevent pneumonia. Your lungs expand as you inhale through the mouthpiece; exhaling into the device expels the air in your lungs. It's difficult at first, but use this device diligently as instructed by your nurse. Restoring lung strength is an important part of recovery.

After an implant or expander procedure, you'll likely go home the same day. You'll be moved to a hospital room if you need to be monitored a bit longer or if you have had an autologous reconstruction.

Managing Pain

Pain is always a concern after surgery, but many women describe post-reconstructive discomfort as more of a dull, heavy feeling than sharp or unbearable pain. A lot depends on the type of reconstruction you've had and your own pain tolerance. To better understand the source of your pain, consider this: You know how annoying a paper cut can be, and that affects only the top layer of skin. Your surgical incision is a paper cut magnified, slicing through skin, fat, and, in some cases, muscle.

Effective pain management addresses not only general postoperative pain at the incision sites but nerve and musculoskeletal pain as well. With improved healing protocols, postoperative discomfort is capably managed and the need for opioids is reduced or eliminated (see sidebar). Oral medication is usually adequate after implant or expander surgery. Flap surgery is more invasive and requires more substantial pain control. Your surgeon may administer a local anesthetic to block nerve pain near the incision site. After surgery, you'll have a small, self-medicating pump to regulate the amount of pain medicine you receive. You can use it when you need it without fear of overdosing. If this adequately controls your discomfort, you won't be as groggy, drowsy, or constipated as you would be with stronger narcotics. When your pain significantly subsides, you'll be switched to oral painkillers. To ensure your comfort, you'll be asked frequently to rate your level of pain.

The trick to managing pain is to stay ahead of it by keeping a constant, even flow of medication in your system. Dose yourself before it becomes unbearable. This is no time to be tough. Patients who control their pain heal faster than those who don't. Fresh incisions are tender, and applying pressure to them, either internally or externally, will hurt. To your sensitized tissues, a sneeze or cough can feel like a grenade going off. Holding your hand or a pillow gently against your incisions will help. Try to support healing incisions in the same way when getting in or out of bed.

Improving Circulation and Movement

Movement improves your circulation, prevents fluid from settling in your lungs, and helps your system return to normal. Slowly and carefully flex and stretch as many body parts as you can without causing pain. Initially, you'll have limited mobility in your arms, and if lymph nodes were removed during your mastectomy, your underarms may be sore. (You'll also receive information about preventing lymphedema and how to recognize its symptoms.) Many movements we take for granted will be difficult and uncomfortable, so be careful and aware of how you move or stretch your body. Your nurse will show you how to perform gentle arm and shoulder exercises to prevent stiffness and regain range of motion. Ask for illustrated instructions that you can take home.

Getting out of bed for the first time will be an effort, particularly if you have an abdominal incision, but it's important to walk around and get your blood circulating, even if just for a few moments. The sooner you become mobile, the sooner you can go home. You'll be encouraged to get out of bed and begin moving around within a few hours after your surgery. It will be difficult and exhausting the first time you get up, but it gets easier as you regain strength.

Bathroom Breaks

A urinary catheter will stay in place until you can walk to and from the bathroom on your own. Constipation is a common problem after general anesthesia.

Enhanced Recovery After Surgery

Many hospitals and surgical centers use Enhanced Recovery After Surgery (ERAS) protocols to shorten hospital stays and help patients safely recover sooner, with less pain and less medication. ERAS recommendations for breast reconstruction include 18 key actions, including the following:

- Allow clear liquids up to two hours before surgery.

- Provide a carb-loaded nutritional drink two hours before surgery.

- Reduce infection by cleaning the surgical area(s) with chlorhexidine (a mild antiseptic) and giving intravenous antibiotics one hour before an incision is made.

- Administer pain-controlling medications before, during, and after surgery to reduce or eliminate the need for opioids.

- Provide medications before and during surgery to reduce the likelihood of post-op nausea and vomiting.

- Emphasize postoperative mobility.

Source: Temple-Oberle C, Shea-Budgell MA, Tan M, et al.; ERAS Society. Consensus review of optimal perioperative care in breast reconstruction: Enhanced Recovery after Surgery (ERAS) Society recommendations. *Plastic and Reconstructive Surgery.* 2017;139(5):1056e–71e.

(Eating lightly the day before your surgery will help to avoid feeling bloated.) Walking, drinking plenty of liquids, and eating sufficient fiber will help get you back on track. Your nurse will provide a stool softener if you need it.

The Rest of Your Hospital Stay

All of your bodily functions must operate normally before you can leave the hospital. Talk with your doctor about staying longer if you don't feel well enough to go home or you develop an infection or other post-op complication. Be sure to have the following when it's time to be discharged:

- post-op instructions, including when you can shower and activities that should be restricted or avoided
- how to care for your incisions
- a list of the warning signs of infection or other problems
- directions for managing your surgical drains (chapter 14)
- prescriptions for pain medication and antibiotics (if you don't already have them)
- after-hours contact information for your surgeon
- a scheduled follow-up appointment with your surgeon

When you've packed up everything you need, and your surgeon has signed your discharge papers, a nurse will help you into a wheelchair and take you outside. (For insurance reasons, patients aren't allowed to walk out of the hospital.) You're on your way home.

Chapter 14

Back Home

Speak to 10 different women who have undergone surgeries and you'll hear 10
distinct stories. Some have wonderful outcomes right away, while others struggle for some time; it's plastic surgery after all. Regardless of the outcome or the
difficulty, women undergoing surgery and reconstruction will be fine. Our bodies
have an amazing ability to heal.

—JANET

After surgery, your definition of a good day will change as you recover and
regain strength. At first, a good day may mean finding a comfortable sleeping
position. That will be redefined when you can stay awake, sit up, respond to
e-mails or texts, and have dinner with your family. Later, a good day will be when
you can lift your arms over your head or go the entire day without pain medication or a nap. One day, your cancer, treatment, reconstruction, and doctor appointments will be behind you. You'll go about your life and forget about your
chest, just as you did before your surgery. That will be an exceptionally good day.

A Timetable for Healing

Once you return home, sleeping or resting will initially take up a large part of
your days. Although you'll be eager to return to your normal routine, don't
rush your recovery. Take it one day at a time, and give in to your need to rest.
Take advantage of the time to write in your journal, catch up on your reading,
enjoy a movie, chat with your loved ones or friends, or nap whenever you feel
the need. Listen to your body and be respectful of your need to heal. As your

body recuperates, so will your energy and spirit. Don't be frustrated when you can't reach the top shelf, pick up your toddler, carry a bag of groceries, or blow-dry your hair. Day by day, you'll get better, and your functionality, strength, and range of motion will improve. How long will it take to get back to normal? Recovery is such a personal matter, and it's different for everyone. A lot depends on your condition before surgery, the type of reconstruction you have—you'll bounce back faster from implant reconstruction than an autologous flap—and how much you do to support the healing process. Here's a general description of what you can expect during the first few weeks. Your recovery may move along faster or take a while longer. Remember to closely follow your surgeon's post-op instructions.

Week 1

You might think that you shouldn't move your arms and shoulders after reconstruction, but the opposite is true. Continuing to do the gentle exercises you learned in the hospital will help prevent stiffness and restore range of motion in your arms and shoulders. Take care to move slowly and carefully—no extensive reaching, stretching, pulling, pushing, or pressing movements, nothing that stresses your tender chest tissue. You'll be advised not to raise your arms above your shoulders or lift anything that weighs more than five or 10 pounds, including your children. You'll quickly discover what you can and can't do (table 14.1). You'll feel tired during your first postoperative week.

Even though you may spend much of the day in and out of bed, you can (and should) take short walks down the hall or around the house to improve your fatigue and prevent muscle atrophy. Take sponge baths or sit in a half-filled tub if you can do that without immersing any incisions until your surgeon says that it's okay to shower. If you're unable to shower but you can't wait to have clean hair, lean your neck carefully over the sink (if you can do it without pain) and have someone do the honors for you. Your clean hair may need to wait a while longer if you can't manage this. Or ask someone to help you use a dry shampoo. Eat small, light meals for the first day or two, especially if your reconstruction included an abdominal incision, to discourage bloating. Postpone coffee and other sources of caffeine, which constrict blood vessels and may delay wound healing, at least until your surgeon gives you the okay to enjoy it again.

You'll have a post-op appointment with your plastic surgeon about a week after your surgery to check your incisions and change your dressing. (You'll

TABLE 14.1 Recovery Do's and Don'ts

INITIALLY, YOU'LL BE UNABLE TO	BUT YOU WILL BE ABLE TO
lift more than 5–10 pounds	take naps
reach over your head	do deep-breathing exercises
sleep on your stomach or surgical side	take daily walks
wash your hair	take approved pain medication
run, lift weights, swim	have meals with the family
wear a regular or underwire bra	stretch and do range-of-motion exercises*
have sex	brush your teeth
return to work	use a computer or mobile device
smoke or drink alcohol	catch up on your reading
drive	let others help you

*Follow your surgeon's instructions regarding when you should restrict and resume certain activities and movements.

need someone to drive you there and back.) Although most of your incisions will have been closed with absorbable sutures, some may need to be removed; that will be done now or in the next week. This is a good time to ask for a copy of your postmastectomy pathology report.

> I always thought napping during the day was such a waste of time. After my surgery, I just gave in to it. I kept a pile of books by the bed. I would wake up, read a little, walk a little, then readjust my pillows and nod off again. How decadent!
>
> —*Mona*

Week 2

You may find that you can do more in the second week, but you're still recovering. After implant surgery, you may be feeling better; and, although you may tire easily, you'll probably be able to stay awake longer during the day. This is the time when it's easy to make the mistake of doing too much too soon. Take

Know When to Contact Your Doctor

It's normal to experience some discomfort, swelling, soreness, and fatigue after surgery. Notify your surgeon, however, if you experience any of the following symptoms:

- chills or fever
- persistent vomiting or nausea
- pale, blue, or cold fingers, toes, or nails
- increased numbness, tingling, or swelling in your arm or fingers
- signs of infection at the incision
- pain that isn't controlled by your prescribed medication

one day at a time. Lengthen your daily strolls. Move slowly and carefully and give yourself time to gradually get back into the swing of things. Everything you do will take longer and use more energy. You're still recovering; never force your body to do something before it's ready. Recovery from autologous reconstruction will take longer. If you've had an abdominal flap, it will be difficult to stand straight or flex your abdomen to sit or get up from a chair or in and out of bed. If you've had a TUG flap, you'll need to continue to limit movement involving your thighs. Follow your surgeon's instructions regarding how and when you should move and stretch your donor site.

I was tired and fuzzy for a few days after my implant reconstruction; I was okay as long as I took my pain pills. I was so much better by the second week that I decided to shop for groceries. What a mistake! In 10 minutes, I was utterly exhausted. I couldn't push the cart one more step. I left it right in the middle of the cereal aisle, got back into my car, and had a good cry.

—*Shelly*

Week 3

By now you should be walking farther and staying up most of the day. You may still need a nap or two to feel more alert and less fatigued. Your incisions should be well on their way to healing, but will still need to be protected. Until they heal, the swelling recedes, and your drains are removed (which may be this week if they haven't already been removed), avoid activities that raise your blood pressure, including sexual activity, because excess blood at the incision can cause more swelling and hinder healing. If your sutures have healed—any surgical glue, tape, or scabs have fallen off without help—and your surgeon gives you the okay, you can begin to gently massage your scars (described in chapter 15).

If you no longer need prescription pain medication, your surgeon may say it's okay to resume driving. First do a test: Sit in a parked car and see whether you're able to open the car door without straining your chest muscles; get in and out, turn the wheel, and be sure that you can comfortably wear your seat belt. If it's too uncomfortable, wait another week before you try again.

Depending on your job and how you heal, you may be able to return to non-strenuous work this week after implant reconstruction. If your reconstruction involved an autologous flap, particularly from the abdomen, you might feel you've hit a recovery plateau about this time. The fatigue, discomfort, and trouble sleeping may catch up with you, and you'll feel weary of it all. You may be able to stand somewhat straighter now, even though your abdomen will still feel tight. Continue taking naps if you need them. Take walks and do your recommended stretching exercises. Tomorrow or the next day (or the day after that), you'll notice an improvement.

Week 4

If your new breasts have healed sufficiently, your surgeon may say it's okay to begin wearing ordinary bras, although you may have to steer clear of underwire

What about Sex?

There's no timetable for resuming sexual activities after a mastectomy and reconstruction because everyone is different. How you heal and how you feel provides a more definitive answer than anything else. Your surgeon will advise when you are physically healed and cleared for intercourse, but you're the one who determines whether you're emotionally prepared for sexual intimacy. Physically, it's important to wait until your swelling has mostly disappeared, your drains have been removed, and you've healed enough, so that you can move without pain or discomfort. Let your body, rather than your libido, tell you when you're ready to "get back in the saddle." (See chapter 16 for more information on intimacy and sex after reconstruction.)

bras for three months or more. If you stopped smoking before your surgery, don't resume until your doctor says it's okay to do so. (You've now been off cigarettes for six to eight weeks—a great start to kick the habit!) You'll probably be able to resume much of your normal routine by this time (if you haven't already), particularly after implant or expander surgery. If you've had a flap procedure—especially a pedicled TRAM—or you've been slow to heal, you may need extra time to get back to performing more strenuous activities and lifting heavy objects. Your abdominal flexibility should continue to improve, but it can take months before the tightness disappears.

For the first couple of weeks after my reconstruction, I was constantly aware of the tightness in my chest, the feeling that something was different. Then, at three weeks, I felt normal, just like I used to before surgery. It was a big deal; I was getting used to the new me. I felt so good. I made plans to go out on my own, but after just a few hours, I was exhausted! I must have overdone it because I needed a nap when I got home; most days I just needed to sit down and relax for a while, and I would feel better. I also realized that it was too soon for me to have been driving on my own. Resting after going out seemed to be the routine until almost five weeks when most of my energy returned. Although I may have felt well during those early weeks, my body was working very hard in the background . . . healing.

—*Leanne*

After my mastectomy with DIEP reconstruction, I stayed in the hospital for six days. My pain was minimal; I was off all pain meds, including ibuprofen, within a week. I ate meals with my family on my first day home and slept in bed—that was difficult since I had to sleep flat on my back for the first three weeks. My healing was aided significantly by all the help I accepted, including meals, preschool rides, and a cleaning service. I was able to care for myself within 10 days of surgery, and I was back to normal within a month. The lifting restriction was the hardest part of the recovery process for me. As a stay-at-home mom, I wasn't able to lift my youngest in and out of the crib.

—*Jenni*

Managing Medication

Consider the following tips to manage your medication, control your pain, and maintain a level of comfort as you recover:

- Take it when you need it. It's more effective to keep a level amount of pain medication in your system than to wait until your pain becomes unmanageable.
- Be prepared. In the first week or two after surgery, your pain may wake you up during the night. Time your medication so you have one dose just before you go to bed. Keep water and saltines or graham crackers by your bed so you won't have to get up (or wake someone else) to take your medicine.

- Taper off. When you begin feeling less pain, you can begin to wean yourself gradually from your pain medicine: take one pill instead of two or a half instead of a whole. When you think you can tolerate something less, switch to Tylenol or another over-the-counter medication your doctor recommends.
- Combat constipation. Pain medications and decreased mobility may leave you irregular, and straining from constipation can cause hemorrhoids and stress abdominal incisions. Proactively increasing your daily fiber intake and staying well hydrated can minimize or prevent the problem. Iron promotes constipation—if you take a multivitamin, use one without iron until your bowels are back to normal. It's a good idea to avoid caffeine for a while. It's a diuretic, and losing fluids contributes to constipation. Frequent walking will also help restore your regularity. If your bowels refuse to cooperate, try a stool softener.
- Don't drive until you no longer take pain medication.
- Avoid alcohol. It exacerbates drowsiness from pain medication and can sometimes interfere with antibiotics.

Dealing with Drains

Surgical drains are soft plastic bulbs with thin, flexible tubing sutured under the skin near the incision (figure 14.1). When the bulb is compressed (the sides are squished together), the drain automatically suctions fluid from the body.

You'll be eager to get rid of these pesky contraptions; however, they aid healing by siphoning off fluids from the surgery sites. Consider what the postsurgical experience was like before someone invented these devices: all that fluid collected by drains would otherwise accumulate in the body, promoting swelling and infection and delaying healing. Until the early 1990s, patients stayed in the hospital until their drains were removed. Today, shorter hospital stays are emphasized and drains are managed at home.

Measuring and Emptying Your Drains

Before you leave the hospital, a nurse will show you how to correctly empty the drains and provide a measuring cup and a daily log to record the amount of fluid collected. You should measure the contents and empty the drains a few

FIGURE 14.1 Surgical drains collect fluids from incision sites.

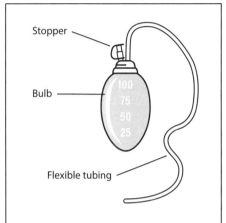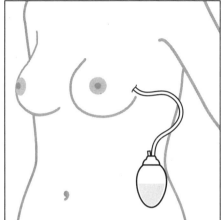

times a day, according to your surgeon's instructions. (This is a good job for your spouse or partner.) Here's what you'll do:

1. Wash your hands thoroughly with soap and water or sanitizing gel.
2. Unpin the drain from your clothing or remove it from your clothing pouch/pocket.
3. Strip the tube to remove any clots (stringy solids): Firmly but gently hold the tubing with one hand where it enters your skin. Press the sides of the tubing together, sliding the fingers of your other hand down the length of it to strip out the fluids and solids.
4. Open the plug at the top of the drain bulb and empty the contents into the measuring container. Be sure to squeeze the bulb to empty it. Note the color and characteristics of the fluid. Initially, it will be bloody, then yellowish, and finally clear. Notify your doctor if the fluid is cloudy, milky, or foul-smelling.
5. Record the time of day and the amount of fluid on the log provided by the hospital.
6. Squeeze the empty bulb flat to expel all the air. Close the plug to create the suction necessary to remove fluids from the incision.

Re-pin the drain to your clothing or place it back in your special pouch/pocket.

7. Flush the fluid down the toilet.
8. Repeat the process with each drain.
9. Rinse out the measuring container—never rinse the tubing; tap water can introduce bacteria—and cleanse your hands again.

Drains are more annoying than painful, but they can cause soreness where they enter the skin. You'll have one in each breast after a mastectomy, one in your armpit if lymph nodes are removed, and one or more at your donor site after an autologous procedure. You can minimize discomfort and awkwardness by immobilizing the drains as much as possible so they don't pull on your skin. Pin the plastic loop on top of each drain to your bra, the inside of your robe or shirt, or slip it over a belt to hold it away from the incision and keep it from swinging or catching on doorknobs or furniture. When you shower, pin the loops to a headband or long shoelace draped around your neck to keep the drains from swinging around. Always position drains just below your incision so they'll work properly. Call your surgeon if you have any telltale symptoms of infection in the skin around the drain tube.

Drains are effective, but they can be lumpy under clothing. Until they're removed, camouflaging your drains, if they make you self-conscious, with an oversized shirt or sweater is your best fashion strategy. Or simply pin your drains to your shirt or waistband. You can also search for "mastectomy drain garment" online, where you'll find plenty of options for camisoles, shirts, and other clothing to hold your drains. Two good examples designed by women who have had a mastectomy are the Marsupial (www.turnerhealth.com), a terrycloth belt with attachable drain pouches, and Pink Pockets (www.pink-pockets.com), peel-and-stick flannel pockets that adhere to any clothing to hold your drains (figure 14.2).

Your surgeon may remove some or all of the drains after several days, or they may need to stay longer, depending on the amount of drainage. Once the level of emptied fluid drops below 30 cubic centimeters (about 1 ounce) for two consecutive days, your surgeon will remove the drains by first snipping the sutures, then quickly pulling the tubing out of your skin. You can reduce any discomfort if you take a big breath and forcibly exhale as the surgeon pulls the tube out.

FIGURE 14.2 The Marsupial terrycloth belt (*left*) and Pink Pockets (*right*) comfortably hold surgical drains.

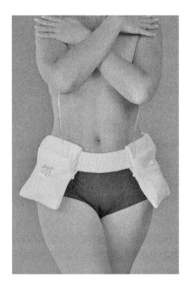 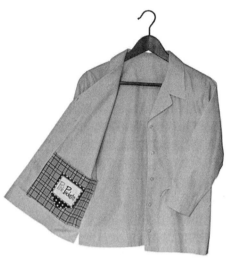

Image for the Marsupial provided by Tony Cane-Honeysett. Image for Pink Pockets provided by Diane LeBleu, Creator of Pink Pockets

Drains were the worst part of my reconstruction. One wouldn't have been so bad, but I had four: one at each breast and two in my hips. One day the tubing caught on a doorknob as I walked by, and it yanked sharply against the incision. That hurt!

—*Kate*

My husband took me to the mall to find a top that would accommodate my drains. I assured him I would be fine, and then I proceeded to get myself stuck inside a blouse while I was alone in the dressing room. I couldn't lift my arms. All I could do was sit on the chair and alternate between laughing and crying. At least 20 minutes went by before I was able to find the perfect amount of yoga, finesse, and frustration to free myself from the shirt. I zipped myself and my drains back into my hoodie and went home to my pillows.

—*Kari*

Tips for an Easier Recovery

Much of your recovery depends on your actions. First and foremost, be relentless in taking care of yourself. Until you recover, you can't return to your roles as mom, spouse, partner, wage-earner, or caretaker. You have one priority now, and that is to heal. *You* have to be number one—not the job, family, or anyone else. You can't expect to come home from the hospital and immediately ramp up to normal speed. You needn't treat yourself like an invalid; just don't overdo it. Be aware of "patient burnout," a malaise that can come out of the blue when you feel sick and tired of being sick and tired, frustrated that you can't do all the things you want to, and you just want to be normal again.

Caring for Your Incision(s)

Initially, treat your incisions with care: Check on them often and keep them warm and dry. Don't smoke, vape, or use tobacco products, which can delay healing. Resist applying lotions, oils, creams, or powders to a healing incision, except something that your physician recommends. Some swelling and/or bruising is to be expected and should improve as the incision heals. Notify your surgeon right away if conditions along the incision and the surrounding area indicate infection (chapter 15):

- pus or cloudy fluid drains
- bleeding
- increased redness, swelling, or pain
- swelling that doesn't improve
- red streaks radiating outward from the incision
- fever over 101° or whatever level your surgeon dictates

Showering

Once your surgeon gives you the go-ahead to get your incisions wet, do so only in the shower. Avoid bathwater, ocean water, swimming pools, saunas, and hot tubs until cleared by your surgeon. For as long as you need to keep your incisions dry, adjust the showerhead so that the water doesn't beat on them. Stand with your back to the water (if you don't have incisions anywhere on the back of your body) or use a handheld showerhead. Be very careful because you may still be weak and your incision won't be completely healed. If you feel too tired to stand, try sitting on a shower chair or asking for help. Wash with gentle, unscented soap, and then lightly pat your incisions dry. Leave the surgical tape or glue in place until it falls off on its own or your surgeon removes it. If you had axillary lymph node dissection, be careful when shaving your underarm, which will be temporarily numb if the sensory nerves were irritated.

Getting In and Out of Bed

Be careful getting in and out of bed. Those simple, automatic movements we take for granted every day will initially be difficult. Think about how you're going to move before you do. Get into bed by first sitting on the edge and then slowly swinging your legs up. Cover your affected breast with one arm and leverage your position with the other. Move up the bed by scooting your behind from side to side until you're reclining against the pillows. To get out of bed after unilateral reconstruction, carefully roll onto your healthy side and use your unaffected arm to leverage yourself into a sitting position.

If you've had a bilateral mastectomy with or without reconstruction, use your legs and abdominal muscles to first bring yourself into a sitting position, and then swing your legs over the side. Plant your feet on the floor and slowly straighten your knees until you're standing. Entry and exit are trickier with an abdominal incision. You'll need someone to help you while you hold one arm over your chest and the other over your abdomen. Many women find it more comfortable to sleep in a recliner that can be easily repositioned. If your bedroom is upstairs, consider sleeping downstairs until you can easily manage the stairs.

The Art of Sleeping Comfortably

Rest and sleep allow your body to direct its resources toward healing, but finding a comfortable position once you get home can be easier said than done. You may be able to sleep on your side after a couple of weeks, but you'll need a bit longer before sleeping on your stomach. You need to sleep on your back or in a semi-upright position, as you did in the hospital, to keep pressure away from your healing breast tissue. This may feel a bit strange at first. One way to rest comfortably in bed is to make a nest of pillows. First, position a firm pillow against the headboard or wall—wedge pillows, a body pillow, or sofa cushions work well—then arrange more pillows in front of it to serve as a backrest. You may find that propping your body this way is more comfortable than lying flat. Once you're in bed, ask someone to reposition the pillows until you're comfortable.

Small pillows can provide extra support wherever you need it: between your knees, under your surgery-side arm (or both arms if you've had bilateral reconstruction), or neck. Elevate your knees after DIEP or TRAM surgery to relieve abdominal tension. A mastectomy pillow that goes underneath your arms and over your chest to protect your incisions can be wonderful. (Search online for "mastectomy pillow.") If you just can't get to sleep or stay asleep, ask your surgeon for a mild sleeping aid.

Sleeping exclusively on your back and spending so much time in bed can cause backaches. Carefully and gently stretch your back to keep it limber. Do isometric exercises in bed, first flexing the muscles along the spine and then releasing them in small concentrated movements. Shrug your shoulders and roll your neck gently from side to side. When you're out of bed, stand straight while you flex your spine, as if you're pushing it against a wall, and then pull it back toward you.

> My husband was afraid of rolling into me, so he slept in our guest room for six weeks after my reconstruction. It was the only time in our marriage when we slept apart, but it helped. I slept better, and he was close enough to hear me if I needed something during the night.
> —*Karina*

Compression Garments

After your surgery, wearing compression garments for several weeks helps to minimize swelling and bruising, accelerate healing, and keep your new breast in place as it heals. (Compression garments may also be required after fat grafting.) It's okay to remove these garments when you shower as long as you put them right back on afterward. Your surgeon will advise when you can switch from a surgical bra to a compression sports bra or a normal bra, and from an abdominal binder (if you had a DIEP, SIEA, or TRAM flap) to SPANX or another type of shapewear.

Diet and Nutrition

Giving your body the nutrition it needs is something you can do to support your recovery and improve your overall health. Focus on eating mostly whole foods, rather than prepackaged, processed, or fast foods. Include lean protein and healthy fats. Keep snacking and high-fat, high-sugar treats to a minimum. Read nutrition and ingredient labels and make good choices. Stay well hydrated to support healing tissue. If you're not sure where to begin, visit www.choose myplate.gov or speak with a nutritionist who can help you create an easy-to-follow plan.

— EXPERT INSIGHT —

How Diet, Fitness, and Smoking Affect Surgery

MINAS CHRYSOPOULO, MD

Wounds need a lot of energy to heal well. Patients need a healthy diet before and after surgery: protein, zinc, and vitamins A and C are crucial for wound healing. The importance of healthy nutrition is emphasized by the link between obesity and postoperative complications. Patients with obesity have thicker adipose (fat) layers with a poorer blood supply. The blood flow and the amount of vital nutrients and oxygen reaching healing tissues is, therefore, less robust. They have much higher rates of infection, wound-healing problems, and hematomas and seromas compared to patients who are not obese. Staying well-hydrated before and after surgery is very important, as dehydration causes the skin and soft tissues to become dry, which negatively impacts healing. Smoking can also prevent healing. Nicotine shrinks blood vessels, depriving tissues of the nutrients and oxygen required for healing. At best, this slows the wound-healing process; at worst, smoking can cause wounds to break down. Many smoking-cessation products contain nicotine and therefore also increase the risk of healing problems. Cigarette smoke contains carbon monoxide, which lowers the level of oxygen in the blood. Since oxygen is vital for healing, it's crucial to quit smoking and avoid all nicotine products before and after surgery to decrease the risk of healing complications. Finally, regular exercise before and after surgery (once cleared by your surgeon) boosts the immune system and is encouraged.

Encourage Healing

Help your body recover by not smoking or vaping, which impede healing. It's also a good idea to refrain from drinking alcohol because it thins the blood. Talk to your surgeon before you use marijuana or other recreational drugs. Listen to your body. Don't be afraid to say "no, thank you" or "not now" if you're not up to a visit or a telephone call. It's good to have time to yourself, to reflect, accept, and just be.

Remember to Breathe

Regularly perform the breathing exercise (or a similar method) described in chapter 12 to relax, reduce anxiety, and manage pain. Continue this practice throughout your recovery and even beyond anytime you feel the need to relax and refocus.

Restore Strength, Flexibility, and Mobility

Gentle, restorative movements that stimulate circulation and restore flexibility are extremely important after a mastectomy, with or without reconstruction, and even more so after radiation therapy. After surgery, it's important to do the right kind of movements, at the right time, and in the right way. Healing takes time, however, and it's important to take things slowly, gradually increasing your physical activity while your body heals. Here are some helpful resources for cancer survivors and postsurgical patients:

- The American Cancer Society website explains and illustrates postmastectomy exercises designed to restore range of motion and recondition your chest, arms, and shoulders (www.cancer.org/cancer /breastcancer/moreinformation/exercises-after-breast-surgery).
- Your YWCA, local hospital, or breast clinic may offer special instruction for postmastectomy rehabilitation.
- If you have difficulty regaining full mobility and range of motion in your arm(s) and shoulder(s), ask your physician for a referral to a physical therapist or certified exercise specialist who specializes in postmastectomy physiology and can create a special restorative exercise program for you.

How you move is just as important as how much you move. Carefully ease into any kind of exercise, avoiding movements that feel too strenuous. It may be helpful to do exercises after a shower when your muscles are warm and relaxed. The tightness across your chest and in your underarms will improve as you continue your exercise program. Begin cautiously, perform all movements gently and with awareness, and never stretch or pull to the point of pain. You might need to refrain from weight-bearing and more strenuous abdominal exercises for up to eight weeks or more after an autologous abdominal flap.

Yoga may condition your body before surgery, but many poses can aggravate your shoulders, arms, chest, or donor sites if they're performed before you've healed sufficiently. Once your surgeon says it's okay to begin or resume yoga—which could be six weeks or more after surgery—start with gentle poses that are most beneficial after a mastectomy and/or reconstruction. (Many yoga studios provide specially designed yoga classes with modified poses for cancer survivors.) Until that time, avoid Downward Facing Dog, handstands, neck postures, and poses that put pressure on sensitive muscles and tissue. Ditto with stretches that are too intense for the abdomen, thigh, hip, or elsewhere after autologous reconstruction. No matter what exercise or movement you do, if it feels weird, uncomfortable, or painful, don't do it.

Optimism Helps You Heal

Just three months after losing his legs in an accident on the track, IndyCar world champion Alex Zanardi was up and walking on artificial limbs. Zanardi said of his recovery, "The good thing is that I've turned the first page of that book. I've finished the first chapter. All of the others are very, very short." That's a positive outlook on recovery. If you can view your reconstruction with the same outlook—the worst is behind you—it will be easier to keep the endpoint in view.

While maintaining a positive outlook isn't always easy, it may help you get back into the swing of things more quickly after your surgery. While it may sound like a cliché, the healing power of positive thinking is widely recognized; so much so that many healthcare providers recommend developing a positive mental attitude to encourage recovery. Pessimism is stressful, hard on the body, and may weaken the immune system, while positive thoughts are believed to prompt physiological changes that strengthen the immune system and decrease pain. If you need help, a mental health specialist can help you:

- keep a positive frame of mind about your recovery
- stay focused on your outcome rather than the process
- be kind to yourself and remain patient during recovery
- realize that even though setbacks may occur, each day brings you closer to getting back to your "normal" life

Seeing Your New Breasts for the First Time

It's not unusual to have conflicting feelings about seeing your new breasts. You'll be expectant and hopeful, waiting to see the outcome of several months of planning, surgery, recovery, and waiting. You may feel anxious about what you'll see as you look down at your chest or into a mirror. The reconstruction photos you saw during your research are no longer important because this is real and personal. These are your breasts, not someone else's. Initially, your breasts may be bruised and swollen and not look the way you'd hoped they would. Don't be surprised if your surgeon proclaims your breasts to be beautiful. Being far more used to this than you are, your surgeon is able to see beyond the swelling and redness to visualize the outcome. Remember that you're a work in progress. This isn't what you'll look like several months or a year from now when you're fully healed and your scars have faded. You've suffered a very personal loss. Give yourself time to come to grips with it and grieve for it, if that feels right. The recovery process is temporary. Hang in there, and know that the worst is behind you.

When I first saw my reconstructed breasts, I burst into tears. They were horrible! My doctor smiled and said my two little ugly ducklings would grow up to be beautiful swans, and he was right. Nine months later, when I look at my breasts now it is hard to imagine they had such an ugly beginning.

—*Holly*

Chapter 15

Dealing with Unexpected Problems

My scar had a big pucker right in the front of my breast. In about 20 minutes, my surgeon reopened the incision, cut away the scar tissue, and sewed it back up. It felt tight for a few weeks, and then it healed and looked better than before.

—DONNA

Unexpected complications and setbacks can develop after any surgery, and breast reconstruction is no exception. While breast reconstruction rarely fails, complications are not uncommon. The fact is, plenty of women who have breast reconstruction have to deal with related problems. Some are temporary bumps in the reconstructive road that are easily improved or resolved; others may require more management, and in some cases, another surgery. Although serious issues are uncommon, any type of surgery carries risk. When problems linger beyond recovery or become severe, corrective steps can and should be taken. You don't have to live with these issues. Most often, they can be resolved during revision surgery or in your surgeon's office. Complications specifically related to expander, implant, and autologous reconstruction are discussed in chapters 6 through 9. This chapter explains common issues that are inherent with surgery.

Inherent Risks of Surgery

Your risk for postoperative problems is greater after more invasive procedures: a mastectomy more so than a lumpectomy, and a mastectomy with breast reconstruction more than a mastectomy alone. Longer autologous surgeries are more likely to have issues than shorter implant procedures. Although most people experience none of these issues after a mastectomy or reconstruction, one or more problems may develop.

Seroma

A *seroma* is similar to a hematoma but involves an accumulation of clear fluid rather than blood under the skin. Seromas are less likely with surgical drains and compression garments; they do sometimes develop soon after surgical drains are removed. Small seromas often resolve on their own as the body resorbs them. Larger seromas can cause significant swelling—you may even hear fluid sloshing when you move. These symptoms may be accompanied by pain, skin discoloration, warmth, or redness. Untreated seromas can harden and become infected, requiring antibiotics. You may need another surgical drain for a few days or your surgeon may need to drain the site with a needle and a syringe if the excess fluid isn't eventually resorbed. If the problem area grows large enough to restrict oxygen supply to the tissue, it may require surgical repair. If you've had an implant procedure and the fluid continues to build up, you might need to have the implant removed and later replaced.

Infection

Skin is the body's natural barrier to infection. Anytime it's opened—with a cut, scratch, or incision—infection has an opportunity to sneak in. Hospitals have well-established protocols to reduce the likelihood of infection. Precautionary procedures (such as maintaining a sterile operating environment, keeping incision sites meticulously clean, and dispensing antibiotics through your IV) help protect you during your surgery. When identified early, most infections respond well to antibiotics. Broader infections can be more difficult and may delay healing. Hospitalization, intravenous antibiotics, and possibly additional surgery to drain off excess fluids may be required for infections that progress. You're more susceptible to infection if you smoke, have diabetes, are obese, or have reduced immune function.[1] Infection is of particular concern when you have tissue expanders or implants, which can become contaminated by bacteria in the bloodstream and lead to capsular contracture. For this reason, some plastic surgeons recommend taking preventive antibiotics before any subsequent invasive procedures, including colonoscopy, cosmetic surgery, and even dental work, including teeth cleaning.

Treating infections that occur with implant-based reconstruction usually involve removing the implant and *debriding* (removing unhealthy tissue) from the pocket, and placing a surgical drain there, followed by a course of antibiotics. A new implant or an autologous reconstruction can be done several weeks later. Infections that develop after autologous reconstruction generally respond well to antibiotics, with no need to return to the operating room. Contact your surgeon immediately if you develop signs of infection: swelling, breast pain, fever, warmth or redness at the incision site, or a discharge from the incision.

My plastic surgeon initially planned to fill the tissue expanders a little after my mastectomy so I wouldn't be completely flat when I woke up. When she attempted to fill them, the breast skin on the right side began to die, so she removed the saline on that side. A week later, I had my first debridement surgery, but the incision popped open again the following week. After another debridement, the incision stayed closed, but my back, stomach, and scar line became red. My entire breast was also red and swollen. I had a cellulitis infection and needed two strong antibiotics for ten days. Then fluid began to leak from my scar, and the surgeon had to remove the expander.

—*Marti*

Delayed Wound Healing

Some people require more time to heal than others, particularly when a weakened immune system or chronic health problem leads to *delayed wound healing*. The incisions of diabetics and smokers, for instance, often take more time to close after surgery than non-diabetics and non-smokers.[2] Slow-healing wounds can often be treated with dressings. If the incision refuses to close, *negative pressure wound therapy* may be used. This involves sealing a special bandage over the wound and attaching it to a gentle vacuum pump that encourages healing by drawing out fluid and infection and pulling the edges of the wound together.

Infection slows the healing process, so take every precaution to prevent it. Keep the area around your incisions scrupulously clean and wash your hands frequently. Your body expends copious amounts of energy during the healing process. You can promote healing by staying hydrated to support blood circulation to the wound and eating a daily variety of nutritious foods, including sufficient protein, healthy mono- and polyunsaturated fats, and antioxidant-rich foods that supply plenty of vitamins.

Bleeding

Excessive bleeding is unlikely, particularly when incisions are made with electrocautery tools that use high-voltage electrical current to cut through soft tissue and seal blood vessels. Still, it's important to heed your surgeon's caution to temporarily discontinue vitamins, herbs, supplements, and medicines that thin the blood. A damaged blood vessel may leak into the surrounding tissue, forming a *hematoma*. Symptoms include pain, a feeling of fullness at the leakage site, and skin that appears dark, as though it's bruised. Your surgeon will want to monitor any hematoma closely because if it grows too large, it could compress tissues and prevent oxygen from reaching the skin, potentially causing infection, a wound that opens or leaks fluid or blood, or necrosis. A hematoma that isn't resorbed may require surgery to reopen the incision, drain the pooled blood, and reseal the blood vessel. You're at higher risk for a hematoma if you have a bleeding disorder or hypertension. Hematomas can also develop if excessive pressure is put on the breast too soon, such as if you compress it too tightly, bump it, or massage it too vigorously.

Blood Clots

A blood clot can be particularly dangerous if it develops in a deep vein in a leg during or after surgery. This *deep vein thrombosis (DVT)* can be serious if a piece of the clot breaks loose and travels to your lungs. This is called a *pulmonary embolism* and it can be life-threatening. Fortunately, the potential for DVT is typically well-managed and the risk related to breast reconstruction is low.[3] Patients are carefully screened for risk factors before surgery, and after surgery, standard practices, including sequential compression devices, encourage blood flow. Frequent walking throughout the day offsets the inactivity during and immediately after surgery, which increases the risk of developing DVT.

Those at higher risk include individuals who are obese, older than age 65, under general anesthesia for more than three hours, have longer hospital stays, or have had a previous surgery 30 days before breast reconstruction. If you're in this category, your surgeon will discuss whether you should receive blood-thinning medication during and after surgery and whether an implant reconstruction is a better option for you. If you're taking tamoxifen, which increases the risk of blood clots, your surgeon may advise you to stop taking it for a week or two before your operation. You shouldn't interrupt or discontinue taking your medication without talking with your oncologist.

Necrosis

Breast skin is fragile after a mastectomy. If it's exceptionally thin after the breast tissue is removed or too many blood vessels that feed the skin are damaged or severed during surgery, it may die from *necrosis*, which is a lack of blood supply. Your surgeon needs to know about this right away. Depending on the extent of the problem, your surgeon may advise a wait-and-see approach or recommend a massage for several weeks to soften the area. A small area of necrosis involving the top layer of skin with healthy skin below (indicating a hearty blood supply) may peel away and heal on its own or it can be surgically removed. If you have tissue expanders, releasing some of the saline may reduce the tension on your skin, giving it "breathing room" to heal.

Your surgeon may apply a topical nitroglycerin ointment to dilate the arteries and veins feeding the skin to increase blood flow. Sessions in a *hyperbaric oxygen therapy* chamber are another way to promote healing for small areas of necrosis. (This treatment is similar to the method of treating deep-sea divers who have decompression sickness.) You breathe pure oxygen in the pressurized space, which your blood then carries to the wound. A larger area of necrosis usually must be removed and may need to be replaced with a skin graft (skin transferred from elsewhere on your body). Your implants or autologous flap may also need to be removed if your breast becomes infected.

A more serious, although less common, problem is the death of a significant portion of the breast skin or an entire tissue flap. Skin that turns black, indicating that all layers of the skin have died, must be removed. In this case, an expander or implant would be exposed to infection and need to be removed. (A layer of acellular dermal matrix beneath the skin may help salvage some implant reconstructions.) Should an entire autologous flap die, which is uncommon, it would also need to be removed. This would require a healing period of several months before a new reconstruction with an implant or another flap could be performed. Risk factors for necrosis include smoking, increased age, being very overweight, and having thin skin or circulatory problems. Previous radiation to the chest or breast also increases the risk of necrosis after a mastectomy.

> My nipple-sparing mastectomy with reconstruction went well. My
> nipples looked good and didn't hurt, but my doctor said some of the
> tissue was dying—about half of the nipple and areola were necrotic—
> so I needed a few sessions in a hyperbaric oxygen chamber. My nipples
> healed after half a dozen sessions. They're a different color and look,
> and I'm okay with that.
>
> —Joanna

> My right DIEP reconstruction was beautiful; my left side was less
> cooperative due to a compromised blood supply. After a lengthy operation and another surgery the following day to try to connect the flap
> artery to a blood vessel in my underarm, my plastic surgeon said we'd
> have to wait and see how my left breast fared. After eight weeks, some of
> the tissue lived and some did not. Compared to my natural-looking
> right breast, my left breast was small, hard, and lumpy; they were far
> from a matching set. During an outpatient surgery, the dead flap tissue
> was cut away, and I was fitted with an expander. I am still waiting before
> exchanging it for an implant. Though I never thought I'd focus so much
> attention and time on my boobs, I realize that in the big picture, fifteen
> months of surgeries, healing, and waiting is not long at all. I waited
> longer for my youngest to sleep through the night when he was a baby!
>
> —Jenni

Lingering Pain

Even though most postreconstruction discomfort gradually disappears, some people experience pain or muscle spasms after their incisions have healed. There's a big difference between ordinary discomfort as healing progresses and subsequent chronic or intense pain. And though you may be content to live with cosmetic flaws, you should always seek help for unrelenting pain. Aside from interfering with your physical, emotional, and psychological well-being, it hinders your immune system's ability to fight disease and infection. Persistent pain can be caused by scar tissue, hematoma or seroma, chemotherapy, or radiation treatment. A lack of appropriate reconditioning may also be the cause. A cycle of pain may continue, for example, when you don't properly rehabilitate your arm and shoulder after surgery: it hurts, you don't use it, it gets worse.

Postmastectomy pain syndrome (PMPS) isn't always discussed as a potential risk of breast surgery, even though it's estimated to affect between 20 and 30 percent of people who have a lumpectomy or mastectomy.[4] Defined as "chronic pain in the anterior aspect of the thorax (the front of the body between the neck and the abdomen), axilla, and/or upper half of the arm beginning after a mastectomy or quadrantectomy and persisting for more than three months after the surgery," PMPS is chronic *neuropathic pain*.[5] It results when nerves that provide sensation to the chest wall, shoulder, upper arm, or underarm are severed or damaged during a lumpectomy or mastectomy. Symptoms may include mild, moderate, or intense burning, throbbing, or tingling in the arm, shoulder, surgical scar, or chest wall. Some women experience shooting pain or itching that can't be satisfied. PMPS may eventually disappear or never go away. Some evidence suggests that psychosocial factors (such as anxiety, interrupted sleep, and assuming the worst will happen) may increase the risk for persistent postmastectomy pain.[6] It can develop immediately or months after any type of breast surgery, but symptoms are more likely to occur after

- a mastectomy
- a lumpectomy that removes tissue from the underarm or the upper outside portion of the breast
- an axillary lymph node dissection (not sentinel lymph node biopsy)
- poorly controlled pain during and immediately after surgery
- radiation therapy after a lumpectomy

PMPS isn't well studied, and regrettably, it's not fully understood or acknowledged. Too often, it can be erroneously diagnosed as ordinary postsurgical pain. It's often identified with a physical exam, testing, and imaging to rule out other potential causes. With no widely accepted standards of definition, criteria for diagnosis, or management guidelines, PMPS can be challenging to treat. Fortunately, the number of women who develop PMPS has declined, possibly because fewer women need axillary lymph node dissection.[7] If you develop unrelenting pain after your surgery, don't give up or tell yourself that you must learn to live with it. You may need a trial-and-error process to find a solution that works. A neurologist can make a correct diagnosis and prescribe the best path forward. If pain persists, ask for a referral to a pain specialist, preferably someone who has experience identifying and treating PMPS. Treatment might include a variety of approaches, including combinations of the following:

- analgesics
- cortisone or anesthetic injections
- acupuncture
- nerve blocks
- fat grafting[8]
- nonsteroidal anti-inflammatory drugs (NSAIDs)
- opioids
- antidepressants and anti-seizure medications
- cognitive-behavioral therapy
- targeted physical therapy, including massage
- regular exercise to release endorphins that block pain signals to the brain
- meditation

Improving Scars

Scarring is a natural part of the body's healing process and an unavoidable side effect of surgery. Tissue scars when the *epidermis*, the outer layer of skin, is damaged—like when you badly burn your finger or get a deep cut. When the *dermis*, the thick tissue beneath the epidermis, is affected—as when a surgical incision is made—the body produces a connective tissue protein called *collagen* to fill in the gaps. It's the body's version of spackle that forms the scar. Scars look different from the rest of your skin because collagen has no sweat glands or pores. When too much collagen is produced, the result is a thicker, more prominent scar.

Why does your friend's mastectomy or donor site scar look better than yours? The appearance of a scar is determined by your age, genetics, ethnicity, the depth of the wound, and how the incision and underlying tissues are sewn together. If you smoke or have poor circulation, inhibited blood flow at the incision site may result in a more obvious scar. Any scars you have from previous surgeries or wounds are a good indication of how your reconstruction scar will heal. What can you do to minimize unsightly scars? Here are a few suggestions to promote healing to make them smoother, flatter, and less noticeable:

- Leave the wound alone. To keep the scar line as thin as possible, try not to fuss with your healing incision or pick at the surgical tape or glue that holds the edges together. Avoid lifting, bending, pulling, or any movement that stretches or puts tension on the incision site, which delays healing and causes scars to widen and stretch.
- Give it time. Mastectomy and reconstruction scars are hard to ignore after surgery, and they never disappear. Most fade to pink after two to three months as collagen and new blood vessels heal the incisions. Scars become thinner white lines in a year or so—it takes that long to heal completely—and eventually fade into the breast skin. On some individuals, scars remain deeply pigmented, bumpy, or raised; in others, they're barely visible.
- Moisturize. A moist wound heals better than a dry wound; but never moisturize a fresh incision, which may invite infection and make the scar worse. Read labels to avoid products that include preservatives, fragrance, or alcohol, which dry the skin. Vitamin E oil may be an adequate moisturizer, but no solid evidence shows that it improves scarring. Your surgeon will advise when you can begin to moisturize and the best products to use and avoid.
- Massage the scar line. Gently rub lotion or cream into the scar with your fingertips helps to stretch and break down fibers beneath the skin. (The lotion makes it easier for your fingertips to glide across your skin.) Begin with a light touch and then progress to deeper and firmer massage, applying pressure along the length of the scar, then across it (figure 15.1). Massage deeply but not to the point of pain. Roll the scar between your fingers each day to keep the tissue soft. Do this two to three times daily for 10 minutes.

- Apply a topical silicone scar management product. When your incisions close, use a scar management product as recommended by your surgeon. Over-the-counter silicone-based sheets and gels won't eliminate scars, but they can improve redness and flatten raised areas. These products must be used consistently—10 to 18 hours a day for several months—for them to have an effect.
- Nourish your body with adequate vitamin C and zinc. Both aid in wound healing and vitamin C also stimulates collagen production. Taking a good multivitamin that includes both should do the trick, or add several servings of citrus, green leafy vegetables, and foods that are high in protein to your daily diet.
- Protect your scars from ultraviolet light. Scars may darken and become hard if exposed to sunlight or tanning beds during the first year after surgery as your tissue heals. Even indirect sun exposure can adversely affect their appearance. Apply a sunblock of SPF 30 or higher with UVA and UVB protection and reapply frequently.
- Re-excise the scar. Surgery can't remove a scar, but it can make it less noticeable.

FIGURE 15.1 Massaging along the scar line (when your surgeon gives you the okay) will leave your scar flatter and more supple. It also helps to moisturize the scar, which helps the healing process and reduces itchiness.

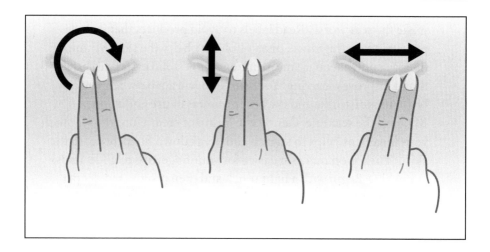

Some people develop large *hypertrophic scars* that rise above the level of the surrounding skin and remain painful or tender. *Keloids* are thick scars that spread into the skin around the incision. Although anyone can develop keloids, they're more common in dark-skinned individuals. (If other family members develop keloids, you're more likely to have them as well.) Let your surgeon know if you're prone to problem scarring so that a different type of suture can be used, which may help. Applying silicone sheeting or gel as soon as an incision is fully healed can also help to prevent or minimize hypertrophic scars and keloids. One or more of the following treatments may be used to reduce the size and improve the appearance of hypertrophic scars and keloids:

- dermabrasion
- laser surgery
- steroid injections
- cryosurgery (extreme cold)
- pressure therapy (with a device worn for several months)
- fat grafts
- excising (removing) the scar and reclosing the incision
- superficial, low-dose radiation therapy

My mastectomy scar is horrible and thick. Even though my doctor revised it, three years later, it's still pretty bad. I knew that was a possibility because I've never scarred well, even from minor cuts. My doctor said it's as good as it's going to get.

—*Jean*

Lymphedema

Removing or radiating axillary lymph nodes creates a lifetime risk of lymphedema—pronounced swelling in the shoulder, arm, or hand on the side of the body that is treated. Chemotherapy, which can scar lymphatic vessels, may also interrupt the lymph system.

Your risk for lymphedema is higher if you have lymph nodes removed *and* radiation therapy; the risk is lower after a sentinel node biopsy. There's no way to predict who will or won't develop lymphedema. It may appear soon after a lumpectomy or a mastectomy, or months or even years later. Lymph nodes that can no longer drain fluid effectively may cause swelling in the arm that may be almost unnoticeable, like fluid retention during your menstrual period. The affected arm may feel heavy, painful, tight, or numb. In extreme cases, the arm becomes enlarged from shoulder to fingertips.

Lymphedema is a chronic condition; it can't be cured. When treated early, however, lifelong management with compression bandages and sleeves, special exercises, and therapeutic massage that gently shifts lymph fluid so that it drains is the best management option. The National Lymphedema Network (www.lymphnet.org) provides information and support for this condition.

Prevention is the best defense. Surgeons who use *axillary reverse mapping* to identify underarm lymph nodes before surgery can identify and remove lymph nodes that drain the breast, which allows them to preserve lymph nodes that drain the arm. This procedure requires additional training and isn't widely used, but may become more common as a result of clinical trials.

It's important to learn how to reduce your risk of lymphedema. Contact your doctor at the first sign of swelling, even mild swelling, in your arm or chest after breast surgery. (Rings or sleeves that suddenly become too tight may be early indications of lymphedema.) If lymphedema develops, request a referral to a certified lymphedema specialist who can show you how to manage it so that it doesn't progress.

My arm, hand, and fingers began to swell right after my mastectomy. I couldn't bend my wrist or straighten my arm all the way, and it throbbed constantly. It was impossible to hold or carry my baby. I suffered for several months until my doctor sent me to a physical therapist who taught my husband how to do a special massage. We've made this a part of our daily routine. I feel better and my husband is happy he can do something to help. The lymphedema is still there; at least it's manageable now.

—*Skye*

Reconstruction Do-Overs

Sometimes revisions aren't enough to fix what's wrong. Although most women don't repeat their reconstruction, it's sometimes done when a reconstruction fails, produces unacceptable results, causes chronic pain, causes unsatisfactory scarring, or is a poor match for the opposite breast after unilateral reconstruction. Do-over surgeries remove the initial reconstruction and leave the chest

Surgeries to Improve Lymphedema Symptoms

You may be a candidate for lymphedema surgery if your condition doesn't respond to conventional, nonsurgical treatment or it progresses to an advanced stage. While the following procedures don't eliminate lymphedema, they may make it more manageable by reducing the amount and frequency of compression management needed. It's important to choose a surgeon who has experience performing these procedures.

- *Lymphatic bypass* restores healthy lymph flow by rerouting and reconnecting damaged lymph vessels to healthy blood vessels.

- *Vascularized lymph node transfer* replaces damaged or missing lymph nodes with healthy nodes from elsewhere in the body. This procedure can be performed simultaneously with DIEP flap breast reconstruction to replace axillary lymph nodes that were previously removed with healthy lymph nodes from the groin.

- *Lymphatic debulking* removes excess skin and fibrous scar tissue in patients with advanced lymphedema. The overall volume of the affected tissue may be reduced with liposuction as an outpatient procedure or with surgery. Compression garments are still needed after surgery.

flat or replace the breasts with a second reconstruction. Having another reconstruction might happen after you've had a chance to heal or years later. Deciding in favor of a total "do-over" can be a decision you easily make; you might be so disappointed or uncomfortable with the reconstructive results that you're willing to go flat or try a different procedure. For some women, though, the decision to endure another surgery and recovery can be agonizingly difficult. You don't necessarily need to return to the surgeon who performed your initial reconstruction. It's a good idea to seek opinions from a couple of other reconstructive surgeons. Your insurance should cover the cost of your re-do procedures, but it's always wise to check with your health insurer before you proceed with surgery. Because autologous reconstruction rarely fails, secondary reconstruction more often removes breast implants, which are more likely to develop issues or fail.

Explant to Flat
Women who have repeated infections, capsular contracture, malfunctions, or concerns about breast implant illness or BIA-ALCL may feel that enough is enough and have an explant surgery to remove their implants. If they don't want to try autologous reconstruction, the implants and surrounding scar tissue are removed, and the incision is closed with an aesthetic flat closure.

Explant to New Implant
People who have explantation often want to try implants of a different size, style, shape, or fill. Replacing an implant may also involve changing from subpectoral to prepectoral or vice versa.

Explant to Autologous Flap
Some women who are dissatisfied with their implant reconstruction or experience implant failure—whether it's from infection, capsular contracture, or another issue—have autologous reconstruction. In a single surgery, the implant is removed, and a new breast is reconstructed with the person's own tissue.

When I decided to have a prophylactic nipple-sparing double mastectomy due to my *BRCA1* gene mutation, I met with some of the best plastic surgeons. Perhaps because I was thin or maybe because the surgeons I selected were more expert at implants, I never contemplated and was never offered any reconstructive options other than implants. My concerns over having a double mastectomy and the changes it would make to my body were far less than my worry of potentially getting cancer. I had the surgery. It left me with round, perky breasts that fit my body nicely. I was grateful and never had any regrets.

For many years, my implants gave me back the breasts that were taken away but I looked better than I felt. My implants were under my pectoralis muscles, which was standard of care at the time. They pulled not only at my chest muscles, but also the muscles in my upper back. The implants progressively became harder and less comfortable. I did a good deal of research, learned about different options, and spoke with women who had chosen other types of reconstruction. After meeting with several plastic surgeons, I felt I had two good choices: have new implants placed over the pectoralis muscles or replace my implants with tissue from my upper buttocks—an SGAP autologous flap. (I wasn't a candidate for a DIEP flap.) While this surgery is more complicated and would scar my upper buttocks, it also offers many benefits.

After careful consideration, I selected an incredibly kind and skilled surgeon and had the SGAP procedure. My 13-year-old implants were removed and replaced with warm, living tissue from my tush. My recovery went more smoothly than I could have imagined and eight months after my surgery, I am so happy with the decision I made. The muscles in the front of my chest, as well as in my upper back, remain where they are meant to be and no longer feel strained. My breasts are soft, and they look and feel natural, and I will never need to have them replaced again. For the second time, I feel grateful and have no regrets.

—*Karen*

Autologous Flap to Flat

On the rare occasion when an entire flap must be removed due to infection or necrosis, women may choose to forego further reconstruction and instead go flat. The flap is removed—akin to performing another mastectomy—and the incision is closed.

Autologous Flap to New Autologous Flap

A tissue flap reconstruction that fails can be replaced with a different autologous flap if that's what the individual prefers. The new flap must be taken from a different donor site than the one that provided the initial flap.

Autologous Flap to Implant

When an autologous flap must be removed, a second reconstruction using breast implants can be performed. If the implants are placed over the muscle, there's no need to create a submuscular pocket. Tissue expansion may be required if the implant is placed under the chest muscle.

Strategies for Minimizing Complications

While you can't eliminate all possibility of postrecovery complications, taking a few precautions beforehand will help minimize your chances of developing issues and cosmetic flaws.

Choose the Most Experienced Plastic Surgeon You Can Find

The skill and experience of your plastic surgeon greatly influences the outcome of your reconstruction. Chapter 18 provides tips for selecting a surgeon.

Manage Your Expectations

Go into surgery with realistic expectations of your outcome, so you won't be surprised when your breast sits too high on your chest or it doesn't match the opposite side. For example, if you decide to proceed with implant reconstruction even though your surgeon warns you of the possibility of complications related to thin or damaged skin after radiation therapy, understand that you have an increased risk of delayed wound healing, necrosis, reoperation, and other complications.

Give Yourself Adequate Time to Heal

Be patient until you're fully healed, because many problems eventually resolve themselves. Reconstructed breasts improve over time. Your reconstruction and scars will look considerably better after a year than they do just two or three months after surgery. What is now a misshapen or asymmetrical breast may be fine once the swelling disappears and your breast settles.

Decide What's Acceptable and What's Not

We are our own harshest critics. Subtle flaws in your breast that are all but invisible to your partner may be objectionable to you. (It's interesting to note that many women who are unsatisfied with their reconstructed breasts say their husband or partner thinks they're just fine.) You might decide you can live with the tiny bulge in your new breast or the wide scar on your abdomen, or you might consider one or both situations unacceptable. After recovery, perhaps you'll feel that you just can't face yet another procedure, and you're willing to accept what you have as good enough. Or you may want to keep trying to correct flaws that are irksome to you.

Take Action

There's no need to suffer in silence. Acknowledging a problem is the first step in improving or correcting it. Though the thought of additional appointments, procedures, and even minor recovery may be unsettling, discuss your dissatisfaction with your surgeon. Your surgeon has likely seen and heard it all before and can determine whether the problem is likely to run its course or deserves additional attention. If your surgeon approached the initial reconstructive process enthusiastically but isn't keen about handling problems after the fact, look for another opinion if you're unhappy with that response to your concerns.

Address Lumps, Bumps, and Bulges

Although a lump is the last thing a cancer patient wants to find in a new breast, it's not uncommon to find a small lump in a reconstructed breast, particularly after flap reconstruction or fat grafting. Discovering a hard spot can be unnerving, especially if you've already been through the breast cancer experience. Most often, it's a bit of fat that has hardened or died. It might also be a suture *granuloma*, scar tissue that forms around the internal sutures that close incisions. Most sutures used for a mastectomy and reconstruction are dissolvable, although your body may have different ideas about that. It will react to any foreign material, even tiny sutures. You may notice a "spitting suture" along your incision; that's a stitch that pokes out through a little bump in the skin. It needs to be removed because once exposed to the air, it may collect bacteria and cause an infection. Your surgeon can easily extract it.

Understand What Can Be Changed and Accept What Cannot

Some problems cannot be fixed. Surgeons can't restore full sensation or eliminate scars, and they may not be able to give you two identical or perfectly symmetrical breasts, especially if you've had radiation therapy. Revision surgery may improve the look of your breast, but it might not get it as close to perfect as you'd hoped. You can always get another opinion about what can be done but at some point, you may need to accept that your reconstruction is as good as it can be.

> Several months after my TRAM reconstruction, I developed what I called my third boob—an A-cup-size lump sticking out above my waistline. My doctor said it was the result of tunneling the flap up under the skin. It did finally shrink, but it took almost a year.
>
> —*B.J.*

Managing Depression, Anxiety, and Unsettled Emotions

Undesirable issues related to losing your breasts and having them recreated aren't always physical. Coping with the confusion, frustration, and uncertainty of a mastectomy with or without reconstruction can be difficult and disruptive. Changes to your appearance and self-image may shake your confidence and self-image and exacerbate existing mental health challenges. Though some days will be better than others, these feelings can wreak havoc on your well-being, life, work, and family. It's important to recognize and confront these feelings, just as you would other health issues before they become detrimental to your health. If you find it difficult to deal with disturbing emotions or they interfere or begin to influence your life, ask your doctor for a referral to a mental health professional who can help you to get back on track with therapy and/or medications. Even when you feel that you're in control and doing well, setbacks can occur. Be kind and patient with yourself when this happens.

Cultivate a Positive Outlook

Maintaining a positive outlook isn't always easy but it may help you get back into the swing of things more quickly after your surgery. It sounds like a cliché, but the power of positive thinking is well studied and supported by research, although it's unclear how or why a positive attitude helps people recover faster from surgery. It may be because compared to feeling anxious or worried, positive thoughts are believed to prompt physiological changes that strengthen the immune system and relieve pain. They also make you feel more in control of the situation. Researchers suspect that those of us who are more positive make better decisions about our health, while negative emotions can weaken immune system responses.

The healing power of positive thinking is widely recognized—so much so that many health experts recommend developing a positive mental attitude to help recovery after surgery. Try massage, music or art therapy, yoga, meditation, and other ways to lift your mood and lighten your spirit. If you need help to achieve and maintain a positive frame of mind about your surgery and recovery, a mental health specialist can help you to

- anticipate your recovery and achieve a more balanced outlook and life
- train yourself to adopt a positive outlook
- focus on what you can do, rather than what you can't
- smile more, even when you don't feel like it (Research shows that smiling lowers elevated blood pressure caused by stress.)
- give yourself a pep talk
- envision what you want to be doing and can do and keep these positive thoughts in mind

Recovering from surgery can be difficult because it temporarily interferes with your regular routine, keeping you from doing things that you want and

How You See Your Body Affects Your Risk of Complications

Researchers have known for some time that psychological factors can influence a person's overall health. One example is that your satisfaction or dissatisfaction with your body before reconstruction can affect how you heal. A small study found that women who had more negative feelings about their body image experienced a higher rate of infections and delayed wound healing after breast reconstruction. The risk of postoperative infection was greater among women who felt unattractive or had low self-confidence. Delayed wound healing was more prevalent in women who were dissatisfied with how they looked in the mirror unclothed and how their bras fit. Women who felt less accepting of their body and felt "less like other women" also had slow-healing wounds. Consulting with a trained therapist who can help you manage these feelings before your surgery may help you heal better, and with fewer problems.

Source: Lewis HC, Hart AL, Fobare A, et al. Preoperative body image factors are associated with complications after breast reconstruction. *Plastic and Reconstructive Surgery*. 2022;149(3):568–577.

need to do. Multiple research efforts link positive thinking and optimism to reduced symptoms, decreased pain, and less stress. Taking the "glass half full" approach—thinking positively instead of negatively—can help you weather recovery as well as possible. How do you do that?

- Try to think optimistically about your surgery: It's treating your breast cancer or reducing your risk for a diagnosis, rather than dwelling on its negative aspects.
- Focus more on the outcome than the process.
- Have confidence in your doctors, surgeons, and healthcare team.
- Be kind to yourself and remain patient as you heal.
- Realize that even though you may have setbacks, each day brings you closer to being fully recovered.

Questions for Your Surgeon

- What possible complications might develop during my surgery or recovery?
- How common are these problems?
- What signs of these issues should I watch for?
- What can I do to help myself recover?
- What can I do before and after my surgery to reduce the likelihood of problems?
- How will any complications be managed or resolved?

Chapter 16

Life after Reconstruction

My husband kept ignoring my reconstructed breast. I couldn't feel much there, but emotionally, it was important to me to include it in our lovemaking. When I mentioned this, he said he was afraid of hurting me. After we talked about it, we both felt relieved, like a huge barrier between us had been broken down.

—ALMA

At last, after months of doctors' appointments, treatment, surgeries, and recovery, your reconstruction journey is over. You've beaten cancer (or taken steps to prevent it), your new breasts are in place, and you're ready to move on. You may feel a wonderful sense of closure as you leave your plastic surgeon's office for the last time. Or you might be sad, particularly if you've come to regard your surgeon as a trusted friend. This isn't unusual. You've spent a lot of time together during your reconstruction, and now your emotional umbilical cord is about to be severed. Now what? Now you experience the sweet relief of returning to your pre-diagnosis life before the tests and treatments began.

Getting Back to Ordinary

It's often said that cancer is a journey. Sometimes we don't realize that until we reach the end of the process and look back. If only hindsight had arrived a little sooner! If you can view reconstruction that way—as an odyssey with an outcome—you'll fare better. When you're uncomfortable, uneasy, or fed up with the mastectomy and reconstruction ordeal, remember it isn't a life sentence. It's a finite experience with a beginning, middle, and end. You'll never forget your mastectomy and reconstruction, but eventually, personal and professional priorities that were shelved during the process will be restored, and your emotional and physical scars will heal. You'll return to a life without surgeons, weird sleeping positions, or checking your breasts throughout the day. Your surgeries and recovery will become distant memories.

It takes time to get used to the idea of losing one or both breasts. Sometimes it takes a lot of tears, too. Your new breasts will be very different from your natural breasts, and that takes some getting used to, even if they look the same. Most of us can't simply flick an emotional switch and go seamlessly from being patients to non-patients. If you're nagged by unease or depression that you just can't seem to shake, even when your reconstruction is completed, consider the following:

- Put your breast cancer and reconstruction in perspective. It's a bit of a platitude, but cancer does change your perspective. Treatment and reconstruction offer positives for those who are open to them.
- Reprioritize and learn—or re-learn—to appreciate life and all it offers. Separate the nickel-and-dime issues, like getting stuck in traffic or burning the toast, from truly serious matters. Figure out what's important in your life and move those things to the top of your priority list. Try not to feel guilty about items that sink to the bottom and don't get done.
- Don't hide from your feelings. Grief and angst come in all sizes. Some people are emotionally strong, taking mastectomy and reconstruction in stride with a Zen-like approach or an "I-don't-have-time-for-this" attitude. Others find it impossible to regain any sense of normalcy. It's okay—and healthy—to react in a way that's natural for you. At some point, though, you'll get tired of being angry, tired of being sad, and tired of having your life put on hold. The best therapy is to acknowledge your feelings and let 'em rip. Then dust off your emotional self and move forward.
- Turn off negative self-talk. It happens to the best of us: sooner or later those dark thoughts creep into our consciousness. When you catch yourself thinking negatively, replace gloomy thoughts with positive affirmations.

- Create an outlet for your emotions. Deal with your feelings before they begin controlling your life and send you into a downward spiral of adverse emotions. Talk to your partner, a trusted friend or family member, a clergyperson, or a local support group. Writing is also therapeutic. Try your hand at poetry or journaling, letting your uncensored thoughts flow freely onto the paper or computer screen.
- Focus on your postreconstruction life. Appreciate the loss you've suffered from your mastectomy but also consider the control you've gained over breast cancer.
- Ask for help. If negative thoughts persist and become more than a temporary funk, consider speaking with a mental health professional who can help you resolve troubling issues.

Realize That Friends Mean Well

Your friends will want the best for you, even when it may not seem that way. While most people you know will be nothing but supportive, some people have a difficult time dealing with illness, surgery, or recovery. Friends may not be able to look you in the eye without crying. You might find yourself comforting them, instead of the other way around. Others may be embarrassed as they struggle for the right thing to say. Some might be unable to accept the fact that you're fine, even after your recovery; they may continue to view you as a victim even when you've returned to your normal routine. Each time they see you, they may ask "How are you?" in a soft, sad voice. Don't be surprised if some folks can't seem to draw their eyes away from your chest. Many are curious about mastectomy and reconstruction. When they realize they're talking to your chest, they may become embarrassed. They're all trying to help in their own way. Just take a deep breath and realize they mean no harm.

Remember to Laugh

Mastectomy and reconstruction certainly aren't funny, but we can always find humor if we look hard enough. Laughter is powerful medicine. It releases endorphins, sending feel-good messages from the brain throughout the body. Studies suggest that laughter boosts the immune system and reduces pain. One little chuckle or a rollicking belly laugh releases lots of tension. Ever noticed how quickly kids rebound from sadness? It may have a lot to do with their capacity for laughter; they seem to laugh quite a bit more than adults. Find ways to laugh each day. Get inspired by exploring Laughter Yoga (www .laughteryoga.org), a combination of relaxation techniques, deep breathing, and laughing that helps to combat stress and anxiety.

Mend Your Mind, Body, and Spirit

Perhaps, like many breast cancer survivors, you feel a new lease on life—one that compels you to find a fresh balance between physical, emotional, and spiritual health. You may be determined to take better care of your body, not because anything you've done caused your breast cancer, but because living with disease gives us such profound gratitude for the bodies we have. For some, the breast cancer/mastectomy/reconstruction experience is reason to reassess or reaffirm beliefs. Perhaps you have a renewed conviction to travel, change jobs, or do many of the things you've always wanted to do but put on the back burner when life got in the way. It's good to look back and reflect. It's even better to look forward and embrace the future.

Consider Helping Someone Else

If you're inclined to share what you've learned from your breast cancer experience, you can help others who face the same issues that are now behind you. Whether you spend an occasional hour or get involved full time, you'll find plenty of opportunities to donate your time and insight.

- Let your oncologist, breast surgeon, and plastic surgeon know that you're happy to be a patient reference and speak with other patients who have questions about the mastectomy and reconstruction experience. Many women will welcome your insight as they consider their postmastectomy choices.
- Become a "Reach to Recovery" volunteer for the American Cancer Society.
- Volunteer at your local breast cancer center or support group. Take part in annual Breast Reconstruction Awareness Day activities.
- Donate or raise money for your local breast cancer organization. There are hundreds, if not thousands, of local fundraisers for breast cancer each year across the country. You'll find all kinds of

worthwhile opportunities to raise funds for the cause. Call your local ACS office or search the internet for "breast cancer charity" or "mastectomy support group" to find ways to make a difference.
- If you've inherited a high-risk genetic mutation or have a strong family history of cancer, consider becoming a FORCE volunteer.

Returning to Work

Returning to work is a significant step on the road back to normal. The workplace can be a positive and caring environment, depending on the level of closeness you share with your co-workers and how much they know about why you've been away. Your relationship with them will dictate how much you tell them about your diagnosis, treatment, and reconstruction. Many women consider their co-workers as extended family. Others prefer not to draw attention to themselves or be treated differently. If you would rather keep your experience private, when someone asks why you were away, you can simply say it was for health reasons, a family issue, or something similar.

You may need to ease back into the work routine, especially as long as the pressures and pace of a full day are too taxing. It all depends on the extent of your recovery and the nature of your job: you'll be able to return to an administrative job sooner than a job as a hospital nurse, a daycare center operator, landscaper, or other physically demanding positions. Perhaps you can work flexible hours or part-time until you're back up to speed. If your workplace is a source of stress and uneasiness, take time to consider how you'll deal with it before you return. You may need more time to recuperate if you feel mentally or physically fatigued.

Dating, Intimacy, and Sex

Your medical team gives you information about what to expect before and after surgery, but they may not explain how it might affect your intimate relationship with your spouse or partner. Whether you're single or married, you may worry about how your reconstructed breast will affect your romantic involvements. After months of treatment, surgeries, and recovery, you may feel disconnected from physical pleasure, and intimacy may feel awkward. Lingering effects of treatment can also take a toll on intimacy long after your stitches dissolve and your incisions heal. It can take time, effort, and patience to resolve these issues and get your love life back on track. Sharing the experience is important to your relationship and will make things easier for both of you.

Lost breast sensation takes some getting used to, particularly if your breasts previously took a starring role in the bedroom. You needn't give up the pleasure of your breasts, but you may need to redefine how you go about it. Even though your reduced or altered sensation may be disappointing, you can still enjoy your partner's touch if you concentrate on areas that still provide pleasure. Explore the "new girls" together, guiding your partner's fingertips over them and directing attention to the areas where you can feel touch, instead of where you don't.

Although you're the one who goes through reconstruction and recovery, your experience affects your partner as well. You may be perfectly comfortable in your postmastectomy body and eagerly slip back into the closeness you experienced before your mastectomy and reconstruction. For some women, it's not that easy. Your partner may assume you'll pick up your relationship where you left off, but it isn't always easy to emotionally snap out of it. Open communication will pave the way for the two of you to be more comfortable with your new breasts. It may be a difficult discussion but it's important to express your feelings and encourage your partner to do the same. Ask for patience if you need more time to become aroused; explain what feels good and what doesn't, rather than what your partner is doing wrong. If necessary, discuss how you can change your sexual repertoire to satisfy you both. Try not to assume that you're perceived as undesirable if your partner doesn't initiate intimacy; he or she may simply be afraid to hurt you or may feel rejected, particularly if you're emotionally distant. Your partner will probably take cues from your attitude and comfort level with your new breasts. If you're comfortable seeing and touching them, your partner probably will be, too.

Take Your Time

You've been through a lot. You may be eager to get your love life back to normal, or you may need more time to restore your sexual health. Allow yourself a period of adjustment to get back in the groove. Take it slowly if you feel shy, uncomfortable, or apprehensive. Rekindle your romantic relationship, letting it develop on its own. Spend time alone together, just being affectionate and doing things you love to do. When you don't feel "in the mood," concentrate on enjoying each other's company. Hold hands as you go for a walk. Start and end each day with a hug. Make time to share a soothing bath or a romantic dinner. Kiss and cuddle before you progress to the main event. Work toward being comfortable with the new you and let nature take its course. Talk to your doctor if you have vaginal dryness or loss of libido, which can be affected by chemotherapy and certain medications.

Seeing yourself with confidence and acceptance can be difficult when you don't look the same, you're unhappy with the shape or size of your new breasts, or you've lost or gained more weight than you like. You might be unhappy because your new breasts don't project the way your natural breasts did and your clothes might not fit in the same way. If you feel uneasy or insecure about your body when you're undressed, wear lingerie (a wide selection of sexy, lacy underwear is available after mastectomy with or without reconstruction). Or turn the lights down or off until you become more comfortable with your new breast. Progress at your own pace. Remember, the brain is the most powerful sexual organ we have. Intellectually, you probably know you're still more than the sum total of your breasts, but it may take a while to believe it. If you continue to feel uncomfortable with intimacy, consider joining a support group or seeking professional guidance; talking with a counselor may be all the help you need to get back to a satisfying relationship.

When Your Partner has a Problem

If your spouse or partner has been supportive throughout your mastectomy and reconstruction, you are truly blessed. Many women find their partners to be a constant source of reassurance, loving them for who they are instead of what's on their chest. If the two of you previously shared a strong bond, your relationship is more likely to weather the stress and emotional upheaval of a mastectomy and reconstruction. If your relationship was already weak, your treatment and reconstruction can bring you closer together or drive you further apart. Some partners are scared silly by the thought of cancer and surgery but hesitant to discuss their feelings. Others may react with denial, refusing to acknowledge your cancer and reconstruction. Some—hopefully, few—may wonder what the big deal is if you're able to have your breast recreated. Early on, ask your partner to accompany you to doctors' visits, participate fully in your research, and support you during recovery.

Navigating New Relationships

Dating presents an interesting dilemma. When and what do you tell your partner-to-be? "Nice to meet you. My left breast came from my belly" or "I'm finally getting my nipples done tomorrow!" may be a bit much when you're introduced. When should you speak up and how much should you say? There's no single right answer to these questions. The best approach is to rely on your instinct to know when the time is right. If your date happens to be talking about a relative's struggle with breast cancer, it might be a logical time to share your own experience. In other cases, it may not come up until it becomes very clear that your relationship is heading to the bedroom. Your comfort with the topic and how you feel about the other person will dictate when you talk about your experience and how much you say. That might be early on or later in your relationship.

I was 30 years old when I was diagnosed with stage 1 breast cancer. My aversion to risk was high. As a *BRCA2* mutation carrier who had already survived ovarian cancer, deciding to have a double mastectomy was relatively easy. Being a single woman, I was initially nervous at the thought of being nude in front of someone for the first time. Between the surgical scars and the capsular contracture from my new breast implants, I felt the need to "warn" my would-be partner before initial acts of intimacy. Talk of cancer too soon and the fear of potentially causing me physical harm scared off suitors. I recognized that if I wanted a different outcome, I would need help. This led me to seek the guidance of a counselor, and after some time I came to realize that I should be proud of my battle scars—I fought cancer twice and was victorious. My newly found confidence required me to not only stop apologizing for my body's differences but to learn to embrace them. My advice to other survivors is simple: cancer treatment requires the assistance of a physician. No one would ever dream of saying "toughen up" in response to a cancer diagnosis. Why should our mental health be any different? It's acceptable and even normal to feel depression or anxiety once the fight for survival has passed. Seeking the help of a professional allowed me to be more comfortable in my skin, which lead to a wonderful relationship with a man I married a couple of years later.

—Anne

Surveillance and Follow-Up after a Mastectomy

After a mastectomy, it's wise to remain vigilant, but you needn't live your life in fear. Recurrence is unlikely, but leftover cancer cells sometimes appear under the skin or on the chest wall. Alert your surgeon immediately if you find a suspicious area or lump in your reconstructed breast, so that the source of the problem—whether it is a calcification, a fragment of dead tissue, or a recurrence—can be identified. A small malignancy in the mastectomy scar or the skin is usually removed and then treated with radiation if that wasn't part of your original treatment. A larger tumor also needs to be removed, but it also indicates that the implant or tissue flap may also be removed. For most women, later reconstructing the breast again may be an option. Systemic therapies, including chemotherapy, may also be recommended.

Monitor Your Reconstructed Breast

Breast reconstruction doesn't affect breast cancer recurrence or new tumors, so it doesn't influence whether you should have continuing mammograms. Your mastectomy, however, does. Because you don't have enough remaining breast tissue to screen after a mastectomy, you no longer need routine screening mammograms of the affected side (or sides, if both breasts were removed). Continued mammograms are advised if you've had a subcutaneous mastectomy (an early type of nipple-sparing mastectomy that left breast tissue at the base of the nipple). Routine mammograms are also recommended after a lumpectomy because you retain most of your breast tissue.

Many surgeons recommend an annual clinical breast exam with a baseline mammogram or MRI after reconstruction, especially if you have a genetic mutation that raises your risk of breast cancer, so that any unusual area can be scanned and compared. If you have reconstruction with silicone implants, the FDA recommends periodic screening for a rupture with MRI or ultrasound five years after your implants are placed and every two to three years thereafter. (This recommendation may change, so it's a good idea to check with your surgeon about when you should be screened.) It's also wise to continue examining your breasts each month. Your doctor may order a diagnostic mammogram, ultrasound, or breast MRI if a lump, inflammation, or another area of concern is found in the skin or on the chest wall during a physical exam. If a medical professional has never shown you how to correctly perform a breast self-exam, ask your doctor or nurse to demonstrate.

Monitor Your Opposite Breast

If you've had one breast removed, it's important to have your remaining breast routinely screened with mammograms and/or breast MRI as recommended by your doctor.

Part V
Finding Answers,
Making Decisions

You've learned about mastectomy, the pros and cons of various reconstruction procedures, and what to expect before, after, and during your surgery. In this section, you'll find practical tips for five important related issues, including

- choosing your breast surgeon and plastic surgeon
- getting a second (and even a third) opinion about your reconstruction
- understanding health insurance coverage and payment issues, including how to appeal a denial
- a checklist for making decisions
- information for your family and friends

Chapter 17

Shopping for Surgeons

My surgeon put me at ease by patiently answering all my questions. He smiled a lot, spoke slowly, and explained several different ways the reconstruction might be done. I felt I was talking to a trusted friend.

—CAMERAN

You have a primary care physician who oversees your health, a team of medical professionals who coordinate your treatment, and specialists when you need them. When it comes to reconstruction, however, your plastic surgeon takes center stage. Selecting your doctors is your right. It's also a responsibility that requires effort on your part. Your choice of plastic surgeons is limited only by the restrictions of your health plan and your willingness to seek out someone whose expertise and manner inspire your confidence.

Competent surgeons can remove a breast. Rebuilding one is more complicated. It takes special skill and experience to artfully tailor reconstruction to each person's unique desire and needs. Choosing an appropriate procedure is important, but selecting the right plastic surgeon is even more critical to your outcome. A good plastic surgeon is an artist and a sculptor; your post-mastectomy chest is the surgeon's canvas and clay. Your new breasts are, quite literally, in that person's hands. The plastic surgeon does the work, but you live with it. Some surgeons are good technicians; some are gifted artists. You want one who is both.

Physicians are humans like the rest of us; and, being human, they have different personalities, skills, and opinions. You probably wouldn't choose the first financial advisor or realtor you interviewed. It's the same with plastic surgeons. Selecting a doctor is one of the most important personal decisions we make; yet, a national survey found that we spend more time choosing a car.[1] You might randomly find a surgeon in the telephone directory or online and feel relieved to let the surgeon tell you which procedure you should have and what size your breasts should be. That's an easy decision, though it's one you might later regret. If you make the commitment to pursue reconstruction, it makes sense to find the most experienced surgeon you can—someone who instills confidence, who makes you feel comfortable, and whose work you admire.

Most plastic surgeons perform only certain procedures; few are qualified and experienced in all methods of breast reconstruction. When surgeons downplay one technique or another, it may be because they feel it's not in your best interest. But it may be because they aren't experienced at performing it. Because most surgeons aren't trained in microsurgical breast reconstruction, the most important factor in any autologous procedure, especially muscle-sparing procedures, is choosing someone who routinely performs these surgeries and is more likely to have reduced surgery intervals, fewer complications, and more experience resolving problems that may occur. During your consultations with plastic surgeons, ask about their experience with the specific procedures that appeal to you and how often they perform them. The only surgeons who are qualified to tell you whether you're a candidate for a particular method of reconstruction are those who routinely perform that procedure. If you're hoping for a DIEP reconstruction, and a surgeon who performs only implant reconstruction suggests you don't have enough belly fat, an experienced DIEP surgeon may disagree. Likewise, a surgeon who only does pedicled TRAM reconstruction isn't the best source of information or advice about muscle-sparing DIEP or stacked flaps. The same goes for implant reconstruction. A plastic surgeon who only offers tissue expander-to-implant reconstruction may not mention direct-to-implant as an option. Even if you eventually choose the surgeon with whom you first consulted, it's worth the time and effort to make sure that surgeon is the one for you. It's like hunting for the right pair of shoes: there's a big selection and not everyone will be a good fit. If at first you don't succeed, keep shopping.

The mastectomy surgeon recommended a plastic surgeon, and that's who I saw. He told me how he would rebuild my breasts and I agreed.

I never thought of looking for other surgeons. Months later, I spoke to another woman who had reconstruction with an entirely different technique that sounded much better. Why didn't my surgeon mention that?

—*Lanie*

Five Characteristics of an Ideal Plastic Surgeon

As you research and consult with different surgeons, look and listen for five important characteristics:

1. Skill. There's no such thing as a typical reconstruction because each person is different. It takes skill and experience to rebuild and fine-tune a breast to get the best possible result. Assess a plastic surgeon's qualifications, photos of their work, feedback from other patients, and your own trust in the information the surgeon provides.
2. Compassion. You're more than a statistic on a chart, and you deserve to be treated respectfully and as an individual. A good surgeon cares about your expectations and willingly clarifies information, is sympathetic to your concerns, and reacts to your anxiety with compassion. Ideally, you want someone who is proficient with both the technical and the non-technical aspects of care—not one or the other.
3. Communication. "My doctor doesn't listen to me" is a frequent complaint in patient satisfaction surveys. Your surgeon should talk with you, not to you, and give you undivided attention. Choose someone who cares about your concerns and pays attention to what you want, rather than someone who dictates how your reconstruction will be handled. The surgeon should explain terms and procedures so that you can understand them and patiently answer your questions even when you ask for something to be repeated. You should feel that you and your surgeon are partners in your reconstruction (table 17.1).
4. Rapport. It's important to find a surgeon who speaks and acts as your team member. You'll have many questions and concerns

TABLE 17.1 Optimal Doctor-Patient Communication

YOUR SURGEON'S RESPONSIBILITIES	YOUR RESPONSIBILITIES
encourage questions	be prepared with specific questions
show empathy and give reassurance	provide accurate and complete information
ask you how much you want to know	be open and honest about your concerns
pause frequently to make sure that you're taking in what's being said	speak up if you need something explained, spelled, or repeated
engage you in shared decision-making	actively participate in decision-making
support your need to do more research and consider your options	understand that not all treatment decisions need to be made immediately

Source: Adapted from table 8.1, "Optimal Doctor-Patient Communication," in Miller KD, Camp M, Steligo K. *The Breast Cancer Book: A Trusted Guide for You and Your Loved Ones.* Johns Hopkins University Press; 2021.

throughout the process, and you need to feel comfortable voicing them. One surgeon may be too aggressive, while another may be too impersonal for your taste. Your surgeon should never be condescending, abrupt, or rude.

5. Honesty. Look for someone who describes what you can realistically expect, rather than what they think you want to hear. If you have your heart set on D-cup implants, the surgeon should tell you whether your skin can hold an implant of that size or be expanded sufficiently to accommodate it. Leaning toward a tissue flap? Your surgeon ought to candidly describe what you can expect from the operation and recovery and how you'll look afterward. Think twice if a surgeon promises "You'll be as good as new" or "Your breasts will be perfect." You should be honest, too. Say what's on your mind rather than what you think a surgeon expects to hear.

I was so put off by my surgeon, I skipped my last appointment. He seemed more interested in me as his "creation" than as a person with cancer. He refused to accept that I didn't want big breasts.

—*Alicia*

I saw three different surgeons, who recommended three different techniques! One wanted to reconstruct my breast with implants, another wanted to use tissue from my back, and the third said I would have better results using my abdominal fat.

—*Betty*

The New and Improved Doctor-Patient Relationship

Physician-patient relationships have dramatically changed in the last decade. Doctors, including surgeons, are generally more open, and patients are more informed. Individuals who learn about their mastectomy and reconstruction options are more engaged in their own care, better equipped to participate in shared decision-making, and have better physical and emotional outcomes. Physicians frequently respond to communication cues from their patients. If you remain silent or ask few questions, your surgeon may be less inclined to share information as liberally as you would like. Tell your surgeon of your preferences: whether you prefer things described in lay terms rather than medical jargon, whether you want to know statistics, and whether you'd like to discuss benefits and risks specifically or generally. Encourage your surgeon to be open and clear about potentially distressing information, even when it's hard to hear.

Beware the Pushy Surgeon

Surgeons may not be the best collaborators if they

- talk at you rather than with you
- tell you only about a single type of reconstruction
- tell you what kind of reconstruction you'll have, rather than explaining options and involving you in the decision process
- assume that you want big breasts
- speak only about the advantages of a procedure and not its disadvantages or risks
- don't appreciate your questions or provide meaningful answers
- pressure you to schedule surgery before you've had time to digest the conversation
- are arrogant, impersonal, or apathetic

Where to Start

For your mastectomy, you'll need a breast surgeon or a surgical oncologist who regularly performs mastectomies. If you want breast reconstruction, you'll also need a plastic surgeon. If you have immediate reconstruction, your breast surgeon will collaborate with your plastic surgeon to plan the best incision placement while removing as much tissue as possible. If you're having a lumpectomy or partial mastectomy, consider searching for an oncoplastic surgeon, a specialist who will remove your tumor and then use plastic surgery techniques to reshape your remaining breast tissue.

An initial referral to a breast surgeon often comes from a primary physician or an oncologist—whomever you see regarding a breast cancer diagnosis or high-risk management. In turn, breast surgeons often provide the names of one or more plastic surgeons for reconstruction. You might also consider these resources:

- If possible, choose a surgeon who specializes in breast reconstruction; some do so exclusively. You may want to think twice about having your new breasts created by a cosmetic surgeon who primarily provides "mommy makeovers," face-lifts, or other cosmetic procedures and seldom performs breast reconstruction.
- Many hospitals, cancer centers, and universities with medical centers have departments devoted specifically to breast cancer surgery, and many have excellent reconstruction staff. Surgeons at National Cancer Institute–designated comprehensive cancer centers tend to be highly qualified and experienced. You can find a list of these centers online at https://www.cancer.gov/research /infrastructure/cancer-centers.
- Hospital and recovery room nurses are great sources of information and often have firsthand experience with surgeons' work.
- It's always nice to have a report from someone who's already been through reconstruction, preferably involving the same technique you're considering. (Personal feedback is always preferable to "eeny meeny miney mo" selection.) Reach to Recovery will put you in touch with a volunteer in your area who'll share their insights into the reconstruction experience and give you feedback about their plastic surgeons. (Your local ACS office can provide information about the program.) You might also ask friends or family who have had a mastectomy with or without reconstruction who they do or don't recommend.
- The Facing Our Risk of Cancer Empowered (FORCE) Surgeon Referral Tool (www.facingourrisk.org) is a patient-based database of surgeons that can be searched by surgeon name, city, state, or type of surgery. It puts you in touch with volunteers who are willing to share their experiences.

- Hop online to the American Board of Plastic Surgery (ABPS) (www
  .abplasticsurgery.org), the primary certifying body for plastic surgeons, to search by ZIP code or name. The site also provides each
  surgeon's credentials and whether they're up to date. All surgeons
  listed in the online search tool of the American Society of Plastic
  Surgeons (ASPS) are ABPS-certified (www.plasticsurgery.org).
- Contact your health insurance company for a list of local surgeons
  in your network. (Your policy may require you to use an in-network
  surgeon, particularly if your healthcare is provided by an HMO.)

Pre-appointment Footwork

Before making an appointment for a consultation, doing a little research and
asking a few questions will help you develop a short list of surgeons with whom
you'd like to consult.

Verify Certification

Believe it or not, physicians don't need to be certified to perform plastic surgery. In most states, any licensed physician can perform plastic surgery. Although board certification doesn't guarantee proficiency, it's the best starting
place. Before you schedule a consultation, verify a surgeon's credentials at the
ABPS or ASPS website. Board-certified plastic surgeons must meet demanding requirements and pass extensive written and oral exams while maintaining
"ethical standing and safe and effective approach to multiple reconstructive
and cosmetic challenges." Certification must be renewed every 10 years. You
might also want to find a reputable surgeon who belongs to the ASPS. While
not a certifying organization, the ASPS requires that members maintain "a rig-
orous set of training and patient safety standards" to qualify for membership.

Start Screening Before You Make an Appointment

As an initial screening step, check surgeons' websites or call their offices to inquire about the following:

- Is the surgeon accepting new patients?
- Does the surgeon accept your health insurance?

- Does the surgeon perform the procedure you prefer?
- What breast reconstruction procedures does the surgeon perform?
- What is the surgeon's hospital affiliation? (It should be an accredited, reputable hospital or cancer care center.)

Schedule a Consultation

After weeding out surgeons who don't take your insurance, don't provide the procedure you want, or don't have the experience you're looking for, you're ready to arrange consultations with the top two or three (or even four) surgeons on your list. Try scheduling an appointment early in the day, if that works for you. This will give you a better chance of seeing the doctor on time. Your appointment time will fly by as the surgeon examines you and describes various reconstructive procedures. Good plastic surgeons keep busy. If you're interested in immediate reconstruction, let the surgeon's office know if your mastectomy date is quickly approaching; they may be able to fit you in. In the meantime, interview other surgeons on your list.

Making the Most of Your Consultation

Your consultation appointment will begin with a review of your cancer diagnosis or treatment, genetic status (if you're pursuing preventive mastectomy), and overall medical history. The discussion should include the reconstructive procedures the surgeon performs and what the surgeon thinks would work well for you (and why) based on your concerns and preferences. The surgeon will check the quality and amount of your breast skin. If you're considering flap reconstruction, the surgeon will determine whether you have sufficient tissue and, if so, which donor site best matches your priorities and preferences. You should also review the surgeon's portfolio of before-and-after patient photos. This will probably reflect only their best work, so ask to see photos of not-so-good reconstructions as well, to get a broader perspective. (Not all surgeons are comfortable showing these or may not make them available, but it doesn't hurt to ask.) Use the following tips to make the most of your limited appointment time.

Come Prepared

Even the best doctor can't explain all the nuances of a procedure or recovery in a single short appointment. Learn as much as you can on your own, and then make a prioritized list of the questions you would most like to have answered during the consultation. When you schedule an appointment, ask whether you should bring your pathology reports, mammograms, or other medical records for review. Then contact your doctor's office or hospital to gather up everything you need.

Don't Be Afraid to Communicate

The most successful consultation is interactive and mutually honest. Describe what you want from reconstruction and voice your concerns. If you would like smaller, larger, or rounder breasts, now is the time to say so. Ask questions to assess and compare the different ways surgeons approach reconstruction. Don't be afraid to speak up if you need something explained, spelled out, or repeated. Ask the surgeon to draw you a picture to clarify a procedure. Inquire about anything that concerns or confuses you, no matter how insignificant it may seem.

Take Notes

Experts say we forget 50 percent of what we hear in a doctor's office. That's not surprising because new information and terms can be overwhelming, especially when you're trying to get used to the idea of a mastectomy and may still be dealing with treatment issues. Jot down or record the key points of your discussion so you can review them later. If you go to your appointment alone, use a tape recorder to capture your conversation. Better yet, bring someone with you. Four ears are better than two. Your appointment buddy can take notes as you focus on listening.

Let It All Sink In

Never feel pressured to make a decision about a surgeon or to schedule a procedure before you leave the office. Take time to carefully consider what you've heard. Discuss your options with your partner or an impartial trusted friend to get another perspective.

The Value of a Second (or Third) Opinion

No single method of reconstruction is right for everyone. There are many techniques, many options, and many opinions. Reconstruction recommendations vary widely, depending on the plastic surgeon's area of expertise and preference. Getting more than one professional opinion isn't a rule or a requirement; it's always a good idea, even if you ultimately decide to go with the original surgeon. Another surgeon's input can be helpful, especially if you're unsure, confused, or conflicted about how to proceed, or you just want validation that the procedure you're considering is your best option. An additional opinion may also inform you of newer reconstructive procedures or techniques that you may not know about. You have nothing to lose and everything to gain by getting a second, if not a third, opinion. Wanting another opinion shouldn't offend a surgeon; it's standard practice with any operation. Contact your health insurance company to determine under what conditions additional consultation appointments are covered. (Most health insurance pays for second opinions.)

It's best to evaluate each surgeon on their own merits. You're the judge of what's best for you. Remember, you're doing the hiring. You needn't feel compelled or coerced to have one surgeon or another do your surgery. If you're uncomfortable with a surgeon for any reason, find someone else.

After much research and window shopping with every consultation, I found a plastic surgeon who was the perfect match for me in every sense. I was immediately struck by his casual demeanor and appreciated his reassurances, availability, track record, and references; yet, it was his striking confidence that won me over. We reviewed many of his before-and-after pictures to gain a real sense of what I wanted. We discussed the expander method at great lengths and mutually felt this route would provide optimal reconstruction for me. He was there for all of my medical needs and always returned my phone calls and e-mails promptly. Most of all, he was an absolute perfectionist and I appreciated his artistic abilities.

—Marie

Tips for Travelers

You're fortunate if you live in a city with experienced reconstructive surgeons. The best reconstructive opportunities aren't always possible locally, particularly if you live in a small town or rural area. If the surgeons and techniques you prefer aren't available nearby, you'll need to decide whether you'll settle for the local surgical expertise or travel for your reconstruction. Even though journeying to another city for your surgery involves more time, effort, and cost—insurance doesn't typically pay for travel and hotel costs, and your out-of-pocket expense may be higher—if you're able to do so, it may be worthwhile to pack up for a few days to get the surgeon and procedure you want.

If your insurance carrier denies a physician who is out of network, the surgeon's office may work directly with them to provide more information or help to appeal the denial. If you're having immediate reconstruction, the office staff may also recommend a breast surgeon with whom the surgeon routinely works, so you won't need to find someone to do your mastectomy. If you can manage it, consider driving, taking a train, or flying in for a consultation and returning home the same day. If that doesn't work, many surgeons offer virtual or telephone consultations: you swap information and provide photos of your breasts and donor site by e-mail and follow up with a video conference. If you like what you hear, you can then arrange an in-person consultation or schedule your mastectomy and/or reconstruction. Once your surgery date is on the calendar, you can complete all the necessary pre-op testing in your hometown, with a copy of the results forwarded to your distant plastic surgeon. As a precaution, you may want to contact a local plastic surgeon or surgical oncologist before your reconstruction to ask whether they'll provide follow-up care if you need it.

It may be hard to fathom traveling across the state or country to have surgery and all that this entails, but many people do. Many reconstructive surgery practices, especially those that practice breast reconstruction exclusively, have patient relations staff who coordinate insurance coverage, manage preauthorization if it's required, facilitate consultation appointments, and recommend nearby hotels that provide patient discounts. They'll also advise you on when you need to be there, how long you'll need to stay before your initial post-op appointment, and when you'll be cleared to return home. If you'll be flying home after reconstruction, arranging for a wheelchair at the airport will help you avoid jostling crowds and long walks through the terminal, and you'll be able to pre-board the airplane.

> I did an enormous amount of research until I found the procedure and doctors that I felt were the best fit for me, which meant traveling about four hours from my home for surgery. I knew recovery would be uncomfortable, and rather than having to make the four-hour drive multiple times, I opted to recover in a hotel. By being away from home I was forced to take it easy, which would never have happened at home, and I was able to truly relax and recover.
>
> —Jess

Questions for Plastic Surgeons

A consultation probably won't be long enough to ask every question that you have, but you'll want to get enough information to decide whether to entrust your care to a particular surgeon. These questions will help you make that decision:

- What are my options for breast reconstruction?

- Which option do you recommend for me and why?

- How many surgeries of this type have you performed and how regularly do you perform them?

- What is your success rate with this procedure?

- Will my underlying health condition (if you have one) affect my reconstruction?

- What are the best and worst results I can expect?

- Will you perform the reconstruction through my mastectomy incision(s)? What other incisions, if any, will I have, and where will they be made?

- How will my nipple and areola be affected by my reconstruction (if you're having a nipple-sparing mastectomy)?

- How many surgeries and office visits will be required, and over what period of time?

- What are the possible side effects and risks of the procedure?

- Do you recommend surgery for my opposite breast for symmetry (if you're having unilateral reconstruction)?

- How long will the surgery take and how long will I stay in the hospital?

- What will my recovery be like and how long will it take before I'm able to return to my normal routine?

- What if I'm unhappy with my results?

- May I see your before-and-after photos of patients who have had this procedure?

- May I speak with a couple of your patients who've had the same procedure?

- Will someone on your staff provide information about traveling for my reconstruction?

Chapter 18

Payment and Insurance Issues

> My insurance company was great. My benefits manual outlined how mastectomy
> and reconstruction were covered. My in-network surgeons performed the proce-
> dure I wanted, and I didn't give it a second thought. I never even saw a bill, so I
> assume everything was paid.
>
> —DAWN

Paying for breast reconstruction is often not straightforward, even when
you have insurance coverage. The Women's Health and Cancer Rights Act
(WHCRA) requires individual and group health insurance plans that cover
mastectomy to also pay for breast reconstruction; some plans are exempt, and
out-of-pocket costs may apply (table 18.1). Government and church plans
and some self-funded plans aren't required to cover mastectomy or reconstruction, although many do. Also known as Janet's Law, the WHCRA is
named for Janet Franquet, a woman who was denied reconstructive surgery
after a mastectomy because her insurance company considered the replacement of a breast to be cosmetic and medically unnecessary. (Her surgeon generously reconstructed her breast for free.) Franquet pursued a lengthy appeals
process, which she eventually won.

The WHCRA also mandates the following for health insurance companies that cover the cost of mastectomy:

- provide usual and customary coverage consistent with existing
  plan benefits (with the same deductibles and co-payments)

TABLE 18.1 Requirements and Limitations of the Women's Health and Cancer Rights Act

REQUIRES INSURERS* TO PAY FOR	DOES *NOT*
all stages of immediate and delayed breast reconstruction	require insurance companies to pay for mastectomy
breast prostheses and special mastectomy bras	apply to certain government, school, and church plans (some do cover mastectomy and reconstruction)
procedures needed to achieve symmetry with the opposite breast after unilateral reconstruction	guarantee coverage for specific types of reconstructive procedures, out-of-network surgeons, or hospitals
treatment for lymphedema and other complications related to mastectomy and/or reconstruction	provide retroactive coverage; if you weren't insured with your current plan before January 1999 or you had your mastectomy before that time, your current insurer isn't obligated to cover your reconstruction now**

*Applies to health insurers addressed by WHCRA that pay for mastectomy.

**If you change insurance companies and your new plan covers mastectomy, it must also pay for your reconstruction.

- provide a description of these benefits whenever an individual health insurance policy is issued
- describe these benefits in the health plan's summary of benefits and coverage provided annually to policyholders

The WHCRA recognizes breast reconstruction as more than cosmetic surgery. It stops short of guaranteeing your absolute choice in the matter—it doesn't set payment rates or guarantee payment for specific procedures, surgeons, or hospitals. Despite the law's title, its protection isn't limited to women or cancer patients. Men are also covered, as are people who have a mastectomy for medical reasons. High-risk individuals who have preventive mastectomies are also entitled to WHCRA reconstruction benefits as long as their health insurer covers a mastectomy. Although the law doesn't extend to Medicare and Medicaid, both government programs cover the cost of prostheses and reconstructive surgery. (Medicaid coverage varies from state to state.) To learn more about your rights regarding breast reconstruction, do the following:

- Search for "WHCRA" at the Department of Labor's Employee Benefits Security Administration website (www.askebsa.dol.gov).
- Visit the Centers for Medicare & Medicaid Services website (www.cms.gov).
- Contact your state health insurance agency or insurance commissioner for information about laws regarding mastectomies and breast reconstruction; some states provide additional protection and benefits, going beyond WHCRA requirements.

Are You Covered?

Dealing proactively with your insurance company before your surgery is a smart move that will help you avoid unpleasant payment surprises. Never assume your health insurance will automatically cover your reconstruction. Check your benefits handbook, plan document, or policy to determine what is covered and what isn't. Call the customer service department if you need further clarification. Your most valuable ally is the insurance specialist in your plastic surgeon's office. This person deals with pre-authorizations, payments, denials, and related issues every day and probably already has experience dealing with your insurance company. The insurance specialist will be familiar with the appropriate codes that insurance carriers require for each and every billable item. The specialist will help you navigate the insurance maze and do much of the footwork to arrange payment with your insurer.

Working Within Your Health Plan

If your health plan covers mastectomy and reconstruction, it must do so under its overall guidelines. You still have to pay any *deductibles* and *co-payments* routinely required for other plan benefits. In other words, if your plan normally pays 80 percent of medical services and you pay the remaining 20 percent, the same schedule applies to your reconstructive expenses. Be sure to follow your plan's process for requesting reconstruction, including pre-authorization.

If your plan generally only pays for services with *in-network* physicians, the same applies to breast surgeons and plastic surgeons. If you have this type of policy, choosing one of these pre-approved surgeons will be to your financial advantage and will limit your *out-of-pocket costs* to whatever deductible and co-pay you're ordinarily responsible for. Healthcare insurers limit services and providers to control costs and increase profits. Their fee schedule is generally based on what they consider to be "usual and customary" charges for a geographic area; this is often only a fraction of a surgeon's "sticker price." In-network providers agree to accept predetermined fees for the services they provide. This is usually much less than what they would customarily charge—they write off the remaining unpaid balance. Your plan may limit your choice of surgeons to those who practice locally or may include surgeons in other cities or states.

Out-of-network providers don't have payment agreements with the insurer and aren't as likely to write off a balance due after receiving an insurance payment. That translates to higher out-of-pocket costs for you.

You may encounter this type of cost if a service related to your mastectomy or reconstruction is performed by an out-of-network surgeon in an out-of-network hospital, whether the surgeon is in your town or a in different city. Costs for a mastectomy and reconstruction vary widely depending on where your surgeon practices and the procedure you choose. (The costs of an implant or DIEP reconstruction in New York and San Francisco are quite different from the cost for the same procedures in Santa Fe or Des Moines.) A surgeon may accept a combination of your insurer's offered payment and your co-pay as payment in full. If not, you may be responsible for paying the difference. It's important to determine your total out-of-pocket expenses before you schedule surgery. If your surgeon advises you to pay in advance and then seek reimbursement from your health insurer, realize your financial risk: your insurance company may compensate you for only a small part of the amount you paid, or none at all.

A percentage of your total out-of-pocket medical expenses may be deductible from your state and federal income taxes, including costs related to your breast cancer treatment, mastectomy, reconstruction, and other health-related expenses you pay during the tax year. Check with a tax professional or see IRS Publication 502 for a complete list of deductible medical expenses.

Appealing When the Answer Is No

Several days after your pre-authorization request, a letter arrives from your insurance company. You're expecting approval but find a refusal instead: your request has been denied. Angry, frustrated, and feeling helpless, people often give up at this point. Is it worth the effort to challenge your insurance company's decision? Yes! You have nothing to lose and so much to gain. Despite federal and state laws protecting a person's right to breast reconstruction, denials occur more frequently than you might imagine. The Affordable Care Act (ACA) protects your right to appeal healthcare denials by employer-sponsored or private health insurance carriers. (The ACA doesn't apply to self-funded, short-term, and certain other health plans, which may have different guidelines for appeals.)

You should know before you begin that attempting to get your insurer to recant can be frustrating and time-consuming. But healthcare organizations aren't perfect—they make mistakes—nor are they invincible. Many people win appeals, and you may be able to do the same, depending on the circumstances. Your health insurer may have received incorrect codes from a billing physician or be unclear or mistaken about why your service was necessary. If the company realizes it's made a mistake or feels it's more cost-effective to grant your request than fight it, the decision may be reversed.

Follow the Process

Challenging a denial is your legal right. You must follow your plan's appeal procedure exactly as it is described in your denial letter and your benefits manual. When you contact your insurance company, request a case manager for your appeal. Your case manager will become familiar with your case, and contacting that person directly will save you the time and hassle of having to go through customer service representatives each time you call. By law, employer-provided insurance plans may have no more than two appeal levels:

- First-level appeals are usually decided by an insurance company claims reviewer and signed off by a medical professional. Unless an obvious coding error or other administrative mistake was made, a denial at this level is unlikely to be overturned. It doesn't hurt to ask your case manager to arrange a call between your plastic surgeon and the medical director who approved the denial or who will be reviewing your appeal. (A surgeon-to-surgeon conversation can improve the chances of having your denial overturned.)
- If your internal appeal is unsuccessful, you can try a second-level appeal, which is considered by a review panel that includes at least one physician in the same specialty you requested—in this case, reconstructive surgery. If your insurance carrier allows it, you can

also try an in-person appeal at this level, which can be more effective than a written appeal.

Focus on the Reason for Denial

Your insurer must state the reason for its refusal in its notification to you. It may be difficult to find rhyme or reason in the logic behind the decision; all health insurance policies are different and coverage varies, depending on many variables. Call your insurance company and request a copy of the medical opinion on which your denial is based; this should be the focus of your request for reconsideration. In most cases, your denial will be based on one of the following reasons:

- "Benefit not provided" means your plan doesn't provide the service you requested. Check your benefits summary to see whether a mastectomy is a covered benefit. If it is, the insurer must also provide coverage for reconstruction. Include a copy of the WHCRA wording with your appeal letter, stating that the denial appears to be in violation of the law.
- "Not medically necessary" is one of the most common reasons for the denial. It means that the insurer doesn't consider your procedure necessary for your continued good health. If your insurer vetoes your request for risk-reducing mastectomy, for example, ask your oncologist, primary care physician, or medical geneticist (or all three) to write letters describing your family history of breast cancer, confirming your high-risk status, and advising that the National Comprehensive Cancer Network, a consortium of cancer experts that establishes guidelines on cancer care and updates them yearly, recommends consideration of risk-reducing mastectomy for women with inherited mutations in the *BRCA1, BRCA2, PALB2, PTEN,* and *TP53* genes. (Additional genes may be added as more data is made available.) Remember that if your insurance company covers mastectomy, it must also pay for reconstruction.

  If your surgeon's office made an administrative error while submitting a claim to your insurer, they should resubmit the claim with the correct codes and describe the procedure as medically necessary rather than cosmetic. If your surgeon recommends a larger breast implant to improve symmetry with your opposite breast, for example, your insurer is likely to reject "patient prefers increased breast size" or "exchange 300 cc breast implant to 400 cc breast implant" as the reason for the procedure. Approval is more likely to be granted when the description clearly states that the revision surgery is necessary to improve asymmetry or other problems related to mastectomy or breast reconstruction. If your plastic surgeon routinely performs breast reconstruction, the surgeon's billing specialist will be familiar with what needs to be submitted. Still, it's a good idea to check when you receive a denial.

- "Out-of-network" is a common reason for rejecting reconstruction requests and one of the most difficult appeals to win, especially if the procedure you're requesting is available from in-network surgeons. Unless you can show that your request is medically necessary, your chance for a reversed denial is slim. If a surgeon in your network provides DIEP reconstruction, your insurer will likely refuse your request to go to an out-of-network surgeon for the same procedure. However, if DIEP is the only procedure for which you're a candidate and your in-network surgeons don't perform DIEP, you have a stronger argument. If you can obtain documentation from an in-network surgeon validating your decision, so much the better.

- "Procedure is experimental" means your carrier doesn't recognize or accept the procedure you requested. The company may be unfamiliar with a particular type of reconstruction, especially newer procedures, and once educated, might reverse its denial. Support your case with peer-reviewed studies and articles in medical journals that prove your requested procedure is established, bona fide, and safe. One other circumstance may work in your favor: if you can show that other insurers cover the procedure you're requesting (your surgeon's billing coordinator can help with this), you may sway the company to change its opinion and, in doing so, both help yourself and pave the way for people who request the procedure in the future.

Build Your Case

The most difficult part of an appeal is crafting your response without letting your frustration and emotions get in the way. Although your reconstruction is a personal matter for you, it's a business decision for your insurance company. And while it's disheartening to have your request refused, this is the time for logic to prevail. Resist the temptation to fire off an immediate angry response. Be aggressively persistent without being hostile. You have a better chance of succeeding if your appeal is concise, clear, and includes fact-based evidence that justifies your position. Don't waste your time reiterating what the insurer already knows. Stick to the issue at hand, focusing on evidence that refutes the reason for rejection.

Start working on your appeal strategy soon after you receive notification of denial. Gather up all the information you need: applicable medical records, supporting letters from physicians, and research materials that help make your case. Top it off with a formal cover letter that includes the following:

- your insurance policy number
- your appeal claim number
- acknowledgment that you've received the denial
- a request for a "physician review," which asks for a review by a plastic surgeon
- a request for reconsideration

Ask for Help

Don't be shy about asking your physicians to provide supportive letters or point you in the right direction for peer-reviewed studies and medical reports on the procedure you want. (They may have sample letters that have worked successfully for other patients.) The nonprofit Patient Advocate Foundation (www.patientadvocate.org) will help you along the way, at no charge, and act as a liaison between you and your insurance company. The organization's website also has sample appeal letters. Triage Cancer (triagecancer.org) is another helpful organization. The Cancer Legal Resource Center's Step-by-Step Guide to Navigating Health Insurance Appeals (thedrlc.org) provides comprehensive instructions on filing an insurance appeal. Facing Our Risk of Cancer Empowered (FORCE) has an online library of sample appeal letters (search for "appeals" at www.facingourrisk.org).

Keep a Paper Trail

Maintaining accurate, organized records is important when you need to pay medical bills, file a claim with your insurance company, or file for financial assistance. It's also a necessity for documenting the medical deductions you itemize on your annual tax returns. Carefully organize all bills, receipts, records, and documents related to your mastectomy, breast reconstruction, and any related issues or problems. Keep copies of all written correspondence and a call log of your conversations with your health insurance company employees, noting the date, time, details of the discussion, and name of the employee. If a discrepancy comes up, you'll have supporting documentation.

When All Else Fails

Once you've exhausted your insurer's appeals process (not before), you can contact the office of your state's insurance commissioner to request an appeal with an independent external reviewer who is empowered to sustain or overrule an insurance company's decision. An external review either upholds your insurer's decision or decides in your favor, and your insurance company is required by law to accept the decision. Your appeal rights may vary, depending on the type of health insurance plan you have and the process required by the state in which you live. Fully insured plans (in which your employer buys health coverage from an insurance company) are regulated by state laws, so any external appeal process is administered by the state. Self-insured plans (your employer pays claims from its own resources, even if it contracts with an insurance company to administer the plan) are governed by federal law. You can learn more about state and federal insurance laws and find information about appeals at the US Department of Health and Human Services website (www.healthcare.gov). Check with your state's department of insurance to learn more about the appeal process.

Help for the Underinsured and the Uninsured

The cost of breast reconstruction can be considerable, especially if you're uninsured or underinsured, or if your healthcare policy requires a high deductible or co-payment. The cost involves fees for surgeons, the anesthesiologist, the hospital or surgical facility, presurgical testing and labs, medications,

Appeal Timeframes

Be sure to submit all paperwork on time to meet the deadlines for each level of appeal, as defined by your insurance policy or your denial notice. Send your appeal by certified mail (or other type of mail that requires a recipient's signature) to the appropriate contact listed in your denial letter. Be aware of these timeframes:

Internal appeal
- You must file within 6 months of receiving the denial.
- Your health insurance company must respond within 30 days regarding services or procedures you haven't had yet.
- Your health insurance company must respond within 60 days regarding services or procedures you've already had.

External review
- You must file a request within 4 months after the date you receive a denial from your health insurer.
- External reviewers must respond no later than 45 days after receiving your request. (They must respond within 72 hours or less after receiving a request for an expedited review.)

medical tests and imaging, and related office visits. For most individuals, breast reconstruction is cost-prohibitive without insurance or financial assistance. One option may be to see what affordable plans are available through the federally run or state-operated Health Insurance Marketplace (www .healthcare.gov) in your area. If you don't have health insurance and you can't afford a mastectomy and/or reconstruction, you may be eligible for assistance programs specifically for mastectomy and reconstruction:

- Contact your local hospital, breast cancer center, or medical teaching university to inquire about plastic surgeons who donate reconstructive services to a few people each year (many surgeons do).
- The Patient Advocate Foundation can direct you to financial assistance programs, resources, and/or co-pay assistance programs.
- Some charitable organizations, including the Alliance in Reconstructive Surgery (AIRS) Foundation (www.airsfoundation.org), My Hope Chest (www.myhopechest.org), and the United Breast Cancer Foundation (www.ubcf.org), underwrite or provide grants for breast reconstruction if you meet certain eligibility requirements.
- Other charitable breast cancer organizations may offer financial help for your surgery.
- Medicare provides health insurance if you meet age and income eligibility requirements.
- Your state's department of insurance can provide information about state-funded health insurance plans for which you may qualify.

If paying out of pocket is your only alternative, many surgeons offer reduced fees and payment schedules for breast cancer survivors. Triage Cancer (www.triagecancer.org) provides a variety of educational information about health insurance options, cancer-related finances, appealing health insurance denials, and other related topics.

I was told by my insurance company's customer service department that my risk-reducing mastectomy wasn't covered under any circumstances. I was so angry, I stomped into my boss's office and told her I thought it was incredibly unfair. She contacted our human resources director, who arranged a call for me with a manager at the insurance company. When I explained my high-risk status, the manager said that sometimes the customer service personnel made mistakes and assured me that my mastectomy and reconstruction would be covered. It was a good thing I pursued this because both procedures were paid for without problems.

—Judy

After seeing my friend's fabulous reconstruction results, I was determined to go to her plastic surgeon, who happened to be out-of-network for me. My health insurance company denied my request. Even though I spent hours talking with people at the insurance company and writing appeals, I couldn't get them to change their minds.

—Trish

Questions for Your Health Insurer

- Does my plan cover my mastectomy? (If the answer is yes, it must also cover reconstruction.)
- How many "second" opinions are covered?
- How should I obtain preauthorization for my surgery?
- Am I limited to in-network surgeons and services?
- If I travel to another surgeon who specializes in a particular technique not available within my network, what expenses will be covered?
- Is there a limit to the amount of coverage provided?
- Is my hospital stay covered? If so, for how many days?
- Will all payments be made directly to providers?

Chapter 19

A Road Map for Making Difficult Decisions

You do as much research as you can by reading and talking to people who have the appropriate knowledge and experience; then you do what's right for you.

—JILL

Reconstruction can be an exciting and terrifying possibility. The decisions you face are complicated and intensely personal. For many people, deciding to have reconstruction is a no-brainer; if they're going to lose their breasts, they want to replace them. Others adamantly don't want or need reconstruction. Some individuals are conflicted about what they should do. No matter what you ultimately decide, no answer is right or wrong. You may have a team of family, friends, support group volunteers, and medical professionals helping you on your mastectomy and reconstruction journey, but you're the one who weighs your options and make decisions that feel right for you.

With a mastectomy looming ahead, you may know precisely how you want to proceed. Or you may be living in a state of uncertainty about what to do and when to do it. Should you have reconstruction? Is a nipple-sparing mastectomy an option you'd like to pursue? Would implants or autologous reconstruction give you a better result? Which alternative has a recovery that meets your priorities? Should you travel for a procedure you can't have locally or for a more experienced surgeon who can offer you a better reconstructive outcome?

FIGURE 19.1 Move forward step-by-step as you make decisions about mastectomy and reconstruction.

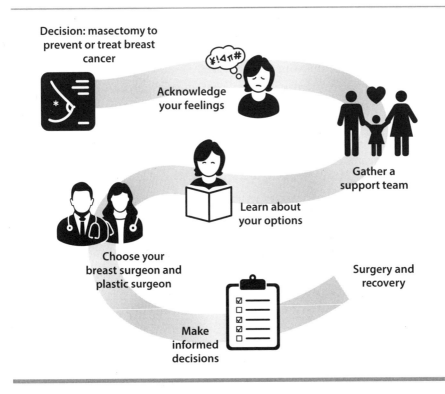

Making informed decisions about a mastectomy and breast reconstruction can help to restore the lack of control you may feel during your diagnosis and treatment. So how do you find answers when you're not even sure of the right questions (figure 19.1)?

Moving in the Right Direction

Making the best decisions may seem like a tall order, considering the many procedures and options to learn about and sort through. With so much to absorb, you may feel as though you're stuck on a merry-go-round of endless terms and concepts. The following tips will help you make your way through the onslaught of information and what-ifs in front of you.

1. Establish a positive attitude. Think of your research as an empowering action rather than an awful chore. Your investigative efforts will help you make a confident decision.

2. Learn about your alternatives. When it comes to surgery (or any medical decision), being informed is always better than being impetuous. Learning about your options gives you something special: the power of choice. Breast cancer isn't a medical emergency for most people. Unless you've been diagnosed with an aggressive breast cancer, taking some time to learn about reconstruction probably won't adversely affect your health, and you needn't make decisions about mastectomy and reconstruction options that you haven't had time to consider thoroughly. You should, of course, discuss this research interval with your medical team. If you're having a preventive mastectomy, you have the luxury of more time to research, learn, and consider. You would probably compare loan rates before financing a home and get to know someone pretty well before marrying them or forming a business partnership. It's only logical to approach a decision concerning your physical and emotional well-being with the same scrutiny. To use a corny football analogy, don't sit on the bench. Suit up and get in the game. Be your own advocate. Gather all the objective, up-to-date information you need, and give yourself time to review and understand it.

3. Recruit a study buddy. Having a research helper saves time and provides a second perspective. Your spouse or partner may be the best person for the task; sharing the experience can help build understanding, commitment, and compassion. Or ask a relative or close friend to assist you.

4. Be patient and persistent. Take things one step at a time. Don't let frustration get you down. Take a break when you think you can't absorb any more information. Have lunch with a friend, spend quality time with the family, get lost in a novel, or go for a walk.

5. Deal with data. Always use credible information sources. As much as possible, weed out the influences of media hype, personal anecdote, and urban myth. Make your decisions based on the facts of a particular procedure and a surgeon's expertise. Ask your surgeon for clarification when you're unclear about something. Stay organized. Keep a binder of your medical records, test results, research,

doctor visits, communications with your health insurance provider, and other related documents.

6. Sort through your options. When you learn that a mastectomy is a certainty, you may already have a particular reconstruction procedure in mind. Even so, it's still wise to consider the many possibilities available to you. Understanding your options will demystify reconstruction, replace the unknown with the expected, and reduce your anxiety about the various ways your breasts can be rebuilt. Along the way, you may discover that reconstruction can give you better breasts than you expected, or that it requires more than you're willing to go through. Work your way through each of your options one by one, eliminating the unacceptable and prioritizing the choices that remain.

7. Know when to stop. At some point, you'll need to assess the data you've gathered and make your decision. If you're still unsure, consider whether it's best to delay your reconstruction.

8. Take time to absorb. Even after you decide to have reconstruction, you may still have doubts. It's not unusual to feel this way. Experts say shock, denial, anger, and depression typically come before acceptance. Meanwhile, life goes on. There's work to be done, a home to manage, perhaps kids to raise, and pets to feed. Give yourself time to let everything sink in and reflect on what you've learned. Try to recognize and manage the strong, unanticipated emotions you may feel so they don't cloud your thinking. If you're unable to reach a conclusion on your own, speak with a counselor or someone you trust who can help you organize your thoughts and help you through the decision-making process.

9. Prioritize what's most important. Your choice of a particular procedure will be influenced by many factors. You may prefer not to have donor site scars from autologous reconstruction, risk complications with implants after radiation therapy, or travel to another city. Your priority might be to have the quickest reconstruction possible. You might not be compelled to replace your breasts at all. Carefully consider the near-term and long-term benefits and limitations of each alternative against your priorities. As you consider all the variables, use a process of elimination to whittle the possibilities down to procedures that interest you and for which you are a candidate.

10. Make your decision. Consider the input of loved ones, trusted friends, other people who have had a mastectomy, and your plastic surgeon; then listen to your instincts. Others may influence what you decide, but you're the one who must go through the surgery and recovery, and you're the one who will live with the results. It's you, after all, who best knows your body. With many options available, the tough decisions—the what, when, where, who, and how of breast reconstruction—are up to you (figure 19.2). Choose the procedure that best matches your lifestyle and personal priorities. Whatever you decide is the right choice.

FIGURE 19.2 Breast reconstruction requires considering several key decisions.

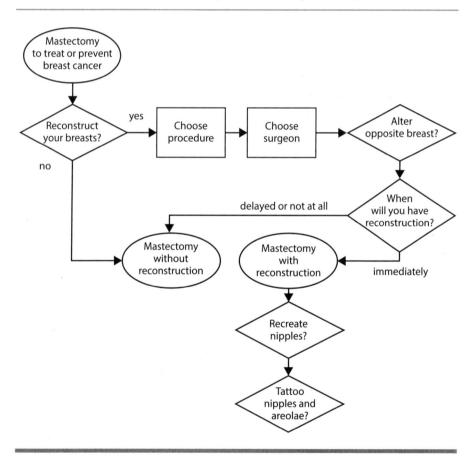

Shared Decision-Making

Although you have the final say regarding your reconstruction—or whether you want to have reconstruction at all—your healthcare team can help you understand important issues and make informed decisions about what's best for you. *Shared decision-making* is a collaborative approach between you, your breast surgeon, and your plastic surgeon. (Your oncologist and other medical specialists may also be involved if you're being treated for breast cancer). Shared decision-making balances your preferences with your surgeon's experience to ensure that you understand the advantages and disadvantages of your options. It also helps you to set realistic expectations and gives you the information and tools you need to make decisions when they need to be made. It can also create a stronger relationship between you and your physicians.

My mother was diagnosed with breast cancer at age 45 and died five years later when I was 16, so my high-risk status raised a host of monsters in my head. I was initially terrified and overwhelmed by the information, and then decided quickly to have a prophylactic mastectomy—I did not want my two children to lose their mother as early as I did. I considered implant reconstruction, the only type available locally, but I was interested in autologous flap reconstruction as soon as I learned about it. I was lucky to connect with someone who had already interviewed several surgeons in my state and nationally who do these procedures and to benefit from her extensive research. The more

I learned about flap surgery, the more I knew it was the best choice for me. Using my own tissue for a more natural look and feel, and not having implants that would need to be replaced down the road were the most important factors. Once I saw a friend's beautiful DIEP flap reconstruction, my fears about the surgery were greatly relieved. I know that combined with nipple-sparing mastectomy, it was the best balance of risk reduction and cosmetic result.

—Sonya

Because of my high inherited risk for breast cancer, having bilateral mastectomy was an easy decision and reconstruction was just part of that process. Two cousins had already been through the process—one had reconstruction, the other didn't. Both seemed happy with their outcomes, which told me there was no right way to go through this decision process; it was an individual choice. Though I had never been fond of my small breasts, I thought I'd be uncomfortable without any reconstruction. Considering all the options, I joked that I was going to the "boob store" to pick out a better pair that was less likely to kill me. Ordinarily, I would never have considered plastic surgery, so I considered this an opportunity to make me feel better about my body. I had lousy odds for breast cancer, but I was going to at least indulge myself with pretty, more proportionate breasts. I knew reconstruction was the right choice for me.

—Jennifer

I agonized over my reconstruction choice, but after thinking and rethinking my options, I ultimately chose implants, because I just couldn't accommodate the childcare and time away from work a flap surgery would require.

—Rachel

Sources of Information and Inspiration

Not so long ago, reconstruction choices were limited, and information was hard to come by. You can now bring an amazing assortment of information and personal experience directly to your desktop or mobile device, if you know where to look for the bits and pieces. Medical reports, journal articles, and personal reconstruction journals can be found on the internet. Before-and-after patient photos can be found on the websites of plastic surgeons and the American Society of Plastic Surgeons (www.plasticsurgery.org). Sorting through all this information can be overwhelming, however; before you know it, you may have spent days in front of your computer yet feel no closer to getting the answers you need. It helps to narrow your search with specific terms. Looking for "direct-to-implant reconstruction" or "PAP flap breast reconstruction recovery," for example, will refine your search. (Put quotation marks around the entire phrase.) Bookmark your favorite websites for easy return.

Mastectomies and reconstruction used to be topics women kept to themselves. While some still prefer to keep their experiences private, many are happy to share the details of their reconstruction and recovery in person, in chat rooms, and on social networking sites. Discussion groups at Susan G. Komen for the Cure (www.komen.org) and the Cancer Support Network (csn .cancer.org) frequently have postings related to reconstruction. The FORCE message boards (www.facingourrisk.org) are some of the most informative and supportive online neighborhoods, particularly concerning reconstruction. Members have been through every imaginable breast cancer and reconstruction experience. No matter where you are in the journey, plenty of previvors and survivors with reconstruction experience who have "been there and done that" are ready and willing to lend a virtual shoulder. Having experienced the same emotional roller coaster and confusion, they can relate to what you're feeling.

One caveat about discussions of mastectomies and breast reconstruction on blogs and message boards: People are often passionate about their reconstruction, whether they're happy or dissatisfied with their results. Realize that other people's experiences won't necessarily be yours, and their choices may not be the best solution for you. Try not to substitute personal opinion for medical advice or use the experiences of just one or two individuals to make your decision. Local support groups can also be helpful. Contact your nearest ACS office, hospital, or breast cancer center to see whether they sponsor reconstruction discussion groups, seminars, or lectures. Your library, bookstore shelves, and online booksellers offer memoirs of individuals who have gone through the same emotional upheaval that you're experiencing.

Patient-Reported Outcomes

BREAST-Q is the most widely accepted method in the United States and many other countries to measure patient outcomes after breast-conserving therapy, mastectomy, and reconstruction. It uses patients' responses to measure expectations, outcomes, and experience related to quality of life and satisfaction with these procedures. Several years of BREAST-Q results show that women prefer

- oncoplastic surgery (lumpectomy) over mastectomy
- nipple-sparing mastectomy over skin-sparing mastectomy
- prepectoral implants over subpectoral implants
- autologous flaps over breast implants

Source: Char S, Bloom JA, Erlichman Z, et al. A comprehensive literature review of patient-reported outcome measures (PROMS) among common breast reconstruction options: what types of breast reconstruction score well? *Breast Journal.* 2021;27(4):322–29; Eltahir Y, Krabbe-Timmerman I, Sadok N, et al. Outcome of quality of life for women undergoing autologous versus alloplastic breast reconstruction following a mastectomy: a systematic review and meta-analysis. *Plastic and Reconstructive Surgery.* 2020;145(5):1109–23.

A Checklist for Making Decisions

- □ go flat or have reconstruction
- □ immediate, delayed, or delayed-immediate reconstruction
- □ skin-sparing or nipple-sparing mastectomy
- □ placement of mastectomy incision(s)
- □ breast implants, autologous tissue flap, or both

If you're considering breast implants:

- □ tissue expansion or direct-to-implant
- □ prepectoral or subpectoral
- □ saline or silicone
- □ round or teardrop
- □ smooth or textured
- □ size and projection
- □ placement of any additional incision(s)

If you're considering autologous reconstruction:

- □ muscle-sparing or muscle-sacrificing
- □ donor site(s)
- □ placement of any additional incisions

Nipple/areola:

- □ nipple reconstruction
- □ nipple/areola tattooing
- □ tattooing only (no reconstructed nipple)
- □ 2-D or 3-D nipple/areola tattoo

Related decisions:

- □ modify your healthy breast (unilateral reconstruction)
- □ choose your breast surgeon
- □ choose your plastic surgeon
- □ pursue a second and even a third option
- □ stay local or travel
- □ investigate/verify authorization of health insurance coverage
- □ identify any deductibles and out-of-pocket costs
- □ seek donated reconstructive services or alternate funding

Chapter 20

Information for Family
and Friends

My family and friends couldn't wave a magic wand and make my recovery disappear, but they did the next best thing. Their thoughtfulness, caring, and constant support saw me through bouts of pain, surgical setbacks, and the tedium of recovery when I was just waiting to get better and get back to normal.

—RACHEL

If someone you care about is facing a mastectomy, breast reconstruction, or both, your support will be a welcome gift. Surgery and recovery can be difficult roads to walk alone. While you can't go through the experience for your loved one, you can rally to their side, providing love and strength to see them through.

Hints for Family Members

For Parents
It's difficult to see your child struggle with life-altering decisions, pain, and anxiety, especially if you've faced a similar situation yourself. You would probably be willing to trade places and spare them the experience if you could. You can help in the weeks before surgery, which can be nerve-wracking for someone facing a mastectomy. Join in as your child researches the options. Read through this book so you'll know what to expect. Help them put their house

in order before surgery and arrange to get things done during recovery. Most importantly, lend a helping hand by supporting whatever decisions they make about mastectomy and reconstruction, even if you disagree. Understand that even though these surgeries aren't life-threatening, they require sacrifice and recovery.

For Siblings

Now is the time to support your sibling, whether you live down the street or across the country. It's not the best time to bring up family grudges or disagreements, but it's the perfect time to let your words and deeds show that you care. Call frequently to make your sibling laugh when they are down. Buy them a pair of nice pajamas (with a front closure) or something that will comfort them in the hospital and when they return home. Bring or send a teddy bear, flowers, or a balloon bouquet. If your sibling is a parent, shift your schedule, if possible, to care for your sibling's children and take them to school, the park, or the movies. Attend their sports activities when your sibling cannot. Be gently supportive. Stay in touch to express your good thoughts and encouragement.

Food for Thought for Partners and Spouses

Unless you've experienced a loved one's surgery and recovery, you may be overwhelmed and feel clueless about how you can best help your partner. This may be frustrating for you, particularly if your usual approach to problems is to try to fix them. You can't fix the situation—you can't change the fact that your partner needs a mastectomy or eliminate their need to heal and recover—yet you can do many things to help them through the experience.

Be a Sounding Board

An old saying goes, "God gave us two ears but only one mouth. Some people say that's because God wanted us to spend twice as much time listening as talking." Listening is a skill, and now, more than ever, your mate will appreciate your sympathetic ear. Give your full attention as your partner expresses concerns and asks your opinion about the many "ifs" involved in mastectomy and reconstruction decisions. Listen to their fears, issues, and questions with an open mind. Consider why they might want to travel to a distant city for reconstruction or why they're leaning in favor of tissue flap reconstruction when implants would be quicker. You don't have to—and shouldn't—make decisions for your partner, but it will be a comfort for them to share ideas with you and know they can confide in you and hear your objective input.

Be a Partner

You may not be able to rescue your partner, but you can join in on the journey. Let your partner know that you're there and that the two of you will go through this physically and emotionally challenging experience together. Be an extra set of ears at doctor's appointments: ask questions, take notes, and look at before-and-after patient photos together. Then discuss what you've learned when you get home. Learn with your partner about reconstructive options and what to expect from recovery so that you can approach these issues as a team. While they are recovering, arrange (and rearrange) pillows so they can rest comfortably. Maybe a gentle back or foot rub would be just the ticket when your partner is down or frustrated. Learn how to empty drains. Your attentiveness will be immensely reassuring. Comfort your partner if they need to have a good cry or to just vent about what they're having to endure. Take time to read *Breast Cancer Husband* by Marc Silver, a revealing look into how a woman's surgery and recovery affect her partner, and tips for coping with the experience.

Be a Communicator

Say yes when friends ask whether they can help. Coordinate a brigade to deliver meals, walk the dog, run errands, and shuttle the kids to and from school and activities. Send e-mail status reports to family and friends so you won't be inundated with calls to check on the patient. Consider using CaringBridge (www.caringbridge.com) or other social networking sites to stay connected.

Be a Cheerleader

Although most people return to their pre-surgery lives after mastectomy and reconstruction without additional problems, the road to recovery is sometimes littered with setbacks. Impatient to have recovery over and done with, your partner may be fragile, fatigued, and anxious, and a small roadblock may seem enormous. Respect your partner's disappointment when their drains need to remain a while longer, their expanders are uncomfortable, or they're coping with an infection. Listen to your partner's concerns and let them know that although these things may feel devastating now, they can be corrected and will get better. Be supportive if they want to pursue corrective action. Let your partner talk when they feel like it, and understand their need for silence when they don't. Be generous with gentle hugs when your partner is angry, impatient, scared, overwhelmed, or frustrated.

Be a Lover

Some people have no problem at all with the transition back to a normal sex life after reconstruction, while others feel irreparably changed. Be patient if your partner's ordeal has left them nervous about intimacy; they may feel insecure about their new breasts or how they look. Use actions and words to offer reassurance that a mastectomy and reconstruction are not the end of your sex life together. Tell your partner that you still desire them and still consider them whole—these are powerful, reassuring words at a time when your partner may question their appeal. Read the section "Dating, Intimacy, and Sex" in chapter 16.

Your partner needs to heal physically and emotionally and may have trouble with one of these things, or both. Realize that while the new breast might feel natural to you, it won't be the same to your partner. They won't have the sensation they're used to in much of the reconstructed breast and may not be able to feel your touch. If the nipples were preserved, they will likely have a different or diminished sensation there as well—and that may change some aspects of your intimacy. Encourage your partner to talk about how they feel, and approach troublesome issues together. Don't be afraid to include their new breasts in your lovemaking; focus on the areas where they have the most feeling.

> When my wife faced mastectomy, I felt a deep and strong conviction that all I wanted was for her to make choices that would most increase her chances of survival, and I would support the decisions she made. Although I knew that I loved her with or without breasts, I was glad that she decided to have reconstruction because I thought it would be

important for her self-image. When the reconstruction was new, I felt her grief when she had no sensation and said that it felt strange when I touched her breasts. I wanted to caress them because they were a part of her; however, I quickly learned to first stroke around and between her breasts where she had felt before touching the area that lacked sensation. In this way, we were both able to appreciate a new intimacy that included her reconstructed chest. Now, 13 years later, I rarely think about the fact that her breasts aren't natural. She has since gained some increased sensation and that is positive for us both.

—Dan

Issues for Caregivers

Whether family member, partner, or friend, if you're acting as a caregiver to someone who is recovering from a mastectomy and/or reconstruction, it helps to understand the scope of recovery and to know what to expect. Be ready to respond to whatever the person needs: cold packs to reduce swelling, a sympathetic ear, or a comforting cup of tea. Help them in and out of bed. Be supportive if setbacks or complications occur. Remain calm and patient, particularly if the person is used to being independent. They may need help getting into the shower or tub, for example, but may not like asking for help. Be patient if the person is abrupt because they're uncomfortable, worried, or frustrated.

If you'll be your partner's primary caregiver, you'll be dealing with two powerful sets of emotions: yours and theirs. Being a caregiver can exact its toll; it's important to balance providing support to the other person and supporting yourself. Keep the end target in mind: the recovery will one day be over. At times, that may be hard for both of you to keep in perspective. Meanwhile, take care of yourself, because the stress and anxiety you feel can easily undermine your health. Eat well, get plenty of rest, and allow yourself to get away for short periods to renew your strength and spirit. Ask a relative or close friend to spend the morning with your partner while you spend some time with family members or friends, tend to errands, or go for a walk. If you feel stressed, find an outlet for your emotions, especially if you're the strong, silent type and it's difficult to talk about your feelings. Speak to another family member, a trusted friend, a clergyperson, or a counselor at your local cancer center. Support groups for partners of cancer survivors, including the National Alliance of Caregiving (www.caregiving.org), can be helpful. Writing about your feelings is also cathartic.

Do's and Don'ts for Friends

As we all know, actions speak louder than words. Besides being practical, actions are a meaningful way to show your feelings, especially if you feel uncomfortable talking about cancer, surgery, or recovery.

Deliver Meals

No matter what type of surgery your friend has had, they won't be spending time in the kitchen anytime soon. One of the most helpful things you can do is to deliver meals that are easily reheated—and offer to recruit neighbors and friends for meal delivery if that hasn't already been done. A hearty soup or stew, pasta, or another main course with a salad and a dessert will be appreciated by the patient and their entire family. It's always nice to throw in extra surprises: a funny card, cute napkins, or treats for pets.

Babysit

If the patient has children, take them out for an afternoon or stay with them during the day. Invite them over for a sleepover with your kids. Take them to school, soccer practice, playdates, and music lessons.

Run Errands

During your friend's recovery, everyday errands and chores that keep a home running smoothly will slide to a halt unless someone else does them. Ask if you can shop for groceries. Stocking your friend's kitchen with the essentials the day before they arrive home from the hospital will be a great help. Drop off and pick up dry cleaning, mow the lawn, or walk the dog (maybe even keep the pooch at your house until your friend recovers). Even if your help isn't initially needed, offer again in a few days.

Entertain and Amuse

Recovery can be tedious between naps. Drop off DVDs, magazines, crossword puzzles, sudokus, and audiobooks by your friend's favorite author. Send flowers or deliver fresh-cut bouquets from your garden. Perhaps nothing lifts the spirits as much as inspiring words. Your friend will appreciate that you took the time to send e-mails and text messages, and even the most committed technophile will enjoy receiving a card in the mail—your friend can reread your friendly words whenever they need a pick-me-up. Don't be afraid to send something humorous; it's good medicine.

Offer Positive Support

Unless you've lost your breasts and then had them rebuilt, there's no way to understand the full impact and intense emotions that go along with the experience. Consider the following guidelines to make sure your well-intentioned words or actions hit the mark:

- Support your friend's decisions. It's hard enough to understand all of the nuances of a mastectomy and reconstruction without having someone second-guess your decisions, especially after the fact. We all make decisions based on our priorities and fears. Respect your friend's decisions, even if you disagree with them.
- Don't avoid all contact because you feel awkward or you're nervous about saying the wrong thing. No matter what's going on in your life at the time, your absence or silence might make it seem as though you don't care or aren't interested, and that may strain your relationship. If you're tongue-tied around your friend and don't know what to say, tell your friend that you're sorry they have to go through this experience and that you're there if they need you. Or simply ask, "How are you doing today?" All conversation doesn't need to revolve around reconstruction and recovery. Talk about the weather, what the kids are up to, or what's going on in the neighborhood—the things you would discuss under other circumstances.
- Temper your contact, avoiding repeated phone calls or text messages throughout the day. Avoid showing up unannounced. Your friend may love a visit; but, on some days, they may not be up to it.
- Try not to be squeamish about surgical details your friend shares with you. Breast reconstruction isn't pretty at first. Try not to grimace or gasp as your friend explains the procedure in graphic detail, opens their shirt to show you the drains, or wants you to see incisions.

Inquire about the surgery, if you're curious, and then respect the extent to which your friend does or doesn't want to share.

- Make eye contact. Sometimes people feel so uncomfortable around recovering friends that they're embarrassed to look them in the eye. Even if you feel nervous, maintaining eye contact will show your friend that they have your undivided attention.
- Be sensitive to the situation. You probably know of others who have had cancer, and you may know of other people who have had reconstruction; but try to avoid comments such as
  - "A co-worker had reconstruction a year ago and she's still in pain."
  - "Why on earth would you go through all that?"
  - "My aunt had breast cancer, too, and she died."
  - "I still don't understand why you just didn't have a lumpectomy."
  - "I can't imagine why you would choose to remove your breasts when you may never develop cancer."

Acknowledgments

Sincere thanks to the many patients, physicians, reviewers, and other individuals who continue to support this book as a resource for people looking for information and answers about mastectomy and reconstruction. A special shout-out to Rose Marie Beauchemin-Verzella, Alex Brody, Lana Hill, Sue Freidman, and everyone who generously shared their experiences. And to the busy plastic surgeons who once again took the time to provide insight and ensure that the technical details in these pages are correct: Minas Chrysopoulo, MD; Frank DellaCroce, MD; Karen Horton, MD; and Joshua Levine, MD. Your ongoing support is a treasured gift.

Glossary

abdominal perforator exchange (APEX) flap. A segment of abdominal skin, fat, and the DIEP artery with a modified method of securing the blood supply to recreate a breast.

acellular dermal matrix (ADM). Sterilized human donor or animal skin used to replace missing tissue.

adjuvant therapy. Treatment given after surgery.

advance directive. A living will and a durable power of attorney.

aesthetic flat closure. A surgical procedure that removes excess breast skin and fat, making the postmastectomy chest smooth and flat against the chest wall.

animation deformity. Visible movement of a breast implant under the chest muscle.

areola. The circle of darkened skin surrounding the nipple.

asymmetry. Uneven size, shape, or position of one breast relative to the other.

autologous flap. An island of skin, fat, tissue, and sometimes muscle that is moved from one location on the body to another to replace missing tissue.

autologous reconstruction. Reconstruction using a person's own tissue.

axillary lymph node dissection (ALND). Removal of underarm lymph nodes to determine whether cancer has spread beyond the breast.

axillary reverse mapping. A procedure that evaluates patterns of fluid drainage from the breast to the lymph node system.

benign. Noncancerous.

bilateral mastectomy. Removal of both breasts.

bilateral reconstruction. Recreation of both breasts after mastectomy.

biopsy. Removal and examination of sample cells, fluid, or tissue.

bottoming out. A condition that occurs when breast implants drop below the inframammary fold.

***BRCA1* and *BRCA2* (BReast CAncer genes 1 and 2).** Genes that, when mutated, significantly increase the risk of developing breast and other cancers.

breast augmentation (augmentation mammoplasty). A cosmetic procedure that increases breast size.

breast cancer. Uncontrolled growth of abnormal breast cells.

breast-conserving therapy (BCT). Lumpectomy followed by radiation therapy.

breast implant. A device filled with saline or silicone gel that replaces missing breast tissue.

breast implant–associated anaplastic large cell lymphoma (BIA-ALCL). A rare type of non-Hodgkin lymphoma linked to textured tissue expanders and textured breast implants.

breast implant illness (BII). A range of symptoms reported by some people who have breast implants.

breast lift (mastopexy). Surgery to reposition a breast higher on the chest.

breast mound. A reconstructed breast without a nipple or areola.

breast prostheses. Breast-shaped forms that are worn to temporarily restore shape and profile.

breast reconstruction. Surgery that uses a manufactured implant or a patient's own tissue to restore breast volume after mastectomy.

breast reduction (reduction mammoplasty). Surgery to reduce the size of the breast.

breast surgeon. A physician who specializes in surgical procedures of the breast.

capsular contracture. Tightening of the scar capsule surrounding an implant.

capsulectomy. Surgery to remove hard scar tissue surrounding an implant.

capsulotomy. A procedure that attempts to compress and break the capsule of scar tissue surrounding an implant.

chemotherapy. Drug treatment that destroys cancer cells.

clinical trial. A controlled scientific study conducted to determine whether a drug or procedure is safe and effective.

cohesive gel. A viscous filling in silicone breast implants.

collagen. Connective tissue protein produced by the body.

computed tomography angiogram (CTA). Imaging technology that views blood vessels.

computed tomography (CT or CAT) scan. An x-ray that produces sectional images of the body.

contralateral prophylactic mastectomy (CPM). Removal of the remaining healthy breast opposite a breast that is removed to treat breast cancer.

co-payment (co-pay). A fixed amount, predetermined by your health insurance policy, that you are required to pay for medical services or prescriptions.

debriding. Surgically removing unhealthy tissue.

deductible. The amount you must pay out-of-pocket for medical expenses or prescriptions before your health insurance begins paying.

deep inferior epigastric perforator (DIEP) flap. A segment of abdominal skin, fat, and the DIEP artery used to recreate a breast.

deep vein thrombosis (DVT). A blood clot that develops in a deep vein.

delayed-immediate reconstruction. Placement of a tissue expander to preserve breast shape and facilitate reconstruction when postmastectomy radiation may be needed.

delayed reconstruction. Surgery to recreate a breast after recovery from mastectomy.

delayed wound healing. When an incision heals more slowly than expected.

dermis. The underlying tissue that supports the skin.

diagonal upper gracilis (DUG) flap. Skin, fat, and muscle taken from the upper inner thigh to recreate a breast.

direct-to-implant ("one-step") reconstruction. Single-stage reconstruction that places a full-sized breast implant immediately after nipple-sparing mastectomy.

dog ears. Puckered skin that forms at the ends of a scar.

donor site. An area of the body that supplies tissue to replace a missing breast.

Doppler probe. A small, portable ultrasound machine that detects blood flow.

duct. The part of the breast that delivers milk to the nipple.

ductal carcinoma in situ (DCIS). Non-invasive cancer that begins in the breast ducts.

durable power of attorney for healthcare. A legal document that identifies the person you designate to make decisions for you if you're unable to do so.

endoscopic latissimus dorsi. A reconstructive procedure that transfers the back muscle to the breast site through the mastectomy incision or a small incision under the arm.

epidermis. The outer layer of skin.

exchange surgery. An operation that replaces a tissue expander with an implant.

explant surgery. An operation that removes a breast implant.

extended DIEP flap. Skin and fat taken from the abdomen and hip to recreate a breast.

extended latissimus dorsi flap. A flap that takes an increased amount of skin, fat, and muscle from the back to create a new breast.

extrusion. A condition in which a breast implant comes through the skin.

fascia. The fibrous tissue covering the muscles.

fat grafting (lipofilling). A surgical process that transfers fat from one area of the body to another.

free flap. A segment of tissue that is cut away from its blood supply and reattached in another area of the body.

free TRAM flap. Skin, fat, and a small portion of muscle taken from the abdomen to recreate a breast.

gel bleed. Droplets of oil that leach through the exterior of silicone breast implants.

gene mutations. Changes in genes that can cause disease and cancer.

general surgeon. A physician who specializes in surgical procedures, including mastectomy.

genetic. Related to or influenced by genes.

genetic counselor. A health professional who is trained to interpret patterns in a family's medical history and estimate an individual's risk for disease.

genetic testing. Examination of a person's DNA to identify gene changes that may increase the risk of disease.

gluteal artery perforator (GAP) flap. Skin and fat taken from the upper buttocks to recreate a breast.

granuloma. A small area of inflamed tissue that develops around sutures.

hematoma. Blood that collects outside the blood vessels.

hernia. The protrusion of an organ through a weakened muscle or tissue.

highly cohesive gel. Semi-solid silicone used in some breast implants.

hybrid breast reconstruction. Combining a breast implant with one or more autologous flaps to recreate a breast after mastectomy.

hyperbaric oxygen therapy. Breathing pure oxygen in a pressurized space to improve blood flow.

hypertrophic scar. A scar that rises above the level of the surrounding skin.

immediate reconstruction. Surgery to recreate a breast as soon as a mastectomy is completed and while the patient is still sedated.

immunotherapy. Treatment that stimulates the immune system to destroy cancer cells.

indocyanine green–based fluorescence. An intravenous medical contrast dye that produces clear images of the blood vessels at the donor site.

inferior gluteal artery perforator (IGAP) flap. Skin and fat taken from the lower buttock to recreate a breast.

inflammatory breast cancer. A rare cancer that develops in the breast skin.

inframammary fold. The crease under the breast.

in-network. A group of healthcare providers and facilities that are contracted with a particular health insurance company to accept predetermined fees for services.

intravenous (IV) line. A thin tube placed in a vein, through which fluids and medications are administered.

invasive breast cancer. Cancer that can spread beyond the breast.

invasive ductal carcinoma (infiltrating ductal carcinoma, IDC). Breast cancer that develops in the lining of the milk ducts and spreads to surrounding breast tissue.

invasive lobular carcinoma (infiltrating lobular carcinoma, ILC). Cancer that develops in the lobules of the breast and spreads to surrounding breast tissue.

keloid. A thick scar that spreads into the skin surrounding an incision.

lateral intercostal artery perforator (LICAP) flap. Skin and fat from the side of the chest near the underarm used to fill out lumpectomy defects.

lateral transverse thigh (LTP) flap. Skin and fat taken from the upper outer thigh to recreate a breast.

latissimus dorsi myocutaneous (LD) flap. Skin, fat, and muscle that is tunneled under the skin from the back to the chest to recreate a breast.

living will. A legal document that states your preference for treatment and resuscitation.

lobes. Glands in the breast that contain milk-producing lobules.

lobules. The parts of the breast that produce milk.

lumbar artery perforator (LAP) flap. Skin and fat taken from the upper hip and waist to recreate a breast.

lumpectomy. Surgery that removes a breast tumor and a border of healthy surrounding tissue.

lymphedema. Swelling in the arm or another extremity caused by excess fluid.

lymph fluid. A clear fluid that carries oxygen, nutrients, and hormones to different parts of the body and removes metabolic waste from cells.

lymph nodes. Small glands that filter impurities in the body.

lymph system. A network of tissues and organs that filter impurities in the body.

magnetic resonance angiography (MRA). Technology that produces clear images of the blood vessels.

magnetic resonance imaging (MRI). A scan that uses magnets to produce images of the body's interior or detect ruptured breast implants.

malignant. Cancerous.

malposition. In the wrong position.

mammogram. An x-ray image of the breast.

mastectomy. Surgical removal of the breast.

mastectomy flaps. Breast skin and underlying fat that remain after mastectomy.

mastopexy (breast lift). Surgery to reposition a breast higher on the chest.

metastasize. The spread of cancer beyond its original location.

microsurgeon. A medical professional who is trained to move tissue from one area of the body to another.

microsurgery. Specialized surgery that uses high-powered magnification to reconnect blood vessels and repair nerves.

modified radical mastectomy. Surgical removal of breast tissue, skin, some or all of the underarm lymph nodes, and the lining over the chest muscle.

muscle-sparing latissimus dorsi flap. Skin, fat, and a portion of muscle taken from the back to recreate a breast.

muscle-sparing TRAM flap. Skin, fat, and a portion of muscle taken from the abdomen to recreate a breast.

necrosis. The death of some or all of the cells in an organ or tissue.

negative pressure wound therapy. Using a medical vacuum to draw out fluid and infection from a wound.

neoadjuvant therapy. Treatment given before surgery.

nerve connector. A conduit that bridges the gap between two cut nerves.

nerve graft. A segment of nerve tissue that bridges the gap between cut or damaged nerves.

neuropathic pain. Pain caused by dysfunctional or damaged nerves.

neurotization. A procedure performed to reestablish sensation.

nipple banking. A procedure performed during mastectomy that stores a person's nipple in their groin until it can be later transferred to their reconstructed breast.

nipple delay. A surgical procedure that improves blood supply to the nipple.

nipple reconstruction. A surgical procedure that recreates the nipple after mastectomy.

nipple sharing. Using part of a healthy nipple to create a new nipple on the opposite breast.

nipple-sparing mastectomy (NSM). Surgical removal of the breast tissue that preserves the nipple, areola, and most of the breast skin.

noninvasive breast cancer. Cancer that doesn't spread beyond the breast.

out-of-network. Healthcare providers and facilities that aren't contracted with a particular health insurance company to accept predetermined fees for services.

out-of-pocket cost. The total amount you pay for medical services not covered by your health insurance.

outpatient. A medical procedure that doesn't require an overnight hospital stay.

pedicled flap. Skin, fat, and muscle that remains connected to its original blood supply and is tunneled under the skin from one area of the body to another.

pedicled TRAM flap. Abdominal skin, fat, and muscle that remains connected to its original blood supply and is tunneled under the skin to the chest to create a new breast.

perforating arteries. Small arteries that run throughout muscle.

perforator flap. A muscle-preserving surgical procedure that transfers skin and fat to another part of the body.

phantom pain syndrome. Itching, tingling, or discomfort where a missing part of the body used to be.

phantom sensation. A perceived feeling from a missing part of the body.

postmastectomy pain syndrome (PMPS). Pain that persists after recovery from mastectomy.

previvor. Someone who has an inherited predisposition to cancer but has not been diagnosed with cancer.

profunda artery perforator (PAP) flap. Skin and fat taken from the upper thigh to recreate a breast.

prophylactic bilateral mastectomy. Surgical removal of both breasts to decrease an individual's high risk of breast cancer.

ptotic. Excessively drooping tissue, as in a "ptotic breast," which occurs when the nipple falls below the inframammary fold.

pulmonary embolism. A blood clot that enters the lung.

pulse oximeter. A device that measures the level of oxygen in blood.

radiation therapy. Treatment with high-energy waves to destroy cancer cells and prevent local recurrence.

radical mastectomy. Surgery that removes the breast tissue, nipple, areola, chest muscles, and underarm lymph nodes.

re-excise. To re-open a wound.

resorb. To absorb again, as when the body reassimilates blood or fluid after surgery or fat after autologous fat grafting.

revision surgery. A surgical procedure that improves the results of an earlier operation.

rippling. Wavelike indentations in breast implants that show under the skin.

risk-reducing mastectomy (RRM). Surgical removal of both breasts to decrease an individual's high risk of breast cancer.

risk-reducing salpingo-oophorectomy (RRSO). Surgical removal of both ovaries and both fallopian tubes to decrease an individual's high risk of ovarian cancer.

rupture. A breach in the shell of a breast implant.

saline. A sterile saltwater solution used to fill tissue expanders and some breast implants.

same-day mastectomy. A mastectomy that is performed as an outpatient procedure.

scar revision. A procedure to improve the appearance of a scar.

sentinel lymph node. The first lymph node to which cancer cells are likely to spread from a tumor.

sentinel lymph node biopsy (SLNB). A minimally invasive surgical procedure to determine whether cancer has spread beyond the breast.

sequential compression devices. Inflatable sleeves placed on a patient's lower legs after surgery to reduce the risk of blood clots.

seroma. A collection of fluid under the skin.

shared decision-making. Collaboration between a patient and their healthcare team while making decisions.

silent rupture. An undetected leak in a silicone breast implant.

silicone gel. A synthetic gel used to fill some breast implants.

skin graft. Healthy skin transferred from one part of the body to another to replace damaged or missing skin.

skin-sparing mastectomy. Surgery that removes the breast tissue, including the nipple and areola, while preserving most of the breast skin.

spirometer. A device that expands the lungs and strengthens breathing after surgery.

sporadic cancer. A cancer that isn't hereditary.

stacked DIEP. Two abdominal flaps of fat and skin combined to recreate a single breast.

subcutaneous mastectomy. An outdated mastectomy procedure that deliberately left breast tissue behind to preserve a patient's nipple and areola.

superficial inferior epigastric artery (SIEA) flap. A segment of abdominal skin, fat, and the SIEA artery used to recreate a breast.

superior gluteal artery perforator (SGAP) flap. A segment of skin and fat taken from the upper buttock to recreate a breast.

surgical drain. A plastic bulb that collects postoperative fluids at the incision site.

surgical flap delay (vascular delay). A surgical procedure that increases the blood supply to an area of tissue before an autologous operation.

surgical oncologist. A physician who specializes in cancer surgery.

survivor. Someone who has been successfully treated for cancer.

symmastia. Breasts that join in the center of the chest.

symmetry. Breasts that are of equal proportion, size, and shape.

targeted therapy. Treatment that restricts or blocks substances that certain cancers need to thrive.

textured breast implant. A breast implant with a roughened exterior.

thoracodorsal artery perforator (TDAP) flap. A segment of skin and fat taken from the side of the chest.

three-dimensional tattooing. A tattoo that uses subtle shading and highlighting to simulate the nipple and areola of a reconstructed breast.

tissue expander. A temporary saline implant that gradually stretches skin and/or muscle to make room for a full-sized implant.

total mastectomy. Surgical removal of the breast tissue, skin, and nipple.

transumbilical breast augmentation. Breast enlargement performed through an incision around the belly button.

transverse rectus abdominis myocutaneous (TRAM) flap. Skin, fat, and an abdominal muscle used to reconstruct a breast.

transverse upper gracilis (TUG) flap. Skin, fat, and muscle taken from the upper inner thigh to recreate a breast.

unilateral mastectomy. Surgical removal of one breast.

unilateral reconstruction. A surgical procedure that recreates one breast after mastectomy.

vascularized lymph node transfer. A surgical procedure that replaces previously removed lymph nodes with healthy nodes.

venous thromboembolism. A blood clot.

vertical profunda artery perforator (VPAP) flap. Skin and fat taken from the upper thigh to recreate a breast.

vertical upper gracilis (VUG) flap. Skin, fat, and muscle taken from the upper inner thigh to recreate a breast.

Women's Health and Cancer Rights Act (WHCRA). Legislation requiring health insurance companies that pay for mastectomy to also pay for prostheses and reconstruction surgery.

Resources

Breast Cancer

American Cancer Society (www.cancer.org)
The Breast Cancer Book by Kenneth Miller, MD, Melissa Camp, MD, and Kathy Steligo
BreastCancer.org (www.breastcancer.org)
National Cancer Institute (www.cancer.gov)
Nationally Designated Comprehensive Cancer Centers (www.cancer.gov/research
    /infrastructure/cancer-centers)
Susan G. Komen Breast Cancer Foundation (www.komen.org)
Young Survival Coalition (www.youngsurvival.org)

Breast Cancer Genetics and Risk

Facing Our Risk of Cancer Empowered (www.facingourrisk.org)
Informed Medical Decisions (www.informeddna.com)
Living with Hereditary Cancer Risk by Kathy Steligo, Sue Friedman, DVM, and Allison
    Kurian, MD, PhD
National Society of Genetic Counselors (www.nsgc.org)

Mastectomy

Amoena (www.amoena.com)
BreastFree (www.breastfree.org)
BreastHealing.com (www.breasthealing.com)
Breast Preservation Foundation (www.breastpreservationfoundation.org)
Flat & Fabulous (www.flatandfabulous.org)
Knitted Knockers (www.knittedknockers.org)
Nearly Me (www.nearlyme.org)
Reach to Recovery (www.cancer.org/treatment/supportprogramsservices/reach-to
    -recovery)
Rub-On Nipples (www.breasthealing.com)
Tender Loving Care (TLC) (www.tlcdirect.org)

Breast Reconstruction

American Society of Plastic Surgeons (www.plasticsurgery.org)
Breast Reconstruction Awareness Day (www.breastreconusa.org)
Cancer Survivors Network (http://csn.cancer.org/forum)
Facing Our Risk of Cancer Empowered (www.facingourrisk.org; search message boards)
Food and Drug Administration (www.fda.gov; search for "breast implants")

Recovery

American Cancer Society (www.cancer.org; search for "exercises after breast surgery")
Annie & Isabel hospital gowns (www.annieandisabel.com)
Elizabeth Pink Surgical Bra (www.mastheadpink.com)
ERAS Society (www.erassociety.org)
Marsupial (www.turnerhealth.com)
National Lymphedema Network (www.lymphnet.org)
Pink Pockets (www.pink-pockets.com)

Coping

Breast Cancer Husband by Marc Silver
Laughter Yoga (www.laughteryoga.org)
Prepare for Surgery, Heal Faster by Peggy Huddleston
Why I Wore Lipstick to My Mastectomy by Geralyn Lucas

Insurance and Payment

Alliance in Reconstructive Surgery (AIRS) Foundation (airsfoundation.org)
CancerCare (www.cancercare.org)
Cancer Legal Resource Center Step-by-Step Guide to Navigating Health Insurance
    Appeals (thedrlc.org)
Insurance Information Institute (www.iii.org)
Medicare (www.medicare.gov)
My Hope Chest (www.myhopechest.org)
Patient Advocate Foundation (www.patientadvocate.org)
Triage Cancer (triagecancer.org)
United Breast Cancer Foundation (www.ubcf.info)
Women's Health and Cancer Rights Act (https://www.dol.gov/agencies/ebsa/laws-and
    -regulations/laws/whcra)

Notes

Chapter 1. Why Mastectomy?

1. Olson JS. *Bathsheba's Breast: Women, Cancer, and History.* Johns Hopkins University Press; 2005.
2. American Cancer Society. Cancer facts and figures 2022. 2022. https://www.cancer.org /content/dam/cancer-org/research/cancer-facts-and-statistics/annual-cancer-facts-and -figures/2022/2022-cancer-facts-and-figures.pdf
3. Lyman GH, Somerfield MR, Bosserman LD, et al. Sentinel lymph node biopsy for patients with early-stage breast cancer: American Society of Clinical Oncology clinical practice guideline update. *Journal of Clinical Oncology.* 2017;35(5):561–64.
4. Lymph Node Surgery for Breast Cancer. American Cancer Society. https://www.cancer.org /cancer/breast-cancer/treatment/surgery-for-breast-cancer/lymph-node-surgery-for -breast-cancer.html
5. Key statistics for breast cancer in men. American Cancer Society. Revised January 12, 2023. https://www.cancer.org/cancer/breast-cancer-in-men/about/key-statistics.html#:~:text =For%20men%2C%20the%20lifetime%20risk,American%20Cancer%20Society
6. Lautner M, Lin H, Shen Y, et al. Disparities in the use of breast-conserving therapy among patients with early-stage breast cancer. *Journal of the American Medical Association Surgery.* 2015;150(8):778–86.
7. Scheepens JCC, van 't Veer L, Esserman L, et al. Contralateral prophylactic mastectomy: a narrative review of the evidence and acceptability. *The Breast.* 2021;56:61–69; Hawley ST, Jagsi R, Morrow M, et al. Social and clinical determinants of contralateral prophylactic mastectomy. *Journal of the American Medical Association.* 2014;149(6):582–89; Nelson JA, Lee IT, Disa JJ. The functional impact of breast reconstruction: an overview and update. *Plastic and Reconstructive Surgery Global Open.* 2018;6(3):e1640.
8. Houssami N, Turner RM, Morrow M. Meta-analysis of pre-operative magnetic resonance imaging (MRI) and surgical treatment for breast cancer. *Breast Cancer Research and Treatment.* 2017;165(2):273–83.

Chapter 2. Considering a Risk-Reducing Mastectomy

1. Domchek SM, Friebel TM, Singer CF, et al. Association of risk-reducing surgery in BRCA1 or BRCA2 mutation carriers with cancer risk and mortality. *Journal of the American Medical Association.* 2010;304(9):967–75; Rebbeck TR, Friebel T, Lynch HT, et al. Bilateral prophylactic

mastectomy reduces breast cancer risk in BRCA1 and BRCA2 mutation carriers: the
PROSE Study Group. *Journal of Clinical Oncology.* 2004;22(6):1055–62.
2. Rebbeck TR, Kauff ND, Domchek SM. Meta-analysis of risk reduction estimates associated
with risk-reducing salpingo-oophorectomy in BRCA1 or BRCA2 mutation carriers. *Journal
of the National Cancer Institute.* 2009;101(2):80–87.

Chapter 3. Going Flat

1. Oliver JD, Chaudhry A, Vyas KS, et al. Aesthetic Goldilocks mastectomy and breast
reconstruction: promoting its use in the ideal candidate. *Gland Surgery.* 2018;7(5):493–95.

Chapter 4. How a Mastectomy Affects Reconstruction

1. Momeni A, Meyer S, Shefren K, et al. Flap neurotization in breast reconstruction with
nerve allografts: 1-year clinical outcomes. *Plastic and Reconstructive Surgery Global Open.*
2021;9(1):e3328; Desai AA, Tecce MG, Christopher A, et al. PC21. Breast flap neurotization
following autologous breast reconstruction: a prospective trial. *Plastic and Reconstructive
Surgery Global Open.* 2022;10(4S):45; Weissler JM, Koltz PF, Carney MJ, et al. Sifting
through the evidence: a comprehensive review and analysis of neurotization in breast
reconstruction. *Plastic and Reconstructive Surgery.* 2018;141(3):550–65.
2. Fu M, Chen Q, Zeng L, et al. Prognosis comparison between nipple-sparing mastectomy
and total mastectomy in breast cancer: a case-control study after propensity score matching.
Annals of Surgical Oncology. 2022;29(4):2221–30; Valero MG, Muhsen S, Moo T-A, et al.
Increase in utilization of nipple-sparing mastectomy for breast cancer: indications,
complications, and oncologic outcomes. *Annals of Surgical Oncology.* 2020;27(2):344–51.
3. Lin A, Shakir A, Garza RM. Staged breast reconstruction before nipple-sparing mastectomy
with reconstruction. *Annals of Breast Surgery.* 2021;5(36); DellaCroce FJ, Blum CA, Sullivan
SK, et al. Nipple-sparing mastectomy and ptosis: perforator flap breast reconstruction
allows full secondary mastopexy with complete nipple areolar repositioning. *Plastic and
Reconstructive Surgery.* 2015;136(1):1e–9e.

Chapter 5. Breast Reconstruction Basics

1. Eltahir Y, Krabbe-Timmerman IS, Sadok N, et al. Outcome of quality of life for women
undergoing autologous versus alloplastic breast reconstruction following mastectomy: a
systematic review and meta-analysis. *Plastic and Reconstructive Surgery.* 2020;145(5):1109–23.
2. American Society of Plastic Surgeons. Plastic surgery statistics report 2020. www
.plasticsurgery.org/documents/News/Statistics/2020/reconstructive-procedure
-demographics-2020.pdf
3. Srinivas DR, Clemens MW, Qi J, et al. Obesity and breast reconstruction: complications and
patient-reported outcomes in a multicenter, prospective study. *Plastic and Reconstructive
Surgery.* 2020;145(3):481e–90e; Panayi AC, Agha RA, Sieber BA, et al. Impact of obesity on
outcomes in breast reconstruction: a systematic review and meta-analysis. *Journal of
Reconstructive Microsurgery.* 2018;34:363–75; Thelwall S, Harrington P, Sheridan E, et al.
Impact of obesity on the risk of wound infection following surgery: results from a

nationwide prospective multicentre cohort study in England. *Clinical Microbiology and Infection*. 2015;21(11):1008.e1–1008.e8.

4. Rifkin WJ, Kantar RS, Cammarata MJ, et al. Impact of diabetes on 30-day complications in mastectomy and implant-based breast reconstruction. *Journal of Surgical Research*. 2019;235:148–59.

5. Castaldi M, George G, Stoller C, et al. Independent predictors of venous thromboembolism in patients undergoing reconstructive breast cancer surgery. *Plastic Surgery*. 2020;29(3):160–68; Song D, Slater K, Papsdorf M, et al. Autologous breast reconstruction in women older than 65 years versus women younger than 65 years: a multi-center analysis. *Annals of Plastic Surgery*. 2016;76(2):155–63.

6. World Health Organization. Tobacco and postsurgical outcomes. January 2020. https://apps.who.int/iris/bitstream/handle/10665/330485/9789240000360-eng.pdf

7. Hart SE, Brown DL, Hyungjin KM, et al. Association of clinical complications of chemotherapy and patient-reported outcomes after immediate breast reconstruction. *Journal of the American Medical Association Surgery*. 2021;156(9):847–55; O'Connell RL, Rattay T, Dave RV, et al. The impact of immediate breast reconstruction on the time to delivery of adjuvant therapy: the iBRA-2 study. *British Journal of Cancer*. 2019;120:883–95.

8. Heeg E, Harmeling JX, Becherer BE, et al. Nationwide population-based study of the impact of immediate breast reconstruction after mastectomy on the timing of adjuvant chemotherapy. *British Journal of Surgery*. 2019;106(12):1640–48.

9. Spera LJ, Cook JA, Dolejs S, et al. Perioperative use of antiestrogen therapies in breast reconstruction: a systematic review and treatment recommendations. *Annals of Plastic Surgery*. 2020;85(4):448–55; Parikh RP, Odom EB, Yu L, et al. Complications and thromboembolic events associated with tamoxifen therapy in patients with breast cancer undergoing microvascular breast reconstruction: a systematic review and meta-analysis. *Breast Cancer Research and Treatment*. 2017;163(1):1–10.

10. Shammas RL, Cho EH, Glener AD, et al. Association between targeted HER-2 therapy and breast reconstruction outcomes: a propensity score-matched analysis. *Journal of the American College of Surgeons*. 2017;225(6):731–39.e1.

11. Chetta MD, Oluseyi A, Zhong L, et al. Reconstruction of the irradiated breast: a national claims-based assessment of postoperative morbidity. *Plastic and Reconstructive Surgery*. 2017;139(4):783–92.

12. Friedrich M, Krämer S, Friedrich D, et al. Difficulties of breast reconstruction—problems that no one likes to face. *Anticancer Research*. 2021;41(11):5365–75; Clemens MW and Kronowitz SJ. Current perspectives on radiation therapy in autologous and prosthetic breast reconstruction. *Gland Surgery*. 2015;4(3):222–31; Kelley BP, Ahmed R, Kidwell KM, et al. A systematic review of morbidity associated with autologous breast reconstruction before and after exposure to radiotherapy: are current practices ideal? *Annals of Surgical Oncology*. 2014;21(5):1732–38.

Chapter 6. Reconstruction with Breast Implants

1. American Society of Plastic Surgeons. Plastic surgery statistics report 2020. https://www.plasticsurgery.org/documents/News/Statistics/2020/plastic-surgery-statistics-full-report-2020.pdf

2. US Food and Drug Administration. Acellular dermal matrix (ADM) products used in implant-based breast reconstruction differ in complication rates: FDA safety communication. March 31, 2021. www.fda.gov/medical-devices/safety-communications/acellular-dermal -matrix-adm-products-used-implant-based-breast-reconstruction-differ-complication

3. Institute of Medicine (US) Committee on the Safety of Silicone Breast Implants. *Safety of Silicone Breast Implants*. National Academies Press; 1999.

4. US Food and Drug Administration. Breast implants—certain labeling recommendations to improve patient communication: guidance for industry and Food and Drug Administration staff. September 29, 2020. https://www.fda.gov/media/131885/download

5. US Food and Drug Administration. Risks and complications of breast implants. June 13, 2022. https://www.fda.gov/medical-devices/breast-implants/risks-and-complications -breast-implants

6. US Food and Drug Administration. Risks and complications of breast implants. June 13, 2022. https://www.fda.gov/medical-devices/breast-implants/risks-and-complications -breast-implants

7. Glicksman C, McGuire P, Kadin M, et al. Impact of capsulectomy type on post-explantation systemic symptom improvement: findings from the ASERF systemic symptoms in women-biospecimen analysis study: part 1. *Aesthetic Surgery Journal*. 2022;42(7):809–19; Wee CE, Younis J, Isbester K, et al. Understanding breast implant illness, before and after explantation: a patient-reported outcomes study. *Annals of Plastic Surgery*. 2020;85(S1 Suppl 1):S82–S86; De Boer M, Colaris M, van der Hulst RRWJ, et al. Is explantation of silicone breast implants useful in patients with complaints? *Immunologic Research*. 2017;65(1):25–36; Balk EM, Earley A, Avendano EA, et al. Long-term health outcomes in women with silicone gel breast implants. *Annals of Internal Medicine*. 2016;164(3):164–75.

8. US Food and Drug Administration. Medical device reports of breast implant-associated anaplastic large cell lymphoma. August 4, 2022. www.fda.gov/medical-devices/breast -implants/medical-device-reports-breast-implant-associated-anaplastic-large-cell -lymphoma; US Food and Drug Administration. Questions and answers about breast implant-associated anaplastic large cell lymphoma (BIA-ALCL). October 23, 2019. https://www.fda.gov/medical-devices/breast-implants/questions-and-answers-about -breast-implant-associated-anaplastic-large-cell-lymphoma-bia-alcl

9. US Food and Drug Administration. Risks and complications of breast implants. June 13, 2022. https://www.fda.gov/medical-devices/breast-implants/risks-and-complications -breast-implants

10. Dijkman HBPM, Slaats I, Bult P. Assessment of silicone particle migration among women undergoing removal or revision of silicone breast implants in the Netherlands. *Journal of the American Medical Association Network Open*. 2021;4(9):e2125381.

11. US Food and Drug Administration. FDA backgrounder on platinum in silicone breast implants. January 18, 2018. https://www.fda.gov/medical-devices/breast-implants/fda -backgrounder-platinum-silicone-breast-implants

Chapter 7. The Expander Experience

1. Walia GS, Aston J, Bello R, et al. Prepectoral versus subpectoral tissue expander placement: a clinical and quality of life outcomes study. *Plastic and Reconstructive Surgery Global Open*. 2018;6(4):e1731.

Chapter 8. Autologous Tissue Flaps

1. Knox ADC, Ho AL, Leung L, et al. Breast reconstruction using the DIEP and pedicled TRAM flaps: a 12-year clinical retrospective study and literature review. *Plastic and Reconstructive Surgery*. 2016;138(1):16–28; Macadam SA, Zhong T, Weichman K, et al. Quality of life and patient-reported outcomes in breast cancer survivors: a multicenter comparison of four abdominally based autologous reconstruction methods. *Plastic and Reconstructive Surgery*. 2006;137(3):758–71.
2. DellaCroce FJ, DellaCroce HC, Blum CA, et al. Myth-busting the DIEP flap and an introduction to the abdominal perforator exchange (APEX) breast reconstruction technique: a single-surgeon retrospective review. *Plastic and Reconstructive Surgery*. 2019;143(4):992–1008.
3. American Society of Plastic Surgeons. Plastic surgery statistics report 2020. https://www.plasticsurgery.org/documents/News/Statistics/2020/reconstructive-procedure-demographics-2020.pdf
4. DellaCroce FJ, Sullivan SK. Application and refinement of the superior gluteal artery perforator free flap for bilateral simultaneous breast reconstruction. *Plastic and Reconstructive Surgery*. 2005;116(1):97–103.
5. Nelson JA, Lee IT, Disa JJ. The functional impact of breast reconstruction: an overview and update. *Plastic and Reconstructive Surgery Global Open*. 2018;6(3):e1640.
6. Yesantharao PS, Nguyen DH. Hybrid breast reconstruction: a systematic review of current trends and future directions. *Annals of Breast Surgery*. 2022;6; Kanchwala S and Momeni A. Hybrid breast reconstruction—the best of both worlds. *Gland Surgery*. 2019;8(1):82–89.
7. Rao S, Stolle EC, Sher S, et al. A multiple logistic regression analysis of complications following microsurgical breast reconstruction. *Gland Surgery*. 2014;3(4):226–31.
8. Chang DW, Wang B, Robb GL, et al. Effect of obesity on flap and donor-site complications in free transverse rectus abdominis myocutaneous flap breast reconstruction. *Plastic and Reconstructive Surgery*. 2000;105(5):1640–48; Rao S, Stolle EC, Sher S, et al. A multiple logistic regression analysis of complications following microsurgical breast reconstruction. *Gland Surgery*. 2014;3(4):226–31.

Chapter 9. Revision Procedures

1. Strong AL, Cederna PS, Rubin JP, et al. The current state of fat grafting: a review of harvesting, processing, and injection techniques. *Plastic and Reconstructive Surgery*. 2015;136(4):897–912; Small K, Choi M, Petruolo O, et al. Is there an ideal donor site of fat for secondary breast reconstruction? *Aesthetic Surgery Journal*. 2014;34(4):545–50.
2. Borrelli MR, Patel RA, Sokol J, et al. Fat chance: the rejuvenation of irradiated skin. *Plastic and Reconstructive Surgery Global Open*. 2019;7(2):e2092; Komorowska-Timek E, Turfe Z,

Davis AT. Outcomes of prosthetic reconstruction of irradiated and nonirradiated breasts with fat grafting. *Plastic and Reconstructive Surgery*. 2017;139(1):1e–9e.

3. Vyas KS, DeCoster RC, Burns JC, et al. Autologous fat grafting does not increase risk of oncologic recurrence in the reconstructed breast. *Annals of Plastic Surgery*. 2020;84(6):S405–S410; Upadhyaya SN, Bernard SL, Grobmyer SR, et al. Outcomes of autologous fat grafting in mastectomy patients following breast reconstruction. *Annals of Surgical Oncology*. 2018;25(10):3052–56; Kronowitz SJ, Mandujano CC, Liu J, et al. Lipofilling of the breast does not increase the risk of recurrence of breast cancer: a matched controlled study. *Plastic and Reconstructive Surgery*. 2016;137(2):385–93.

Chapter 12. Preparing for Surgery

1. World Health Organization. WHO tobacco knowledge summaries: tobacco and postsurgical outcomes. January 20, 2020. https://www.who.int/publications/i/item/9789240000360

2. Beecher SM, Woods JFC. Tamoxifen use in microvascular breast reconstruction and its effect on microvascular complications: a systematic review and meta-analysis. *Annals of Breast Surgery*. 2021;5(14); Parikh RP, Odom EB, Yu L, et al. Complications and thromboembolic events associated with tamoxifen therapy in patients with breast cancer undergoing microvascular breast reconstruction: a systematic review and meta-analysis. *Breast Cancer Research and Treatment*. 2017;163(1):1–10.

3. Makaryus R, Miller TE, Gan TJ. Practice guidelines for preoperative fasting and the use of pharmacologic agents to reduce the risk of pulmonary aspiration: application to healthy patients undergoing elective procedures: an updated report by the American Society of Anesthesiologists Task Force of Preoperative Fasting and the use of pharmacologic agents to reduce the risk of pulmonary aspiration. *Anesthesiology*. 2017;126(3):376–393.

Chapter 15. Dealing with Unexpected Problems

1. John Hopkins Medicine. Surgical Site Infections. https://www.hopkinsmedicine.org/health/conditions-and-diseases/surgical-site-infections

2. World Health Organization. Smoking greatly increases risk of complications after surgery. January 20, 2020. https://www.who.int/news/item/20H01H2020-smoking-greatly-increases-risk-of-complications-after-surgery#:~:text=Smoking%20distorts%20a%20patient's%20immune,nutrients%20for%20healing%20after%20surgery; Villines, Z. How does diabetes affect wound healing? *Medical News Today*. Updated May 8, 2022. https://www.medicalnewstoday.com/articles/320739

3. The American Society of Breast Surgeons. Consensus guideline on venous thromboembolism (VTE) prophylaxis for patients undergoing breast operations. https://www.breastsurgeons.org/docs/statements/Consensus-Guideline-on-Venous-Thromboembolism-VTE-Prophylaxis-for-Patients-Undergoing-Breast-Operations.pdf

4. American Cancer Society. Post-mastectomy pain syndrome. https://www.cancer.org/treatment/treatments-and-side-effects/physical-side-effects/pain/post-mastectomy-pain-syndrome.html#:~:text=How%20common%20is%20PMPS%3F,breast%20or%20the%20underarm%20area

5. Merskey, H. (Ed.) Classification of chronic pain. Descriptions of chronic pain syndromes and definitions of pain terms. Prepared by the International Association for the Study of Pain, Subcommittee on Taxonomy. *Pain*. 1986;Supplement 3:S1–226.

6. Belfer I, Schreiber KL, Shaffer JR, et al. Persistent postmastectomy pain in breast cancer survivors: analysis of clinical, demographic, and psychosocial factors. *The Journal of Pain*. 2013;14(10):1185–95; Mejdahl MK, Andersen KG, Gärtner R, et al. Persistent pain and sensory disturbances after treatment for breast cancer: six year nationwide follow-up study. *BMJ*. 2013;346:f1865.

7. Wang L, Guyatt GH, Kennedy SA, et al. Predictors of persistent pain after breast cancer surgery: a systematic review and meta-analysis of observational studies. *Canadian Medical Association Journal*. 2016;188(14):e352–e361; Schreiber KL, Martel MO, Shnol H, et al. Persistent pain in postmastectomy patients: comparison of psychological, medical, surgical, and psychosocial characteristics between patients with and without pain. *Pain*. 2013;154(5):660–68.

8. Alessandri-Bonetti M, Egro FM, Persichetti P, et al. The role of fat grafting in alleviating neuropathic pain: a critical review of the literature. *Plastic and Reconstructive Surgery Global Open*. 2019;7(5):e2216.

Chapter 17. Shopping for Surgeons

1. Dalessio, J. Americans research cars more closely than doctors. *Huffington Post*. October 26, 2012. https://www.huffpost.com/entry/research-cars-doctors-americans-time_n_2023197

Index

Page numbers in **boldface** refer to figures.

abdominal flap reconstruction, 130–33
abdominal flaps, 124–32
abdominal perforator exchange (APEX)
    flap, 128
ABPS (American Board of Plastic
    Surgery), 278
ACA (Affordable Care Act), 31, 290
Accolate, 103
acellular dermal matrix (ADM), 1, **84**,
    84–85, 319
acetaminophen (Tylenol), 106, 201
ACS. *See* American Cancer Society
adjuvant therapy, 70, 319
ADM (acellular dermal matrix), 1, **84**, 84–85
advance directives, 196, 319
Advil (ibuprofen), 201
aesthetic flat closure, 34, **35**, 319
aesthetics, 97–98, 253; procedures to
    improve appearance, 148–90. *See also*
    symmetry
Affordable Care Act (ACA), 31, 290
age, 10, 69, 167
AIRS (Alliance in Reconstructive Surgery)
    Foundation, 296
ALCL (anaplastic large cell lymphoma),
    breast implant–associated (BIA-
    ALCL), 94, 115, 320

alcohol, 199–200, 208, 226
Aleve (naproxen), 201
Allergan, 80, 94
Alliance in Reconstructive Surgery (AIRS)
    Foundation, 296
ALND (axillary lymph node dissection),
    12, 17–18, 319
American Board for Certification in
    Orthotics, Prosthetics, and
    Pedorthics, 39
American Board of Plastic Surgery
    (ABPS), 278
American Cancer Society (ACS), 11, 31,
    42, 234, 305; Reach to Recovery
    volunteers, 261, 277
American Society of Clinical Oncology
    (ASCO), 17
American Society of Plastic Surgeons
    (ASPS), 278, 305
anaplastic large cell lymphoma (ALCL),
    breast implant–associated
    (BIA-ALCL), 94, 115, 320
anesthesia, 13, 213–15
anesthesiologists, 213–14, 294
animation deformity, 98, 107,
    154–55, 319
Annie and Isabel hospital gowns, 203

antibacterial soap, 210
antibiotics, 114, 204, 226, 238
anxiety, 201, 213, 254–57
APEX (abdominal perforator exchange) flap, 128
areola(s), 11, 319; checklist for making decisions about, 307; preserving, 50; removing, 14, 34, 49; tattooing, **63**, 182–86, **183**
Arimidex, 71
Aromasin, 71
aromatase inhibitors, 71
art therapy, 255
ASCO (American Society of Clinical Oncology), 17
Ashkenazi Jews, 23–24
aspirin, 180, 201
ASPS (American Society of Plastic Surgeons), 278, 305
asymmetry, 98, 136–37, 155, 319. *See also* symmetry
ATM gene, 24
attitude, 235, 255, 259, 263, 300. *See also* positive thinking
augmentation mammoplasty. *See* breast augmentation
autoimmune conditions, 92–94
autologous reconstruction, 46–47, **104**, 116; with abdominal flaps, 130–33; advantages of, 119; basics of, **117**, 117–20; with buttock flaps, x, **138**, 138–39, **139**, 140, 251; checklist for making decisions about, 307; comparison with breast implant reconstruction, 60–61; definition of, 319; with DIEP flaps, 125–28, **126**, 131–32, 144, **145**, 225, 242, 304; disadvantages of, 119–20; explant to autologous flap, 250–51; with GAP flaps, 134, 137–40; indications for,

116; intervals for, 132, 134; with LD flaps, 134, **141**, 142; with LICAP flaps, 134; options, 120; with PAP flaps, 134–35, **135**, **136**; patient insights, 116, 128; preoperative imaging, 122–23; radiation and, 73; removal of, 251; replacement with a new flap, 252; replacement with an implant, 252; revisions for, 159–60; secondary, 252; with SGAP flaps, 138–39, **139**, **145**, 154, 251; with stacked DIEP flaps, 144, **145**; with TDAP flap, 134; with thigh flaps, 136–37; traditional procedures, 120; with TRAM flaps, **129**, 131–32, 254; with TUG flaps, 134, **135**; typical timeline, 117–18; weight gain before, 118
autologous tissue flaps, 61, 116–47; from the abdomen, 124–32; from the back, 124, 140–42; basics of, **117**, 117–20; from the buttocks, 124, 137–40, **138**, **139**; definition of, 319; donor sites, 132–44; from the hips, 124, 142–43; muscle-sacrificing, 123–24; muscle-sparing, 120–24; potential problems and fixes, 144–46; stacked, 144; from the thighs, 124, 134–37, **135**
axillary lymph node dissection (ALND), 12, 17–18, 319
axillary reverse mapping, 248, 319

babysitting, 197, 313
back flaps, 124, 140–42
BCT. *See* breast-conserving therapy
Beauchemin-Verzella, Rose Marie, 186
belly button, 125, 130, 162, 168
BIA-ALCL (breast implant–associated anaplastic large cell lymphoma), 94, 115, 320
BII (breast implant illness), 92–94, 320

bilateral mastectomy, 12–13, **14**; definition of, 319; length of procedure, 37; patient insights, 138–39, 154–55, 304; prophylactic, 28, 138–39, 250–51, 324. *See also* mastectomy

bilateral reconstruction, 60, 319; with breast reduction, 173, **174**; immediate, **52**, 52–54, **54**, 87–91, **89**, **145**, **174**; with SGAP flaps, 138–39, **139**; with stacked flaps, 144, **145**. *See also* breast reconstruction

Biocell implants (Allergan), 94

biopsy, 319; sentinel lymph node, 12, 15–17, 325

biopsy scars, 34, 49

bleeding, 199, 240

blood clots, 69, 71, 201, 240–41

body image, 236, 256

bottoming out, 100, 319

bras: after implant reconstruction, 97; insurance coverage and limitations, 287; mastectomy, 39, 112, 287; surgical, 203

BRCA1 and *BRCA2* (*BReast CAncer 1 and BReast CAncer 2*) genes, ix, 23–24, 29–30, 291; definition of, 319; estimated lifetime risk of cancer with mutations, 26–28; patient insights, 37–38, 250–51, 265; testing for mutations, 31

breast(s): anatomy of, **9**, 9–10; modifying, 166–77; monitoring, 266–67; preoperative mapping of, 197; projection of, 45, 82–83, **83**; ptotic, 53–54, **54**

breast augmentation (augmentation mammoplasty), 167–70; average intervals, 169; breastfeeding after, 176; definition of, 319; with fat transfer, 169–70; with implants,

167–69; incisions for, 167–68, **168**; recovery from, 168–70; transumbilical, 167–68, 326

breast cancer, ix–xi, 10–11; definition of, 319; family history of, ix, 19, 24, 27–28; hereditary, 23, 25–30; high-risk genes, 23–24; inflammatory, 11, 322; invasive, 10, 322; lifetime risk of, 18–19; in men, 18–19; noninvasive, 10, 324; patient insights, 265; prevalence of, 8; resources on, 327; screening for, 10, 171; surgery for, 11–19; surveillance for, 266–67; treatment of, 70–74

Breast Cancer Husband (Silver), 310, 328

Breast Cancer Patient Education Act, 62

breast-conserving therapy (BCT), 11–13; definition of, 319; vs. mastectomy, 19–21

breastfeeding, 45, 176, 182

BreastFree, 40

breast implant(s), 60–61, 80–83; aesthetic issues, 97–98; breast augmentation with, 167–69; and cancer, 94–95; checklist for making decisions about, 307; considerations for, 92; definition of, 319; direct-to-implant reconstruction, 87–91, **89**; expert insights, 89–90; explanation, 93–94, 158, 250; FDA black box warning and labeling, 92, 97; "gummy bear," 1, 80–81; history of, 1; ID cards, 96; leaks, 157; malposition of, 100, **101**, 156; patient insights, 79, 90, 113–14, 154, 250–51, 304; positioning, 84, 95, 107, 113; potential problems and fixes, 97–105; prepectoral placement of, 83, **84**, 84–86, 90; radiation and, 72–74; reconstruction with, 60–61, 72–73, 77, 79–106, 152–57, 222–23,

breast implant(s) (*cont.*)
250–51, 304; removal of, 158, 250–51;
replacement of, 154, 250–51; safety
of, 91–95; saline, 80–81, 92;
screening, 266–67; shape and surface
of, 81–82, **82**; silicone gel, 80–81, 92;
size and projection of, 45, 82–83, **83**,
157; subpectoral placement of, 83,
85–86, **87**, 251; textured, 81–82,
93–94, 326; "Things to Consider
Before Getting Implants" (FDA), 92;
tissue expander-to-implant
reconstruction, 85–87, **87**;
warranties, 96
breast implant–associated anaplastic large
cell lymphoma (BIA-ALCL), 94,
115, 320
breast implant illness (BII), 92–94, 320
breast lift (mastopexy), 170–73, **172**;
average intervals, 169; breastfeeding
after, 176; definition of, 320, 323;
patient insights, 166; recovery
from, 173
breast lobes, 9, **9**, 322
breast lobules, 322
breast mounds, 61, **63**, 86, 111, **183**;
definition of, 320; patient insights,
154–55
breast prostheses, 39–41, **40**; custom,
40–41; definition of, 320; insurance
coverage and limitations, 287; paying
for, 42
BREAST-Q, 306
breast reconstruction, 76–147; with
abdominal flaps, 130–33;
advancements, 1–2; autologous,
46–47, 60–61, 73, **104**, 116–20,
154–55, 159–60, 250–52, 307, 319;
basics of, 5, 59–74; bilateral, **52**, 52–53,
60, 87–91, **89**, 138–39, **139**, 144, **145**,
319; with breast implants, 60–61,
72–73, 77, 79–106, 152–57, 222–23,
250–52, 304; with buttock flaps, x,
138, 138–39, **139**, 140, 251;
complications, 237–57, 287;
coordination with treatment, 70–74;
decision-making, 2–3, 34, 298–307;
definition of, 320; delayed, **66**, 66–68,
125–26, **126**, 287, 320; delayed-
immediate, **73**, 74, 320; with DIEP
flaps, 125–28, **126**, 131–32, 144, **145**,
225, 242, 304; direct-to-implant
(one-step), 87–91, **89**, 321; early
planning, 56–58; effects of
mastectomy on, 44–47; explant to
autologous flap, 250–51; explant to
new implant, 250; final touches,
178–90; follow-up, 193; with GAP
flaps, 134, 137–40; hospital
experience, 212–18; hybrid, 143–44,
322; immediate, **52**, 52–54, **54**, 57,
64–67, **66**, 322; incision design, 57;
information for family and friends,
308–15; insurance issues, 286–97; key
decisions, 302, **302**; with LD flaps,
134, **141**, 142; with LICAP flaps, 134;
life after, 258–67; after lumpectomy,
64; for men, 65; monitoring your
reconstructed breast, 266–67;
one-stage, 1; opposite breast
modification, 166–77; options,
60–62; with PAP flaps, 134–35, **135**,
136; patient insights, 44, 59, 68, 71,
90–91, 112, 128, 132, 138–39, 154–55,
179, 195, 205–6, 212–13, 219, 222–25,
232, 236, 242, 250–51, 254, 258,
272–73, 275, 304, 311–12; patient-
reported outcomes, 306; payment
issues, 62, 286–97; plastic surgeons
for, 276–77; potential problems and

fixes, 97–105; preparation for surgery, 195–211; procedures to improve symmetry, shape, and appearance, 148–90; reasons to choose, 60; recovery from, 97, 130–32, 219–36; resources on, 328; revision procedures, 151–65; secondary, 248–52; with SGAP flaps, 138–39, **139**, **145**, 154, 251; strategies for minimizing complications, 252–54; with thigh flaps, 136–37; timing, 64–68; tissue expander-to-implant, 85–87, **87**; traditional approach, 61, **63**, 120; with TRAM flaps, **129**, 129–32, 254; with TUG flaps, 134, **135**; typical timeline, 87–88; unilateral, 166–67, 307, 324. *See also* autologous reconstruction; surgeons

breast reduction (reduction mammoplasty), 54, 173–75, **174**; average intervals, 169; breastfeeding after, 176; definition of, 320; patient insights, 175; recovery from, 175

breast surgeons, 15, 214; definition of, 320; questions to ask, 22, 43, 49, 58; selecting, 276–78. *See also* surgeons

breast tissue, **9**, 9–10

breathing exercise, 201–3, 234

Burney, Fanny, 7–8

buttock flaps, 124, 137–40, **138**, **139**; breast reconstruction with, x, 134, 138–39, **139**; patient insights, 138–39, 251

cancer: breast implants and, 95; hereditary, 23; ovarian, 265; skin, 95; sporadic, 23, 325. *See also* breast cancer

CancerCare, 42

Cancer Legal Resource Center, 293

Cancer Support Network, 305

capsular contracture, 82, 98, **101**, 102–3, 114, 155; definition of, 320; recurrent, 103

capsulectomy, 103, 155, 320

capsulotomy, 155, 320

caregivers, 312

CDH1 gene, 24

Centers for Medicare & Medicaid Services (CMS), 288

certification of surgeons, 278

cesarean delivery, 126

CHEK2 gene, 24

chemotherapy, 46, 70–71, 109, 151, 320

children: babysitting, 313; communication with, 205–6, 211; passing high-risk genes to, 24

Chrysopoulo, Minas, 233

cleavage, 81; improving, 155, 159, **161**

clinical trials, 320

clothing: compression garments, 232; hospital gowns, 203; after implant reconstruction, 97; mastectomy drain garments, 228, **229**; patient insights, 112; preparing for surgery, 203–4, 208; shapewear, 232. *See also* bras

cohesive silicone gel, 80–81, 99–100, 320

collagen, 189, 244–45, 320

communication, 309–10; documentation of, 294; guidelines for offering positive support, 314–15; with your children, 205–6, 211; with your family and friends, 310; with your surgeon, 273–74, 280

complications after surgery, 237–57, 287

compression garments, 136, 140, 163, 170, 203, 232

computed tomography angiography (CTA), 122, 197, 320

computed tomography (CT or CAT)
scan, 320
constipation, 216–18, 226
consultations with surgeons, 279–81;
preparation for, 280; questions to ask,
284–85; scheduling, 279; tips to make
the most of your appointment time,
279–81
contralateral prophylactic mastectomy
(CPM), 21, 167, 320
co-payment (co-pay), 42, 288–89, 320
coping resources, 328
cosmetic issues: after breast
reconstruction, 97–101, 154; after
mastectomy, 34, **35**
costs, 294–96; out-of-pocket, 31, 288,
324. *See also* payment issues
counseling, genetic, 25, 30–32; paying for,
30–31; questions to ask, 32
CPM (contralateral prophylactic
mastectomy), 21, 167, 320
CTA (computed tomography
angiography), 122, 197, 320
CT or CAT (computed tomography)
scan, 320
custom breast prostheses, 40–41

dating after breast reconstruction,
262–65
DCIS (ductal carcinoma in situ), 10, 19, 321
debriding, 239, 320
decision-making, 2–3; about breast
reconstruction, 34, 60, **73**, 302, **302**;
checklist for, 307; patient insights,
298, 304, 311–12; resources on, 30,
304–5; about risk-reducing
mastectomy, 29; road map for,
298–307, **299**; shared, 303, 325
deductibles, 288, 320
deep breathing, 201–3

deep inferior epigastric perforator (DIEP)
flap, 124, **125**, 125–28; breast
reconstruction with, 125–28, **126**,
131–32, 144, **145**, 225, 232, 242, 304;
definition of, 320; extended, 128,
321; patient insights, 128, 225, 242,
304; stacked, 128, 144, **145**, 325;
variations, 127–28
deep vein thrombosis (DVT), 240–41,
320
delayed-immediate reconstruction, **73**,
74, 320
delayed reconstruction, **66**, 66–68;
definition of, 320; with DIEP flaps,
125–26, **126**; indications for, 67–68;
insurance coverage and limitations,
287; patient insights, 68, 71
delayed wound healing, 239–40, 320
DellaCroce, Frank J., 56
depression, 254–57
dermis, 244, 321
Device Identification Cards, 108
diabetes, 69, 114, 141, 198, 238
diagonal upper gracilis (DUG) flap, 136
DIEP flap. *See* deep inferior epigastric
perforator (DIEP) flap
diet, 198, 233
direct-to-implant (one-step)
reconstruction, 87–91, **89**;
considerations for, 88; definition of,
321; expert insights, 89–90; patient
insights, 90–91
dog ears, 34, 146, 159, 321
donor sites, autologous, 117, 132–44, 321.
See also specific sites
donor site scars, 125; from hip flaps,
142–43; from LD flaps, **141**; patient
insights, 138–39, 154–55; from thigh
flaps, 134–35
Doppler probes, 122, 214, 321

double mastectomy. *See* bilateral mastectomy

drains. *See* surgical drains

drugs, recreational, 200, 234. *See also* medications

ductal carcinoma, invasive/infiltrating (IDC), 11, 322

ductal carcinoma in situ (DCIS), 10, 19, 321

DUG (diagonal upper gracilis) flap, 136

durable power of attorney for healthcare, 196, 321

DVT (deep vein thrombosis), 240–41, 320

Elizabeth Pink Surgical Bra, 203

embolism, pulmonary, 240–41, 324

emotional health, 259–60; management of, 254–57; positive thinking, 209, 255–57, 259, 300; after surgery, 258–62; before surgery, 201; tips for maintaining, 202

Employee Benefits Security Administration, 288

employment: returning to work, 111, 262; scheduling time off, 200

endoscopic latissimus dorsi flap, 141–42, 321

Enhanced Recovery After Surgery (ERAS) protocols, 217

epidermis, 244, 321

exchange surgery, 112–14, 321

exercise: after breast reconstruction, 136, 152, 216, 223, 232, 235; during expansion, 110; postmastectomy, 37, 95, 216, 234–35; before surgery, 198–99

expanders. *See* tissue expanders

expectations, 252

expert insights, 51–52, 56–58, 89–90, 186, 233

explant surgery, 158; definition of, 321; explantation, 93–94; explant to autologous flap, 250–51; explant to flat, 250; explant to new implant, 250

extended DIEP flap, 128, 321

extended latissimus dorsi flap, 141–42, 321

extrusion, 100, 115, 156, 321

Facing Our Risk of Cancer Empowered (FORCE), x, xi, 30, 262, 305; appeal letters, 31, 293; *Living with Hereditary Cancer Risk*, 30; Surgeon Referral Tool, 277

family history, ix, 19, 24, 27–28

family members: communicating with, 205–6, 211, 310; hints and information for, 308–9

fascia, 125, 321

fat grafting (lipofilling), 1, **35**, 154–55, 160–64, **161**; advantages of, 164; definition of, 321; disadvantages of, 164; patient insights, 90, 151, 154–55; procedure, 161–62; questions to ask, 165; recovery from, 163; safety of, 163

FDA. *See* Food and Drug Administration

Feeling Whole Again, 187

Femara, 71

financial assistance: for genetic counseling, 30–31; for mastectomy and prostheses, 42; for mastectomy and reconstruction, 296; resources on, 42, 328; for risk-reducing mastectomy (RRM), 30–31. *See also* payment issues

fitness, 198–99, 233

Flat & Fabulous, 41

flat chests: aesthetic flat closure, 34, **35**, 319; autologous flap to flat, 251; explant to flat, 250; mastectomy without reconstruction, 33–43, **35**, 67

flat denial, 36
fluorescence, indocyanine green–based, 197, 322
follow-up after surgery, 266–67
Food and Drug Administration (FDA), 91–92, 94–95, 101; black box warning and labeling for breast implants, 92; "Labeling for Approved Breast Implants" search recommendation, 97; MedWatch Safety Information and Adverse Event Reporting Program, 92; recommendations for imaging silicone implants, 99–100, 266–67
FORCE. *See* Facing Our Risk of Cancer Empowered
four-dimensional (4-D) nipple reconstruction, 185
Franquet, Janet, 286
free flaps, 123, 321
free TRAM flaps, 130, 132, 321
Friedman, Sue, ix–xi
friends, 260; do's and don'ts for, 313–15; information for, 308–15

GAP flap. *See* gluteal artery perforator (GAP) flap
gel, highly cohesive silicone, 80, 322
gel bleeds, 100–101, 156, 321
gene mutations, 10, 23–24, 291, 321
general surgeons, 8; definition of, 321; questions to ask, 22, 43. *See also* surgeons
genes, high-risk, 24
genetic counseling, 25, 321; paying for, 30–31; questions to ask, 32
genetics resources, 327
genetic testing, ix, 25–26; definition of, 321; paying for, 30–31

gluteal artery perforator (GAP) flap, 124, 137–39; breast reconstruction with, 134, 137–40; definition of, 321. *See also* inferior gluteal artery perforator (IGAP) flap; superior gluteal artery perforator (SGAP) flap
Goldilocks mastectomy, 38
gracilis muscle, 124, 135–36, **136**, 326
granuloma, 254, 321
"gummy bear" breast implants, 1, 80–81

hair removal before surgery, 208
Halsted, William, 8, 56
healing: delayed wound healing, 239–40, 320; life after reconstruction, 258–67; optimism for, 235–36; patient insights, 219, 224–25; timetable for, 219–25, 253; ways to encourage, 234; wound healing, 246
health insurance, 2, 286–97; appeal letters, 31, 293; authorization for services, 196; co-payments (co-pays), 42, 288–89, 320; deductibles, 288, 320; denials of coverage, 289–95; patient insights, 286, 296–97; resources on, 287–88, 293, 328
Health Insurance Marketplace, 296
health matters, 68–70
hematoma, 240, 322
HER2 protein, 71–72
Herceptin (trastuzumab), 71–72
hereditary cancer, 23, 25–30
hernia, 126, 128, 146; definition of, 322; repairing, 159
highly cohesive silicone gel, 80, 322
highly cohesive silicone gel implants, 80–81
hip flaps, 124, 142–43
home recovery, 219–36
hormone therapy, 19, 71

Horton, Karen, 89–90
hospital admission, 212–13
hospital care, 212–18; Enhanced Recovery
    After Surgery (ERAS) protocols, 217;
    insurance coverage and limitations,
    287; out-of-network facilities, 289;
    patient insights, 212, 225
hospital discharge, 16, 215, 218
Huddleston, Peggy, 201
humor, 260–61
hybrid breast reconstruction, 143–44, 322
hydration, 208–9, 211
hygiene: preparing for surgery, 209–10;
    after surgery, 231–32
hyperbaric oxygen therapy, 241–42, 322
hypertrophic scars, 247, 322

ibuprofen (Advil, Motrin), 201, 225
IDC (invasive/infiltrating ductal
    carcinoma), 11, 322
Ideal, 80
identification (ID) cards: expander Device
    Identification Cards, 108; implant, 96
IGAP (inferior gluteal artery perforator)
    flap, 137, **138**, 322
ILC (invasive/infiltrating lobular
    carcinoma), 11, 19, 322
imaging: of dense breasts, 9; preoperative,
    122–23, 197; of silicone implants,
    99–100
immediate reconstruction, 57, 64–67;
    benefits of, 65–66, **66**; bilateral, **52**,
    52–54, **54**, 87–91, **89**, **145**, **174**;
    definition of, 322; delayed-immediate,
    73, 74, 320; patient insights, 51
immunotherapy, 322
implants. *See* breast implant(s)
incisions: autologous reconstruction, 120;
    breast augmentation, 167–68, **168**;

caring for, 230; mastectomy, 45, 57;
    nipple-sparing, **50**, 50–51; skin-
    sparing, 49, **49**. *See also specific procedures*
incision scars. *See* scars and scarring
indocyanine green–based fluorescence,
    197, 322
infection, 114, 205; after reconstruction,
    238–40; signs of, 230, 239
inferior gluteal artery perforator (IGAP)
    flap, 137, **138**, 322
infiltrating/invasive ductal carcinoma
    (IDC), 11, 322
infiltrating/invasive lobular carcinoma
    (ILC), 11, 19, 322
inflammatory breast cancer, 11, 322
information for family and friends, 308–15
information sources, 304–5
inframammary fold, 45, 322
in-network providers and facilities, 322
inspiration, 304–5
Institute of Medicine, 91
insurance. *See* health insurance
intimacy, 209, 262–65
intracapsular rupture, 100–101
intravenous (IV) line, 213
invasive breast cancer, 10, 322
invasive/infiltrating ductal carcinoma
    (IDC), 11, 322
invasive/infiltrating lobular carcinoma
    (ILC), 11, 19, 322

Janet's Law. *See* Women's Health and
    Cancer Rights Act
JCPenney, 40–41
journaling, 201, 204

keloids, 247, 322
Knitted Knockers, 40
Komen, Susan G., 31, 305

LAP (lumbar artery perforator) flap, 124, 142–43, 322

lateral intercostal artery perforator (LICAP) flap, 124, 142; breast reconstruction with, 134; definition of, 322

lateral transverse thigh (LTP) flap, 136

latissimus dorsi myocutaneous (LD) flap, 124, 140, **141**; breast reconstruction with, 134, **141**, 142; definition of, 322; endoscopic, 141–42, 321; extended, 141–42, 321; muscle-sparing, 141–42, 323; variations, 141–42

laughter, 260–61

LD flap. *See* latissimus dorsi myocutaneous (LD) flap

LICAP flap. *See* lateral intercostal artery perforator (LICAP) flap

life after reconstruction, 258–67

lipofilling. *See* fat grafting

liposuction, 154–55, 162

living will, 196, 322

Living with Hereditary Cancer Risk (Steligo, Friedman, and Kurian), 30

lobular carcinoma, invasive/infiltrating, 11, 19, 322

love handles, 137, 142–43, 160

LTP (lateral transverse thigh) flap, 136

lumbar artery perforator (LAP) flap, 124, 142–43, 322

lumpectomy, 11–13; comparison with mastectomy, 19–21; definition of, 322; fat grafting after, 160; indications for, 13; reconstruction after, 64

lymphatic bypass, 249

lymphatic debulking, 249

lymphedema, 18, 247–48; definition of, 323; early indications of, 248; health insurance coverage for treatment of, 287; patient insights, 248; risk of, 18; surgeries for, 249

lymph fluid, 9, 323

lymph nodes, 9, **9**; axillary lymph node dissection, 12, 17–18, 319; definition of, 323; sentinel lymph node biopsy, 12, 15–17, 325; vascularized transfer of, 249, 326

lymph node surgeries, 15–18

lymphoma, 94–95, 115, 320

lymph system, 15, 323

magnetic resonance angiography (MRA), 197; definition of, 323; preoperative, 122

magnetic resonance imaging (MRI), 10; definition of, 323; before mastectomy, 21; after reconstruction with silicone implants, 81, 99–100, 266–67

male mastectomy, 18–19

malposition, 100, **101**, 156, 323

mammograms, ix–xi, 10, 323

mammoplasty: augmentation, 167–70, 319; reduction, 54, 173–75, **174**, 176, 320

mapping: axillary reverse, 248, 319; preoperative, 197

Marsupial, 228, **229**

massage, 110, 255; for necrosis, 241; scar line, 245, **246**

mastectomy, 7–8, 13–14; bilateral, 12–13, **14**, 28, 37, 138–39, 154–55, 304, 319, 324; comparison with lumpectomy, 20; contralateral prophylactic, 21, 167, 320; definition of, 323; early planning, 56–58; effects on reconstruction, 44–47; expert insights, 56–58; financial assistance for, 42, 296; follow-up, 266–67; Goldilocks, 38; history of, 7–8; with immediate reconstruction, 67; incision, 45, 57; indications for, 13–14; insurance coverage and limitations, 286–87; insurance issues, 291; length of procedure, 37; vs. lumpectomy, 19–21; male, 18–19; modified radical, **15**, 323; nipple-sparing, 1, 50–58, 90–91, 242, 304, 324; partial, 11–13; patient insights, 7, 23, 33, 37–38, 44, 106, 110–11, 113–14, 138–39, 154–55, 195, 205–6, 225, 242, 248, 250–51, 296–97, 304, 311–12; postmastectomy pain syndrome (PMPS), 243–44, 324; prevalence of, 8; radical, 8, 12, 14, **15**, 324; rationale for, 7–22; resources on, 327; risk-reducing, ix–x, 23–32, 138–39, 250–51, 291, 296–97, 325; same-day, 16, 325; sew-in pockets, 39; skin-sparing, **49**, 49–50, 325; subcutaneous, 325; surgeons, 276–78; total, 12, 14, **15**, 326; unilateral, 12–13, **14**, 37, **126**, **172**, 324; what to expect, 34–38; without reconstruction, 33–43, **35**, 67

mastectomy bras, 39, 112, 287

mastectomy drain garments, 228

mastectomy flaps, 84, 323

mastectomy pillows, 232

mastopexy. *See* breast lift

Medicaid, 287

Medicare, 287, 296; coverage for breast prostheses and mastectomy bras, 42; coverage for breast reconstruction, 31; coverage for genetic counseling, 31; coverage for genetic testing, 31; coverage for postmastectomy complications, 287

medications: discontinuing before surgery, 201; for pain, 215–16, 225–26; post-op prescriptions, 204; preparing for surgery, 210; tips to manage, 225–26

meditation, 110, 255

MedWatch Safety Information and Adverse Event Reporting Program, 92

men: breast cancer in, 18–19; breast cancer risk, 26–27; breast reconstruction for, 65; as husbands, 195, 258; mastectomy for, 18–19

mental health, 235–36, 265

mental health specialists, 255, 265

Mentor, 80

metastasis, 15, 323

microneurorrhaphy, 47

microsurgeons, 121, 197, 323

microsurgery, 323

mind-body techniques, 201, 328

mobility, 234–35

modified radical mastectomy, 12, 14, **15**, 323

Montgomery tubercles, 186

Motrin (ibuprofen), 201

movement, 216; getting in and out of bed, 231; restorative, 234–35

MRA. *See* magnetic resonance angiography

MRI. *See* magnetic resonance imaging

multivitamins, 246

muscle relaxants, 103, 111

muscle-sacrificing flaps, 123–24. *See also specific flaps*

muscle-sparing flaps, 120–24. *See also specific flaps*

muscle-sparing LD flaps, 141–42, 323

muscle-sparing TRAM flaps, 130; breast reconstruction with, 132; definition of, 323

music therapy, 255

My Hope Chest, 296

nail polish, 207
Napoleon, 7–8
naproxen (Aleve), 201
National Alliance of Caregiving, 312
National Cancer Institute, 277
National Comprehensive Cancer
    Network, 291
National Lymphedema Network, 248
National Society of Genetic
    Counselors, 25
necrosis, 115, 146, 188–89, 241–42;
    definition of, 323; patient insights,
    242; risk factors for, 242; treatment
    of, 159–60, 241–42
negative pressure wound therapy,
    239–40, 323
neoadjuvant therapy, 70, 323
nerve conduits, 47–48, **48**
nerve connectors, 47–48, 323
nerve grafts, 47–48, 323
neuropathic pain, 243, 323
neurotization, 47–48, **48**, 323
New Attitude, 187
new relationships, 265
nipple(s), **9**; Paget's disease of, 19;
    positioning, 53–54, **54**, **174**, 188;
    prosthetic, 187; removing, 34, **35**,
    188; repositioning, 173, 188; Rub-On
    Nipples, 187
nipple banking, 56–58, 182, 323
nipple collapse, 187
nipple delay, 55–56, 323
nipple grafts, 189
nipple reconstruction, 178–82, **181**, **183**;
    advantages of, 179; checklist for
    making decisions about, 307;
    definition of, 323; disadvantages of,
    179–80; 4-D, 185; nonsurgical
    alternatives, 187; patient insights,
    178–79, 188–89; problems and fixes,

187–89; with skin grafts, 181–82;
    typical intervals for, 181
nipple sharing, 182, 323
nipple-sparing mastectomy (NSM), 50–58;
    candidates for, 53; definition of, 324;
    expert insights, 51–52; history of, 1;
    with immediate direct-to-implant
    reconstruction, 87–88, **89**; with
    immediate reconstruction, **52**, 52–54,
    54; incisions, **50**, 50–51; patient
    insights, 51, 90–91, 242, 250–51, 304;
    and ptotic breasts, 53–54, **54**, **174**;
    what to expect, 55
nipple tattooing, **63**, 182–76, **183**; color
    selection, 183–84; expert insights,
    186; patient insights, 188–89; 3-D
    tattooing, 184–85, **185**, 188
noninvasive breast cancer, 10, 324
Nordstrom, 40–41
Not Putting on a Shirt, 41
NSM. *See* nipple-sparing mastectomy
nutrition, 198, 233

obesity, 68, **69**, 118, 198, 233
oncologists, 31, 70–71, 74, 291; patient
    insights, 68, 71; surgical, 64,
    276, 325
oncoplastic surgery, 64
one-step reconstruction. *See* direct-to-
    implant reconstruction
operating room, 213–14
opposite breast modification, 166–77
optimism, 235–36
out-of-network providers and facilities,
    287, 289, 292, 324
out-of-pocket costs, 31, 288, 324
outpatient procedures, 16, 20, 67, 86,
    112, 324
ovarian cancer, 23, 29, 265, 324
oxygen therapy, hyperbaric, 241–42, 322

Paget's disease of the nipple, 19
pain: lingering, 242–44; neuropathic, 243, 323; phantom, 324; postmastectomy pain syndrome (PMPS), 243–44, 324
pain management, 201; patient insights, 106, 110–11, 132, 222–23, 225; post-op, 204; after surgery, 215–16; tips for managing medications, 225–26; with tissue expanders, 110–11
PALB2 gene, 24, 291
PAP flap. *See* profunda artery perforator (PAP) flap
parents, information for, 308–9
partners, information for, 309–12
Patient Advocate Foundation, 42, 292, 296
Patient Decision Checklist, 92
patient insights, 7, 23, 33, 44, 51, 56, 59, 68, 71, 79, 90–91, 106, 112–14, 116, 128, 132, 138–39, 141, 151, 154–55, 166, 175, 178–79, 188–89, 195, 205–6, 212–13, 219, 224–25, 229, 239, 242, 247–48, 250–51, 265, 271–75, 281, 283, 286, 296–98, 304, 308
patient-reported outcomes, 306
patient rights, 62
payment issues, 286–97; assistance programs, 296; out-of-pocket costs, 288–89; paying for breast reconstruction, 62; paying for genetic counseling, 30–31; paying for mastectomy and prostheses, 42; paying for mastectomy and reconstruction, 296; paying for risk-reducing mastectomy (RRM), 30–31; resources on, 328. *See also* health insurance
pectoralis muscles, 83–85, **84**, 87, 106, **117**; animation deformity, 154; patient insights, 90, 250–51

pedicled flaps, 123, 324
pedicled TRAM flaps, **129**, 129–30, 132, 324
perforating arteries, 121, 126, 324
perforator flaps, **121**, 121–23, 324
pertuzumab (Perjeta), 71–72
phantom pain syndrome, 324
phantom sensations, 46–47, 324
philanthropy, 261–62
physical therapy, 132, 142, 234
physicians. *See* surgeons
pigmentation, 188
Pink Pockets, 228, **229**
plastic surgeons: certification of, 278; ideal characteristics, 273–74; patient insights, 272–73, 281, 297; questions to ask, 105, 115, 147, 165, 177, 190, 284–85; resources on, 277–78; selecting, 252, 271–85
PMPS (postmastectomy pain syndrome), 243–44, 324
Poland syndrome, 59
positioning, breast implant, 84, 95, 107, 113; malposition, 100, **101**, 156, 323
positioning, nipple, 53–54, **54**, 173, **174**, 188
positive support, 314–15
positive thinking, 209, 255–57, 259, 300
postmastectomy boutiques, 40–41
postmastectomy exercises, 234–35
postmastectomy pain syndrome (PMPS), 243–44, 324
postmastectomy rehabilitation, 234–35
postoperative (post-op) care, 214–18
postoperative (post-op) instructions, 218
power of attorney for healthcare, durable, 196, 321
pregnancy, 133
preoperative (pre-op) care, 212–13
preoperative (pre-op) evaluation, 196
preoperative (pre-op) imaging, 122–23, 197

preoperative (pre-op) instructions, 195, 200, 209–10
preoperative (pre-op) mapping, 197
preparing for surgery, 195–211, 328
prepectoral breast implant placement, 83, **84**, 84–86, 90
prescriptions. *See* medications
previvors, 24, 324
profunda artery perforator (PAP) flap, 124, 135, **135**; breast reconstruction with, 134–35, **135**, **136**; definition of, 324
prophylactic mastectomy: bilateral, 28, 138–39, 250–51, 324; contralateral, 21, 167, 320; patient insights, 30, 138–39, 250–51
prostheses, 38–41, **40**, 320; insurance coverage and limitations, 287; patient insights, 112; paying for, 42; tips for buying, 41; where to shop, 40–41
prosthetic nipples, 187
PTEN gene, 24, 291
ptotic breasts, 53–54, **54**, 324
pulmonary embolism, 240–41, 324
pulse oximeters, 213, 324

radiation therapy, 72–74, 234–35, 324
radical mastectomy: definition of, 324; history of, 8; modified, 12, 14, **15**, 323
Reach to Recovery, 39, 261, 277
recliners, 200
reconstruction. *See* breast reconstruction; nipple reconstruction
recovery: abdominal flap reconstruction, 130–32; breast augmentation, 168–70; breast lift, 173; breast reduction, 175; do's and don'ts, 221; Enhanced Recovery After Surgery (ERAS) protocols, 217; fat grafting, 163; at home, 219–36; life after reconstruction, 258–67; patient insights, 128, 219, 222–25, 232, 283, 308; preparation for, 206–7; reconstruction with autologous flaps, 128, 130–32, 134, 140, 142; reconstruction with implants, 95–97, 222–23; resources on, 328; revision procedures, 154; tips for, 230–35; when to contact your doctor, 222
recreational drugs, 200, 234
rectus abdominis muscles, 124, **125**
reduction mammoplasty. *See* breast reduction
re-excision, 45, 324
Reforma, 187
rehabilitation, postmastectomy, 234–35
relationships: doctor-patient, 275; new, 265
relaxation, 201, 211
resorption, 160, 324
resources, 327–28; for decision-making, 30, 304–5; for financial assistance, 42, 328; for going flat, 41; for health insurance, 287–88, 293, 328; for information and inspiration, 304–5; for selecting plastic surgeons, 277–78
returning to work, 262
revision surgery, 61, 98, 149, 324; after autologous reconstruction, 159–60; with fat grafting, 160–64, **161**; patient insights, 151, 154–55, 237, 247; procedures, 151–65; questions to ask, 165; after reconstruction with implants, 152–57; for scars, 34, **35**, 137, 325. *See also* secondary reconstruction
rippling, breast implant, 84, 86, 98–99, 156, 325; patient insights, 90
risk-reducing mastectomy (RRM), ix–x, 28–30, 291; definition of, 325; indications for, 28; patient insights, 23, 138–39, 250–51, 296–97; paying

for, 30–31; risk of cancer recurrence after, 50
risk-reducing salpingo-oophorectomy (RRSO), 29–30, 325
RRM. *See* risk-reducing mastectomy
RRSO (risk-reducing salpingo-oophorectomy), 29–30, 325
Rub-On Nipples, 187
ruptures: of breast implants, 81, 96, 99–101, **104**, 157; definition of, 325; silent, 99–100, 325; of tissue expanders, 114

safety: of breast implants, 91–95; of fat grafting, 163
saline: adding to tissue expanders, 107–9, **108**; definition of, 325
saline breast implants, 80–81, 92; comparison with silicone implants, 81; patient insights, 154; rupture, 99, **104**
salpingo-oophorectomy, risk-reducing (RRSO), 29–30, 325
same-day mastectomy, 16, 325
scar revision, 34, **35**, 137, 325
scars and scarring, 244–47; biopsy, 34, 49; donor site, 125, 134–35, 138–39, **141**, 142–43, 154–55; gluteal, 116; hypertrophic, 247, 322; keloids, 247, 322; mastectomy, 37–38, 49, 51, **66**; patient insights, 37–38, 51, 116, 138–39, 154–55, 237, 247; suggestions to promote healing, 245–46, **246**; uneven or poorly healed, 144–46
scar tissue, 74, 81–82, 94–95, 99–100
SCC (squamous cell carcinoma), 95
secondary reconstruction, 248–52; autologous flap to flat, 251; autologous flap to new flap, 252; explant to autologous flap, 250–51; explant to flat, 250; explant to new implant, 250

second (or third) opinions, 281
self-care, 204, 208–9
self-image, 236, 256, 311–12
self-talk, 259
sensation(s), 46–47; losing and regaining, 46–48; patient insights, 90, 138–39, 311–12; phantom, 46–47; postreconstruction, 90–91, 138–39; restoration of, 47–48, **48**
sensory nerves, 46
sentinel lymph node biopsy (SLNB), 12, 15–17, 325
sentinel lymph nodes, 15, 17, 325
sequential compression devices, 214, 325
seroma, 85, 140, 142, 238, 325
sew-in mastectomy pockets, 39
sexual activity: patient insights, 258, 311–12; after reconstruction, 262–65, 311–12; during recovery, 224; before surgery, 209
SGAP flap. *See* superior gluteal artery perforator (SGAP) flap
shapewear, 232
shared decision-making, 303, 325
shopping for surgery, 203–4
showering, 110, 180, 209–10, 230–31
SIEA (superficial inferior epigastric artery) flap, 124, **125**, 127, 325
Sientra, 80
silent rupture, 99–100, 325
silicone breast implants, 80–81, 92; comparison with saline implants, 81; ruptures, 99–100; safety of, 91–95; screening, 266–67
silicone breast prostheses, 40, 42
silicone gel, 80–81, 325; cohesive, 80–81; highly cohesive, 80–81, 322
silicone gel bleeds, 100–101, 156, 321
Silver, Marc, 310, 328
Singulair, 103

skin cancer, 95

skin grafts: definition of, 325; nipple reconstruction with, 181–82

skin-sparing mastectomy, 49, 49–50; definition of, 325; incisions, 49, 49

sleep, 209, 231–32; napping, 221; patient insights, 221, 225, 232

SLNB (sentinel lymph node biopsy), 12, 15–17, 325

smoking, 70, 146, 180, 199, 233

smoking cessation, 199

smooth exterior breast implants, 82

Spectrum implant, 113

spiritual health, 261

spirometers, 215, 325

spitting sutures, 254

sporadic cancer, 23, 325

SPY Elite, 197

squamous cell carcinoma (SCC), 95

stacked flaps, 128, 144, 145, 325

Steligo, Kathy, x

Step-by-Step Guide to Navigating Health Insurance Appeals (Cancer Legal Resource Center), 293

STK11 gene, 24

strength training, 234–35

subcutaneous mastectomy, 325

subpectoral breast implant placement, 83, 85–86, 87, 251

subpectoral tissue expanders, 110–11

superficial inferior epigastric artery (SIEA) flap, 124, 125, 127, 325

superior gluteal artery perforator (SGAP) flap, 137–39, 138, 144; breast reconstruction with, 138–39, 139, 145, 154, 251; definition of, 325; patient insights, 138–39, 154–55, 251

supplements, 201

support groups, 261–62, 305, 312

Surgeon Referral Tool (FORCE), 277

surgeons: breast, 15, 22, 43, 58, 214, 320; consultations with, 279–81; cosmetic, 277; doctor-patient relationship, 275; general, 8, 22, 43, 321; ideal characteristics, 273–74; in-network, 286; microsurgeons, 121, 197, 323; optimal doctor-patient communication, 274; out-of-network, 282, 287, 289, 292, 297; patient insights, 271–75, 281, 283, 297; plastic, 105, 115, 147, 165, 177, 190, 271–85; pre-appointment footwork, 278–79; pushy, 276; questions to ask, 22, 43, 49, 58, 105, 115, 147, 165, 177, 190, 257, 284–85; resources on, 277–78; screening, 278–79; second (or third) opinions, 281; selecting, 252, 271–85; tips for travelers, 282–83

surgery: autologous flap procedures, 60–61; for breast cancer, 11–19; diet and, 233; Enhanced Recovery After Surgery (ERAS) protocols, 217; exchange, 112–14, 321; explant, 158, 250–51, 321; fitness and, 233; for lymphedema, 249; lymph node, 15–18; microsurgery, 323; oncoplastic, 64; opposite breast modification, 166–77; patient insights, 195, 205, 213, 219; paying for, 30–31; post-op care, 214–18; pre-op care, 212–13; pre-op evaluation, 196; pre-op instructions, 195, 200, 209–10; pre-op mapping, 197; preparation for, 195–211; recovery from, 219–36; to reduce breast cancer risk, 29–30; revision procedures, 61, 149, 151–65, 324; risk-reducing, 30–31; risks of, 238–42; secondary reconstruction, 248–52; smoking and, 233. See also specific procedures surgical bras, 112, 170, 203

surgical drains, 34, 226–29, **227**; definition of, 325; mastectomy drain garments, **229**; measuring and emptying, 227–28; patient insights, 154, 229

surgical flap delay (vascular delay), 122–23, 325

surgical oncologists, 64, 276–77, 325

surveillance, 266–67

survivors, 325

Susan G. Komen for the Cure, 31, 305

sutures, spitting, 254

symmastia ("uniboob"), 100, **104**, 157, 325

symmetry: definition of, 325; modifying for, 166–77; patient insights, 166; procedures to improve, 64, 148–77, 287; with prostheses, 39. *See also* aesthetics

tamoxifen, 71, 201

targeted therapy, 71–72, 326

tattooing, nipple and areola, **63**, 178, 182–86, **183**; advantages of, 179; color selection, 183–84; disadvantages of, 179–80; fading, 188; patient insights, 188–89; problems and fixes, 187–89; 3-D, 184–85, **185**, 188, 326; typical intervals in, 181

TDAP (thoracodorsal artery perforator) flap, 124, 134, 142, 326

textured breast implants, 81–82, 93–94, 326

textured tissue expanders, 94, 115

thigh flaps, 124, 134–37, **135**

thoracodorsal artery perforator (TDAP) flap, 124, 134, 142, 326

three-dimensional (3-D) tattooing, 184–85, **185**, 188, 326

thromboembolism, venous, 69, 326

timing, 64–68; appeal timeframes, 295; intervals in autologous

reconstruction with abdominal flaps, 132; intervals in autologous reconstruction with other flaps, 134; intervals in breast modification procedures, 169; intervals in nipple reconstruction and tattooing, 181; intervals in tissue expansion, 109; scheduling consultations, 279; scheduling time off, 314–15; timetable for healing, 219–25, 253; typical timeline with autologous flaps, 117–18; typical timeline with implants, 87–88, 97

tissue expanders, 60–61, 106–15; definition of, 326; Device Identification Cards, 108; exchange surgery, 112–14; filling, 107–9, **108**, 111; patient insights, 106, 110–14, 239, 242, 281; potential problems and fixes, 114–15; radiation and, 72–73; ruptures, 114; Spectrum expander/ implant, 113; subpectoral, 110–11; textured, 94, 115; traveling with, 108

tissue expander-to-implant reconstruction, 85–87, **87**

tissue expansion, 85–86, 111–12; indications for, 87; patient insights, 111–12; sample intervals for, 109; tips for relief, 109–11

tissue flap reconstruction. *See* autologous reconstruction

tissue flaps: autologous, 116–47; free, 123, 321

total capsulectomy, 103

total mastectomy, 12, **15**, 326

TP53 gene, 24, 291

TRAM flap. *See* transverse rectus abdominis myocutaneous (TRAM) flap

transumbilical breast augmentation, 167–68, 326

transverse rectus abdominis
myocutaneous (TRAM) flap, ix,
124, 129–30; breast reconstruction
with, **129**, 129–32, 224, 232, 254;
definition of, 326; free, 130, 132,
321; muscle-sparing, 130, 132, 323;
patient insights, 132, 254; pedicled,
129, 129–30, 132, 324; variations, 130
transverse upper gracilis (TUG) flap, 124,
135, **135**; breast reconstruction with,
134, **135**, 222; definition of, 324;
variations, 136
trastuzumab (Herceptin), 71–72
traveling: for surgery, x, 196, 282–83; with
tissue expanders, 108
Triage Cancer, 293, 296
TUG flap. *See* transverse upper gracilis
(TUG) flap
tummy tuck, 127
Tylenol (acetaminophen), 106, 201

ultrasound, 10; preoperative, 122; after
reconstruction with implants,
99–100, 266–67
ultraviolet light, 246
underinsured care, 294–97
underlying conditions, 69–70
unexpected problems, 237–57
"uniboob" (symmastia), 100, **104**, 157, 325
unilateral mastectomy, 12–13, **14**, **126**,
172; definition of, 324; length of
procedure, 37. *See also* mastectomy
unilateral reconstruction: checklist for
making decisions about, 307;
definition of, 324; options for
opposite breast, 166–67. *See also*
breast reconstruction
uninsured care, 294–97
United Breast Cancer Foundation, 296

US Department of Health and Human
Services, 294
US Department of Labor, 288

vascular delay (surgical flap delay),
122–23, 325
vascularized lymph node transfer,
249, 326
venous thromboembolism, 69, 326
vertical profunda artery perforator
(VPAP) flap, 135
vertical upper gracilis (VUG) flap,
136, 326
vitamins, 201, 233, 240, 245–46
volunteering, 261
VPAP (vertical profunda artery
perforator) flap, 135
VUG (vertical upper gracilis) flap, 136, 326

warranties, 96
weight gain, 118
weight loss, 68
WHCRA. *See* Women's Health and
Cancer Rights Act
Winchester, David J., 51–52
Women's Health and Cancer Rights Act
(WHCRA), 42, 65, 166; definition of,
326; requirements and limitations,
286–87; resources on, 288
work: returning to, 111, 262; scheduling
time off, 200
wound healing, 246; delayed, 239–40, 320
wrinkling, breast implant, 84, 98–99, 156

yoga, 90, 114, 198–99, 229, 235, 255
YWCA, 234

Zanardi, Alex, 235
zinc, 233, 246

About the Author

Kathy Steligo is a coauthor of *The Breast Cancer Book*, *Living with Hereditary Cancer Risk*, and *Confronting Chronic Pain*. A two-time breast cancer survivor, Kathy has had breast reconstruction twice.